Population HEALTH

Population HEALTH

Principles and Applications for Management

Rosemary M. Caron

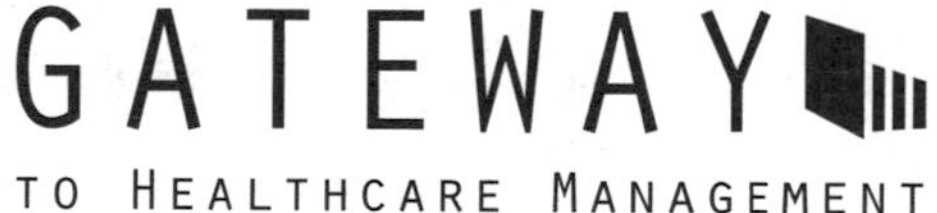

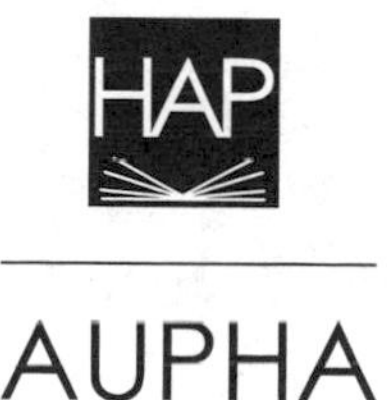

Health Administration Press, Chicago, Illinois
Association of University Programs in Health Administration, Washington, DC

Your board, staff, or clients may also benefit from this book's insight. For more information on quantity discounts, contact the Health Administration Press Marketing Manager at (312) 424-9450.

This publication is intended to provide accurate and authoritative information in regard to the subject matter covered. It is sold, or otherwise provided, with the understanding that the publisher is not engaged in rendering professional services. If professional advice or other expert assistance is required, the services of a competent professional should be sought.

The statements and opinions contained in this book are strictly those of the author and do not represent the official positions of the American College of Healthcare Executives, the Foundation of the American College of Healthcare Executives, or the Association of University Programs in Health Administration.

21 20 19 18 17 5 4 3 2 1

Library of Congress Cataloging-in-Publication Data

Names: Caron, Rosemary M., author. | Association of University Programs in Health Administration, issuing body.

Title: Population health : principles and applications for management / Rosemary Caron.

Description: Chicago, Illinois : Health Administration Press; Washington, DC : Association of University Programs in Health Administration, [2017] | Includes bibliographical references and index.

Identifiers: LCCN 2016050399 (print) | LCCN 2016051576 (ebook) (print) | LCCN 2016051576 (ebook) | ISBN 9781567938616 (print : alk. paper) | ISBN 9781567938630 (xml) | ISBN 9781567938647 (epub) | ISBN 9781567938654 (mobi) | ISBN 9781567938623 (ebook)

Subjects: | MESH: Epidemiologic Measurements | Public Health—methods | Health Status Indicators

Classification: LCC RA427 (print) | LCC RA427 (ebook) | NLM WA 950 | DDC 362.1—dc23

LC record available at https://lccn.loc.gov/2016050399

The paper used in this publication meets the minimum requirements of American National Standard for Information Sciences—Permanence of Paper for Printed Library Materials, ANSI Z39.48-1984. ♾™

Acquisitions editor: Janet Davis; Project manager: Michael Noren; Cover designer: Brad Norr; Layout: Westchester Publishing Services

Found an error or a typo? We want to know! Please e-mail it to hapbooks@ache.org, mentioning the book's title and putting "Book Error" in the subject line.

For photocopying and copyright information, please contact Copyright Clearance Center at www.copyright.com or at (978) 750-8400.

Health Administration Press
A division of the Foundation of the American College of Healthcare Executives
One North Franklin Street, Suite 1700
Chicago, IL 60606-3529
(312) 424-2800

Association of University Programs in Health Administration
1730 M Street, NW
Suite 407
Washington, DC
(202) 763-7283

To my blessings and inspiration—
John, Aidan, Isabella Rose, Liam;
my parents, Arthur and Rosanna; and my sister, Michelle.

To my other blessing, mentor, colleague, and friend—
Professor Emeritus Lee Seidel, Department of Health Management and Policy,
College of Health and Human Services, University of New Hampshire.

BRIEF CONTENTS

DETAILED CONTENTS

+Refer to Fleming text

PREFACE

Population health describes a population-based approach to population-oriented health issues, based on an examination of interactions among multiple determinants of health over the population's life course with the aim of developing affordable, effective, and replicable outcomes. Further, a population health approach encompasses patterns of health determinants, the measurement of resultant health outcomes, and those outcomes' distribution in the population, as well as the policies that influence health determinants (Kindig and Stoddart 2003). Thus, population health requires an effective integration of the public health and healthcare systems.

A passage from *Toward a Healthy Future: Second Report on the Health of Canadians*, by the Federal, Provincial, and Territorial Advisory Committee on Population Health (1999, vii), describes the intersection of the public health and healthcare systems and, I would argue, highlights the need for further integration of these systems:

Why is Jason in the hospital?
Because he has a bad infection in his leg.

But why does he have an infection?
Because he has a cut on his leg and it got infected.

But why does he have a cut on his leg?
Because he was playing in the junk yard next to his apartment building and there was some sharp, jagged steel there that he fell on.

But why was he playing in a junk yard?
Because his neighbourhood is kind of run down. A lot of kids play there and there is no one to supervise them.

But why does he live in that neighbourhood?
Because his parents can't afford a nicer place to live.

But why can't his parents afford a nicer place to live?
Because his Dad is unemployed and his Mom is sick.

But why is his Dad unemployed?
Because he doesn't have much education and he can't find a job.

But why . . . ?

The health of populations is complex, and multiple determinants—both those within our control and those not within our control—have a powerful impact. The interventions implemented to improve health must involve multiple stakeholders, and resources must be affordable, available, and effective to address the inequities in the community. If an intervention to address health inequality is not effective at a reasonable cost, then the intervention will be out of reach for many populations to consider. Furthermore, the metrics for monitoring a population's health outcomes differ from the metrics that would be used to measure an individual person's health outcomes.

A population health approach involves a new way of delivering healthcare to populations. In our reformed healthcare system, this "new way of doing business" requires that healthcare providers be reimbursed for keeping their patients healthy as opposed to being compensated for the volume of sick patients treated. Thus, when taking this approach, we must consider the role of health determinants in the population, the associated health outcomes, and the way we measure those outcomes. The principles and skills that administrators and practitioners need as they monitor, assess, and manage the health of populations in our newly reformed healthcare system are described in the three sections of this textbook.

Population Health: Principles and Applications for Management examines, in great detail, topics that are pertinent to the education and practice of public health and healthcare management in today's dynamic environment. Representative topics include core functions of public health, public health system organization, the basic science of public health, how to assess the health of communities, the role of managerial epidemiology, ways of improving the health of populations, and the contribution of data to this process, as well as the management of the health of diverse populations.

In addition, the chapters of *Population Health* use real case studies to educate today's students about the unique challenges and innovative approaches to promoting the health of populations. The case studies highlight examples of public health and healthcare practice that occurred in different situations, such as the international Ebola outbreak, a nationwide foodborne illness, and a local investigation of a pediatric fatality related to lead poisoning. Educational methodologies complement the case studies to impart the knowledge and skills required of today's healthcare manager and public health professional, presenting a roadmap for a population health approach.

This book is a detailed resource that presents evidence-based approaches useful to instructors and students as they learn how to promote health, prevent disease, and navigate the public health and healthcare challenges of an ever-changing environment. The lessons and topic areas within the text are timeless and offer a framework that can be expanded upon by instructors based on their own experiences. Although public health and healthcare crises can and will change over time, the key concepts and lessons provided within this book are essential to our efforts to improve the health of populations.

References

Federal, Provincial, and Territorial Advisory Committee on Population Health. 1999. *Toward a Healthy Future: Second Report on the Health of Canadians*. Ottawa, Canada: Minister of Public Works and Government Services Canada.

Kindig, D., and G. Stoddart. 2003. "What Is Population Health?" *American Journal of Public Health* 93 (3): 380–83.

Instructor Resources

This book's Instructor Resources include a test bank; presentation PowerPoint slides; answer guides to the book's discussion questions, exercises, and assignments; and resource lists.

For the most up-to-date information about this book and its Instructor Resources, go to ache.org/HAP and browse for the book's title or author name.

This book's Instructor Resources are available to instructors who adopt this book for use in their course. For access information, please e-mail hapbooks@ache.org.

ACKNOWLEDGMENTS

I would like to acknowledge my colleagues from the worlds of academia, public health, and healthcare practice for providing the experiences that have contributed to my work, first as a public health practitioner and currently as a professor of health management and policy.

The writing of this book has offered me the opportunity to reflect on my own preparation, both academically and professionally, to work as a public health practitioner and educator. I gratefully acknowledge my mentors at Regis College, the Geisel School of Medicine at Dartmouth, the Boston University School of Public Health, and the Harvard School of Public Health for the rigor their academic programs offered and the training in inquiry and research they so expertly delivered. I also thank my faculty colleagues at the University of New Hampshire for their mentoring and encouragement as I strive to continually perfect my teaching, research, and service responsibilities.

I would also like to acknowledge my colleagues at the Manchester (New Hampshire) Health Department and the New Hampshire Department of Health and Human Services, for these are the organizations where I learned to practice public health.

Education doesn't always take place in the classroom, and I have enjoyed teaching and learning from students in diverse environments. I have especially enjoyed working with students who are passionate about improving the delivery of public health and healthcare services. I appreciate my students—both those I have had the pleasure to teach and learn from and those I have yet to meet—and I value the chance to share the experience of learning to make our populations healthier.

Further, I am grateful to Janet Davis at Health Administration Press for her excitement and encouragement as I developed and wrote this book. Janet's expert listening skills, Tulie O'Connor's expert content review, and Michael Noren's expert editing ability—and their joint attention to detail—have resulted in this book being presented in a format of which I could not be more proud. Thank you.

Last but not least, as any author knows, writing a textbook is a labor of love. This book is the product of many hours spent conducting research, developing content, writing, formatting, editing, and so on. I am grateful for the opportunity to create a textbook that has the potential to shape the knowledge, attitudes, and behaviors of future healthcare administrators and public health professionals, and I have not taken this task lightly. Because of the time commitment required for this book, I have had to sacrifice time with my family. My family is supportive of all that I do, and I am blessed that they encourage me and are most proud of my achievements. I could not have accomplished this body of work without their love, encouragement, and reassurance. I am forever grateful to them for understanding and appreciating my drive to improve the delivery of healthcare and public health services via teaching undergraduate and graduate students, for these students will work toward preventing disease, promoting health, and protecting the health of populations for a long time to come.

Rosemary M. Caron

SECTION 1

PRINCIPLES, SKILLS, AND APPLICATIONS

CHAPTER 1

PUBLIC HEALTH: ORGANIZATION AND FUNCTION

"A public health professional is a person educated in public health or a related discipline who is employed to improve health through a population focus."

—Institute of Medicine (2003)

Learning Objectives

After completing this chapter, you should be able to

- define *public health* and identify its mission,
- describe the core functions of public health and how they relate to the ten essential services of public health,
- list the three types of disease prevention efforts,
- describe the organization of the public health system,
- compare and contrast the public health and healthcare systems,
- describe one public health initiative, and
- define *population health*.

Introduction

public health system
The public, private, and voluntary entities that contribute to the delivery of essential public health services within a jurisdiction. The system may include government, public health departments, physician offices, emergency response personnel, community health clinics, schools, and charity organizations.

The **public health system** is essential to ensuring a healthy population. This chapter describes the mission of public health, discusses the essential services this system provides, and highlights the greatest public health achievements accomplished to date. Although public health is vital to our everyday lives, we often do not actually think about how it keeps us healthy. This chapter will demonstrate how public health influences our health on a daily basis. Lastly, the chapter will examine the movement, in the age of healthcare reform, toward the integration of the healthcare and public health systems—which is at the center of the concept of population health.

The general population often thinks of public health as "healthcare for the poor." However, providing the poor with access to healthcare is only one aspect of the public health function. The comprehensive approach that the field of public health uses to keep the general population healthy is often misunderstood or underappreciated. This chapter will examine the organization and function of the public health system.

Public Health Defined

health
A state of complete physical, mental, and social well-being—not merely the absence of disease.

public health
The field concerned with advancing society's interest in maintaining conditions in which people can be healthy; also, the science and art of preventing disease, prolonging life, and promoting physical health and efficiency through organized community efforts.

The World Health Organization (WHO), in the preamble of its constitution, defines ***health*** as "a state of complete physical, mental, and social well-being and not merely the absence of disease or infirmity" (WHO 1946). The Institute of Medicine (IOM)—now the National Academy of Medicine—defined ***public health*** as "fulfilling society's interest in assuring conditions in which people can be healthy" (IOM 1988, 7). C. E. A. Winslow (1920, 30), a leader in public health in the early part of the twentieth century, provided a more comprehensive definition that is still cited today:

> Public health is the science and art of preventing disease, prolonging life, and promoting physical health and efficiency through organized community efforts for the sanitation of the environment, the control of community infections, the education of the individual in principles of personal hygiene, the organization of medical and nursing service for the early diagnosis and preventive treatment of disease, and the development of the social machinery which will ensure to every individual in the community a standard of living adequate for the maintenance of health.

This definition highlights the multidisciplinary nature of the field, which is necessary for preventing disease, prolonging life, and promoting health. The overarching goal of public health is to ensure conditions—that is, living and working conditions—in which people in various geographic settings (e.g., neighborhoods, census tracts, communities, cities and towns, states, regions, counties) can be afforded the opportunity to live a healthy life. Winslow's definition elaborates on how we are to accomplish this mission via "organized community efforts," "the organization of medical and nursing services," and "the development of the social machinery"—functions of a public health system that are still practiced today (Winslow 1920).

The History of Public Health

Narrowly considered, public health was originally thought to consist of the measures implemented by a community to protect the population from infectious diseases. In fact, a late-1700s outbreak of yellow fever—a viral disease transmitted by infected mosquitoes and most commonly found in South America and Africa (Centers for Disease Control and Prevention 2016)—prompted the development of the first boards of health in major cities, including Philadelphia; Boston; Baltimore; New York City; Washington, DC; and New Orleans. These events were followed by the sanitation movement of the mid-1800s, which led to the improvement of living conditions and the development of a type of public health organization in major cities (Pfizer Global Pharmaceuticals 2006).

For Discussion: New York City Street Scene

Look at this late-1800s Jacob Riis photo of a New York City neighborhood, and identify the obvious and potential public health threats. We do not typically see this type of living environment in the United States today. Why do you think that is?

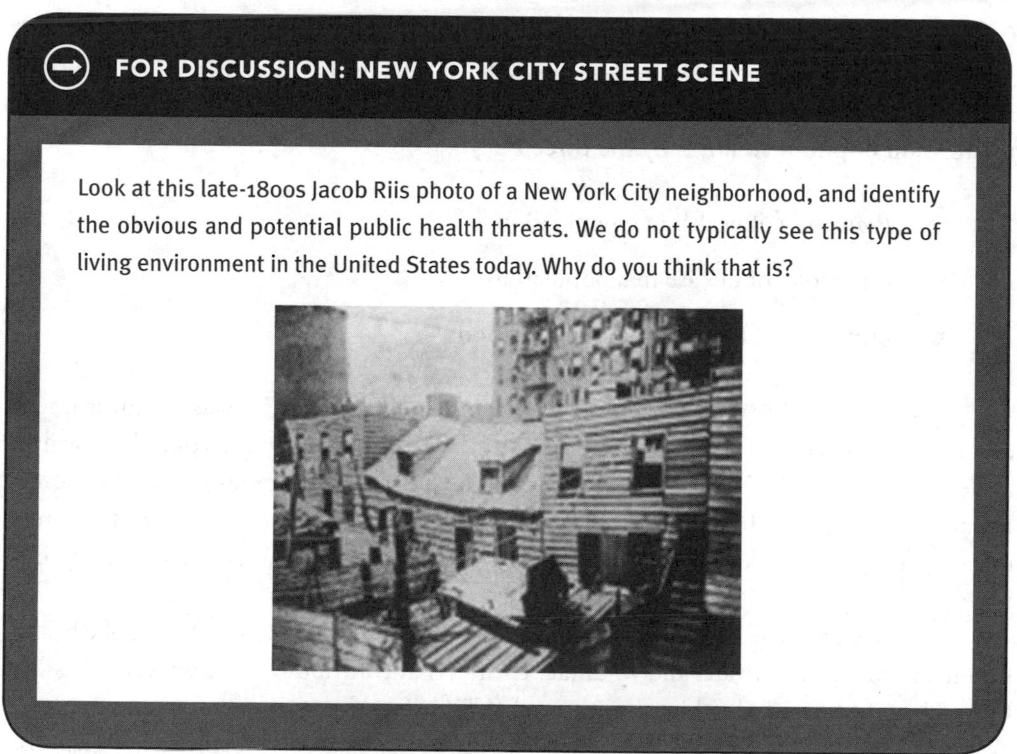

The rich history of public health in the United States dates back to the eighteenth century, when President John Adams signed a law providing for the care and relief of sick and injured merchant seamen in US ports (Pfizer 2006). The resulting marine hospitals were later organized into the Marine Hospital Service, which eventually became the US Public Health Service. The position we know today as the surgeon general was created to administer the Marine Hospital Service.

The focus of public health has expanded as our society has become more complex. Public health today is responsible not only for preventing infectious diseases, as was the case centuries ago, but also for ensuring safe living and working environments, preventing lifestyle- and behavior-related diseases, and preparing communities for emergencies, to name a few examples.

For those interested in reading more about the history of public health, George Rosen's *A History of Public Health* (Johns Hopkins University Press, 1993) offers a comprehensive overview of significant historical contributions to the field. In addition, the US Department of Health and Human Services maintains a website featuring biographies of past surgeon generals (www.surgeongeneral.gov/about/previous/index.html).

The Public Health Mission, Infrastructure, and Essential Services

The mission of public health can be described as health promotion, disease prevention, and protection of populations so they can live a healthy life. A helpful way to remember the mission of public health is by the **three *Ps***:

- *Promotion* of health in a population
- *Prevention* of disease in a population
- *Protection* of the health of a population

To achieve this mission, public health operates at various levels of government and in different sectors (i.e., private and nonprofit). The core functions of public health, as described by the IOM (1988), are **assessment**, **policy development**, and **assurance**. Because no single health agency can execute all these core functions by itself, we rely on a complex network of community-based agencies and organizations to carry out the mission.

The **Centers for Disease Control and Prevention (CDC)** defines the public health system as "all public, private, and voluntary entities that contribute to the delivery of essential public health services within a jurisdiction" (CDC 2014). The system may comprise local and state governmental public health departments, physician offices, emergency response personnel, community health clinics, charity organizations, schools, recreation facilities, and more.

three Ps
The three parts of the mission of public health: the *promotion* of health in a population, the *prevention* of disease in a population, and the *protection* of the health of a population.

assessment
The public health function that involves systematic collection, analysis, and reporting on the health status of a community.

policy development
The public health function that uses scientific knowledge and a shared process to create and implement policies that are protective of the public's health.

assurance
The public health function of confirming that agreed-upon health services are provided and effective.

Centers for Disease Control and Prevention (CDC)
A health protection agency in the United States.

Exhibit 1.1
The Public Health System

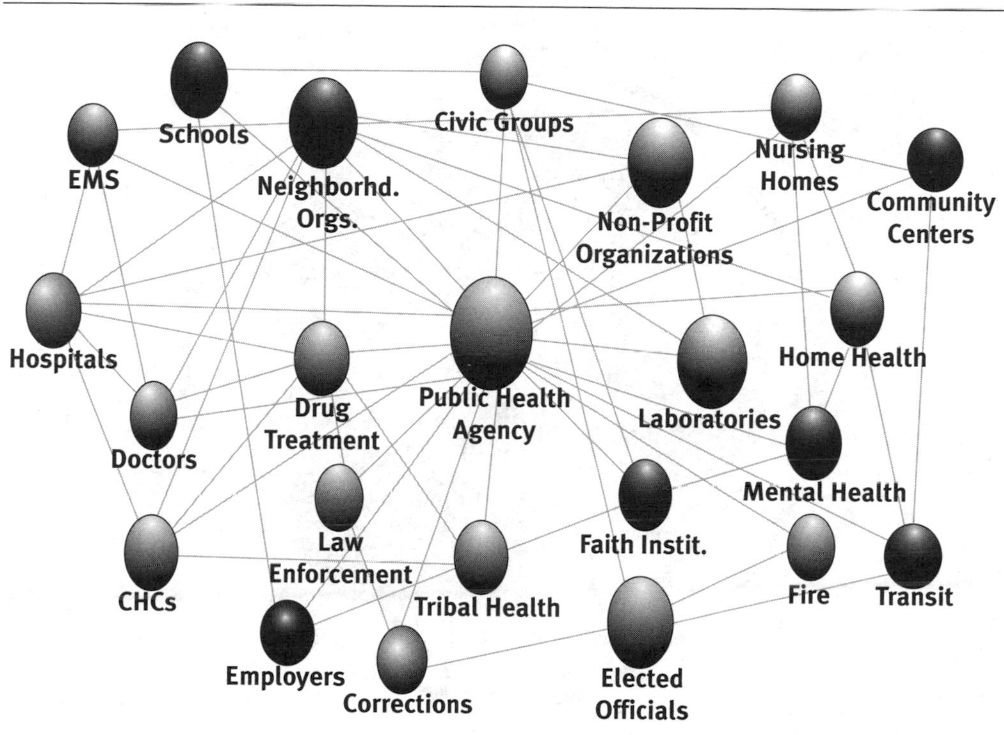

Note: EMS = emergency medical services; CHCs = community health centers.
Source: Reprinted from CDC (2014).

Exhibit 1.1 shows an illustration, as proposed by the CDC, of the organizations, institutions, and agencies—and their working interrelationships in the community—that make up the public health system.

The CDC outlined the structure of the public health system and further described the activities that public health systems should undertake to prevent disease and promote health in communities. These activities are known as the ten **essential public health services (EPHS)**, and they are displayed in the diagram in exhibit 1.2. The EPHS are aligned with the core functions of public health—assessment, policy development, and assurance—in that each service is categorized according to the core function it fulfills. For instance, the diagram shows that the "Monitor Health" service corresponds with the "Assessment" core function.

essential public health services (EPHS)
The public health activities that all communities should undertake to prevent disease and promote health.

The CDC's (2014) detailed descriptions for each essential service are summarized in the sections that follow.

Exhibit 1.2
The Ten Essential Public Health Services

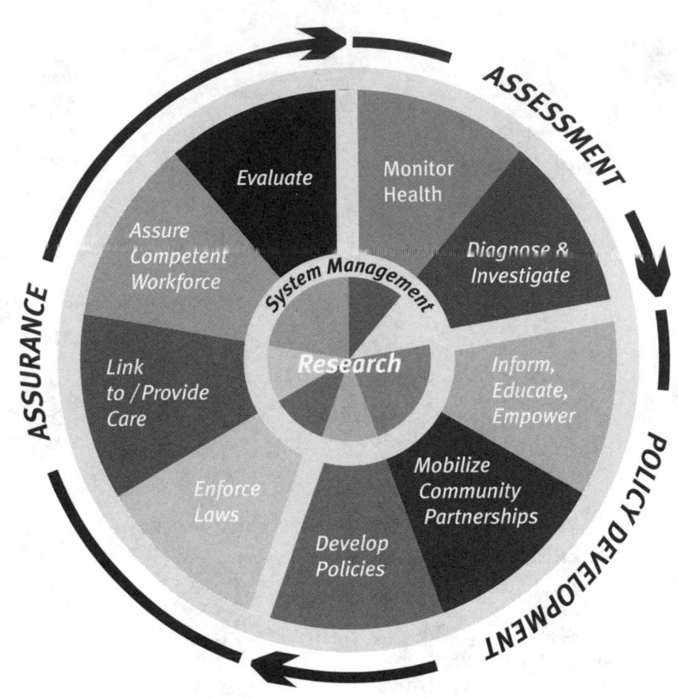

Source: Reprinted from CDC (2014).

EPHS #1: Monitor Health Status to Identify and Solve Community Health Problems

EPHS #1 provides answers to the questions, "What's going on in our state/community?" and "Do we know how healthy we are?" It incorporates the following elements (CDC 2014):

- "Accurate, periodic assessment of the community's health status," which includes
  - identification of health risks and determinants of health, and the determination of health service needs;
  - attention to vital statistics and health status indicators of high-risk groups; and
  - identification of community assets that support the local public health system (LPHS) in promoting health and quality of life
- "Use of appropriate methods and technology, such as geographic information systems (GIS), to interpret and communicate data to diverse audiences"

- "Collaboration among all LPHS components, including private providers and health benefit plans, to establish and use population health registries, such as disease or immunization registries"

EPHS #2: Diagnose and Investigate Health Problems and Health Hazards in the Community

EPHS #2 responds to several questions: "Are we ready to respond to health problems or threats?" "How quickly do we find out about problems?" "How effective is our response?" It involves the following concerns (CDC 2014):

- "Timely identification and investigation of health threats," including "disease outbreaks, patterns of infections, chronic diseases, injuries, environmental hazards," and more
- "Availability of diagnostic services, including laboratory capacity," to conduct rapid screening and high-volume testing
- "Response plans to address major health threats"

EPHS #3: Inform, Educate, and Empower People About Health Issues

EPHS #3 responds to the question, "How well do we keep all segments of our state/community informed about health issues?" It incorporates the following (CDC 2014):

- "Health information, health education, and health promotion activities designed to reduce health risk and promote improved health"
- "Health communication plans and activities such as media advocacy and social marketing"
- "Accessible health information and educational resources"
- "Health education and health promotion program partnerships with schools, faith-based communities, work sites, personal care providers, and others"

EPHS #4: Mobilize Community Partnerships and Action to Identify and Solve Health Problems

EPHS #4 considers the question, "How well do we truly engage people in state/community health issues?" It involves the following tasks (CDC 2014):

- "Identifying potential stakeholders who contribute to or benefit from public health" and increasing those stakeholders' awareness of the value of public health
- "Building coalitions, partnerships, and strategic alliances to draw upon the full range of potential human and material resources to improve community health"
- "Convening and facilitating partnerships and strategic alliances among groups and associations (including those not typically considered to be health-related) in undertaking defined health improvement projects, including preventive, screening, rehabilitation, and support programs."

EPHS #5: Develop Policies and Plans That Support Individual and Community Health Efforts

EPHS #5 addresses the questions, "What policies in both the government and private sector promote health in our state/community?" and "How well are we setting health policies?" It includes the following elements (CDC 2014):

- "Effective local public health governance"
- "Development of policy, codes, regulations, and legislation to protect the health of the public and to guide the practice of public health"
- Systematic planning at the LPHS and state levels for health improvement in all jurisdictions
- "Alignment of LPHS resources and strategies with community health improvement plans"

EPHS #6: Enforce Laws and Regulations That Protect Health and Ensure Safety

EPHS #6 considers the question, "When we enforce health regulations, are we technically competent, fair, and effective?" It incorporates the following (CDC 2014):

- "Assurance of due process and recognition of individuals' civil rights in all procedures, enforcement of laws and regulations, and public health emergency actions taken under the board of health or other governing body's authority"
- "Review, evaluation, and revision of laws and regulations designed to protect health and safety, reflect current scientific knowledge, and utilize best practice for achieving compliance"

- "Education of persons and entities obligated to obey and agencies obligated to enforce laws and regulations," with the aim of encouraging compliance
- "Enforcement activities in a wide variety of areas of public health concern under authority granted by local, state, and federal rule or law," including such areas as abatement of nuisances, animal control, childhood immunizations, food safety, housing code, protection of drinking water, school environment, solid waste disposal, tobacco control, and enforcement activities during emergency situations

EPHS #7: Link People to Needed Personal Health Services and Assure the Provision of Healthcare When Otherwise Unavailable

EPHS #7 addresses the question, "Are people in my state/community receiving the health services they need?" It involves the following concerns (CDC 2014):

- "Assuring the identification of populations with barriers to personal health services"
- "Assuring identification of personal health service needs of populations with limited access to a coordinated system of clinical care"
- "Assuring the linkage of people to appropriate personal health services through coordination of provider services and development of interventions that address barriers to care (e.g., culturally and linguistically appropriate staff and materials, transportation services)"

EPHS #8: Assure a Competent Public and Personal Healthcare Workforce

EPHS #8 answers the questions, "Do we have a competent public health staff?" and "How can we be sure that our staff stays current?" It involves the following elements (CDC 2014):

- "Education, training, and assessment of personnel (including volunteers and other lay community health workers) to meet community needs for public and personal health services"
- Use of efficient licensure processes for professionals
- "Adoption of continuous quality improvement and life-long learning programs that include determinants of health"

- "Active partnerships and strategic alliances with professional training programs to assure community-relevant learning experiences for all students"
- "Continuing education in management and leadership development programs for those charged with administrative/executive roles"

EPHS #9: Evaluate Effectiveness, Accessibility, and Quality of Personal and Population-Based Health Services

EPHS #9 considers several important questions: "Are we meeting the needs of the population we serve?" "Are we doing things right?" "Are we doing the right things?" It incorporates the following (CDC 2014):

- "Assurance of ongoing evaluation and critical review of health program effectiveness, based on analysis of health status and service utilization data"
- "Assurance of the provision of information necessary for allocating resources and reshaping programs"

EPHS #10: Research for New Insights and Innovative Solutions to Health Problems

EPHS #10 addresses the question, "Are we discovering and using new ways to get the job done?" It incorporates the following public health research activities (CDC 2014):

- Initiating research
- Participating in research done by others
- Reporting results
- Implementing policy based on the results

The "Wheel" of Public Health Services

Students should take the time to review and understand the significance of the "wheel" of EPHS, shown in exhibit 1.2. The wheel provides the blueprint by which public health acts in every community (with possible variations based on infrastructure and available resources). Notice that "Research" is at the center of the circle, meaning that, in order to implement these ten essential services and core functions of public health, the work must be grounded in research. In other words, public health research findings inform how the system carries out its services and functions. Furthermore, when thinking about the functions and services illustrated in exhibits 1.1 and 1.2, notice the different areas of knowledge, skills, and disciplines required to ensure a healthy population.

The Community Tool Box (2016), an online resource developed by the University of Kansas (KU) Work Group for Community Health and Development and its partners, offers examples of how the EPHS are practiced in daily public health work. For example, "Informing the public about an epidemiological outbreak investigation in the community" is presented as an example of EPHS #2 ("Diagnose and investigate health problems and health hazards in the community"), and "Maintenance of a sanitary restaurant environment for public well-being" is an example of EPHS #6 ("Enforce laws and regulations that protect health and ensure safety"). The Community Tool Box represents part of the KU Work Group's role as a designated World Health Organization Collaborating Centre for Community Health and Development.

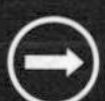

FOR DISCUSSION: PUBLIC HEALTH PRACTICE IN THE COMMUNITY

The field of public health is multidisciplinary in nature and requires collaboration among community organizations and agencies that, on first glance, may appear to have nothing in common. Consider this example: An urban community is experiencing elevated rates of teenage pregnancy. The community also lacks places where adolescents can engage in recreational activities after school, and the parks that do exist are home to gang violence. How do you think teenage pregnancy and violence are related in this example? What community organizations should be involved to help address this public health problem? (Explain your rationale.) Describe two approaches that these identified community organizations should implement to prevent gang violence and teen pregnancy.

The Distinction Between Public Health and Healthcare

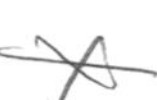

Because the health of a population differs from the health of an individual, public health and healthcare professionals approach their work differently. For example, the public health practitioner's work focuses on the prevention of disease and promotion of health in the population as a whole. In contrast, the healthcare provider addresses health at the individual level by diagnosing and treating one person's medical condition. The "treatment" utilized in public health includes interventions that could be educational or policy-based in nature, for example. Meanwhile, healthcare focuses on classic diagnosis and treatment.

> *"Healthcare matters to all of us some of the time; public health matters to all of us all of the time."*
>
> —C. Everett Koop, former US Surgeon General (What Is Public Health? 2014)

Healthcare provides the diagnosis and treatment, whereas public health addresses the assurance of access to those services. Thus, public health and healthcare should be viewed as complementary health systems that collaborate to help develop the healthiest population possible. Goldsteen, Goldsteen, and Graham (2011, 5) state, accurately, that "public health shares with the clinical professions a fundamental caring for humanity through concern for health." In public health practice, health is achieved via disease and injury prevention, and this prevention can be categorized into three types (Fos and Fine 2000):

primary prevention Prevention efforts concerned with eliminating risk factors for a disease.

secondary prevention Prevention efforts that focus on early detection and treatment of disease.

tertiary prevention Prevention efforts aimed at minimizing disability associated with advanced disease.

1. **Primary prevention** is concerned with eliminating risk factors for a disease. An example of primary prevention might involve providing health education and immunizations.
2. **Secondary prevention** focuses on early detection and treatment of disease (subclinical and clinical). An example of secondary prevention might include a screening such as a colonoscopy or a mammogram.
3. **Tertiary prevention** attempts to eliminate or moderate disability associated with advanced disease. Examples of tertiary prevention might include physical therapy or diabetic foot checks.

Healthcare focuses mainly on secondary and tertiary prevention, when a disease has already occurred and a person is attempting to detect it early so treatment may be initiated (secondary prevention) or working to minimize further disability (tertiary prevention). Public health works in these areas of secondary and tertiary prevention through such efforts as providing access to medical visits, ensuring health literacy among the population, and promoting cultural competence among healthcare providers. The administration of immunizations is an example of an area in which healthcare and public health overlap in prevention, because immunizations are intended to prevent the development of disease (primary prevention). Another example of primary prevention is health education, which can inform people about disease risk factors and prevention methods. These examples highlight the potential for integration of the public health and healthcare systems that are often viewed as distinct.

Exhibit 1.3
The Ten Greatest Public Health Achievements in the Twentieth Century

1. Immunizations
2. Motor vehicle safety
3. Workplace safety
4. Control of infectious diseases
5. Declines in deaths from heart disease and stroke
6. Safer and healthier foods
7. Healthier mothers and babies
8. Family planning
9. Fluoridation of drinking water
10. Tobacco as a health hazard

Source: CDC (2013).

Public Health Achievements and Initiatives

An ongoing debate between the public health and healthcare systems has involved which field is more responsible for the increased life expectancy that Americans experience today. Many are surprised to learn that public health, rather than medical advancements, is the greater contributor. The CDC (2013) states that "public health is credited with adding 25 years to the life expectancy of people in the United States" in the twentieth century. In 2010, the average life expectancy in the United States was 76.2 years for males and 81.0 years for females (Murphy, Xu, and Kochanek 2013)—a significant increase from the 1900 life expectancy of 47.9 years for males and 50.7 years for females (Arias 2012).

The CDC (2013) has identified what it considers the ten greatest achievements in public health in the twentieth century, and those achievements are listed in exhibit 1.3. "These advances have been largely responsible for increasing the lifespan of populations; over 25 of the 30 years [of increase in life expectancy] can be accredited to public health initiatives, while medical advances account for less than 4 years" (What Is Public Health? 2014).

Notice that the twentieth-century public health achievements listed in exhibit 1.3 largely represent issues that we, as members of the public, have come to expect as standard today. Our increased life expectancy and enhanced quality of life are the result of continued improvements in such areas as nutrition, housing, and environmental hygiene. We should continue to allocate resources to promote healthy workplaces and a reduced maternal and infant mortality rate; however, more focused efforts could be directed toward, for example, reducing premature and low-weight births among African American women and providing safer work environments for hazardous occupations. At the same time, we must stay vigilant to researching and preparing for new threats to the public health system in the twenty-first century, such as antimicrobial resistance, food safety, violence, global pandemics, and obesity, to name a few.

The following sections highlight noteworthy public health initiatives at the national, state, county, and local levels.

Exhibit 1.4
Healthy People 2020: Mission and Goals

Mission

Healthy People 2020 strives to:

- Identify nationwide health improvement priorities.
- Increase public awareness and understanding of the determinants of health, disease, and disability and the opportunities for progress.
- Provide measurable objectives and goals that are applicable at the national, state, and local levels.
- Engage multiple sectors to take actions to strengthen policies and improve practices that are driven by the best available evidence and knowledge.
- Identify critical research, evaluation, and data collection needs.

Overarching Goals

- Attain high-quality, longer lives free of preventable disease, disability, injury, and premature death.
- Achieve health equity, eliminate disparities, and improve the health of all groups.
- Create social and physical environments that promote good health for all.
- Promote quality of life, healthy development, and healthy behaviors across all life stages.

Four foundation health measures will serve as an indicator of progress towards achieving these goals:

- General health status
- Health-related quality of life and well-being
- Determinants of health
- Disparities

Source: Reprinted from Healthy People (2016a).

National Public Health Initiative: Healthy People

Healthy People (2016a), an initiative within the US Department of Health and Human Services, provides a model framework to guide health promotion and disease prevention efforts. It uses ten-year plans to develop benchmarks and monitor progress for achieving a healthy population. The mission and goals of Healthy People 2020, the fourth edition of the ten-year plan, are outlined in exhibit 1.4.

Healthy People 2020 has 42 topic areas with more than 1,200 objectives. A smaller set of objectives, called Leading Health Indicators (LHIs), has been chosen "to

Exhibit 1.5
Healthy People 2020: Leading Health Indicator Topic Areas

LHI's

Access to health services
Clinical preventive services
Environmental quality
Injury and violence
Maternal, infant, and child health
Mental health
Nutrition, physical activity, and obesity
Oral health
Reproductive and sexual health
Social determinants
Substance abuse
Tobacco

Source: Healthy People (2016b).

communicate high-priority health issues and actions that can be taken to address them" (Healthy People 2016b). These LHI topic areas are listed in exhibit 1.5.

Goldsteen, Goldsteen, and Graham (2011, 191) write: "Healthy People has been a highly influential initiative for assessing the health of the nation and, by implication, the performance of the public health system. The Healthy People initiative acknowledges that even though the agenda is national, the improvements will come through local actions, which will then affect the state, regional, and national outcomes reports."

Healthy People is the core initiative for prevention efforts across the US Department of Health and Human Services. Exhibit 1.6 lists several other prevention programs currently being administered at a national level.

Exhibit 1.6
Examples of National Prevention Programs

Let's Move! Campaign
National Action Plan for the Prevention, Care, and Treatment of Viral Hepatitis
National Action Plan to Improve Health Literacy
National Action Plan to Prevent Healthcare-Associated Infection
National Action Plan to Reduce Racial and Ethnic Health Disparities
National HIV/AIDS Strategy
President's Food Safety Working Group
Tobacco Control Strategic Action Plan
US National Vaccine Plan

Source: CDC (2015).

FOR DISCUSSION: HEALTHY PEOPLE 2020

The framework offered by the Healthy People 2020 initiative provides an action plan by which states and local communities can select which Leading Health Indicators to address based on the communities' health status, economic resources, and personnel. States can compare their progress relative to prior years or to similar states, and they can observe the nation's progress toward the vision of "a society in which all people live long, healthy lives" (Healthy People 2016a). Review the EPHS, discussed earlier in the chapter, in light of the Healthy People 2020 initiative. Which services do you think apply to the successful implementation of Healthy People 2020? Explain your rationale.

State Public Health Initiative: Healthier Wisconsin Partnership Program

The Healthier Wisconsin Partnership Program (HWPP) is part of a Medical College of Wisconsin endowment titled Advancing a Healthier Wisconsin. The endowment—which was established as a result of the state's health insurance plan, Blue Cross & Blue Shield United of Wisconsin, converting to a for-profit stock insurance corporation—aims to address public health issues affecting the population of the state. HWPP provides funding to academic and community-based partners who plan to jointly address public health issues in three core areas: infrastructure to transform health improvements, affected populations, and health focus areas (Kerschner and Maurana 2012). A list of proposals funded through the program shows a variety of project types, reflecting the diversity of public health issues faced by the state of Wisconsin (Advancing a Healthier Wisconsin Endowment 2016).

County Public Health Initiative: County Health Rankings & Roadmaps Program

Another useful tool to promote health in the community is the County Health Rankings & Roadmaps program, a collaboration between the Robert Wood Johnson Foundation and the University of Wisconsin Population Health Institute (County Health Rankings & Roadmaps Program 2016).

The County Health Rankings report health information for every county in every US state. The rankings examine factors that influence health, such as income, high school graduation rate, unemployment rate, access to healthy food, teen births, and obesity. The

County Health Roadmaps complement the County Health Rankings. Once a community has assessed its rankings (with information available at www.countyhealthrankings.org), the community and its public health partners can decide which health issues pose the most significant challenge and which health issues are feasible to address given the community's available resources and economic and political climate. The community and public health stakeholders work together to assess needs and resources, communicate, act on what is important (which may require policy development), and evaluate the actions taken.

Local Public Health Initiative: Neighborhood Health Improvement

Often, serious health problems and unstable social conditions are concentrated in a relatively small number of distressed areas of urban communities. One such community is Manchester, the largest city in New Hampshire. With a 2010 census population of 109,565, Manchester represents more than 8 percent of the state's total population.

The Manchester Health Department (MHD) closely examined the health status of the community's residents and identified eight neighborhoods that "have been shown to share significantly higher rates of overall neighborhood deprivation and poor health outcomes such as higher rates of coronary heart disease mortality, violent crime, expectant mothers with late or no prenatal care, adolescent pregnancies, lead poisonings, childhood obesity, pedestrian accidents and fatalities, uncontrolled asthma, and substandard housing as compared with other neighborhoods" (MHD 2014).

To address these conditions, the MHD, along with other public health system partners, proposed a "**collective impact**" approach. Research has contrasted collective impact strategies with traditional "isolated impact" strategies (Kania and Kramer 2011, 2013), finding that "successful collective impact initiatives typically have five conditions that together produce true alignment and lead to powerful results: a common agenda, shared measurement systems, mutually reinforcing activities, continuous communication, and backbone support organizations" (MHD 2014, 56). The community of Manchester and its public health partners are working collaboratively to reduce the impact of persistent public health issues.

collective impact
An approach to problem solving that involves organizations from different sectors agreeing to address a specific issue using a common agenda, aligning their efforts, and using the same measures for success.

Another example of a collective impact approach is Shape Up Somerville, an anti-obesity campaign in Somerville, Massachusetts. The citywide program aims "to reduce obesity by engaging schools, city government, civic organizations, community groups, businesses, and other people who live in, work in, and visit the city" (Collective Impact Forum 2013). The effort has had a significant impact through programming, policy work, and physical infrastructure improvements.

FOR DISCUSSION: A DAY IN THE LIFE

Consider the "typical day" described below and discuss the role that public health plays to keep you healthy and safe.

7:00 am

Your alarm clock rings, and you roll out of bed. You turn the faucet to brush your teeth, and fluoride-enriched water flows out. Despite being reluctant to commute to work this morning, you have slept well.

7:30 am

Before you leave the house, you have a balanced, nutritious breakfast. The milk, orange juice, and coffee you prepare have all been inspected and approved as ready for human consumption. The same goes for your bread, bagels, cereal, bananas, or any other breakfast food you choose.

8:00 am

You hop in the car for your daily commute to work and buckle your seatbelt. As you are driving, you can be assured that public health experts have conducted research that has led to improved traffic safety laws.

9:00 am

Your workday has begun. The air filters provide the office with clean air. Public health experts who researched the effects of proper posture on chronic musculo-skeletal injuries developed your office chair with ergonomics in mind. The over-head lights have been designed to provide just the right amount of light to keep you awake during work while also reducing depressive symptoms.

12 noon

At lunch, you go for a brisk walk. The CDC encourages adults to get at least 30 minutes of activity each day. Regular exercise can help you

- control weight;
- control high blood pressure;
- reduce risk for Type 2 diabetes, heart attack, and colon cancer;
- reduce symptoms of depression and anxiety;

(continued)

- reduce arthritis pain and disability; and
- reduce risk for osteoporosis and falls.

5:00 pm
You go to meet friends or work colleagues for an early dinner. You open the restaurant door, and before being seated, you catch a glimpse of the city or county certificate of approval. The certificate signifies that your chosen restaurant serves clean food.

8:00 pm
Before reading a best-selling novel and falling asleep, you decide to watch some television. The evening newscaster mentions the latest study into the effects of smoking on lung cancer and another study about the latest data released for a new cancer drug. The Food and Drug Administration announced approval of a new medication to treat asthma, and public health experts are handling possible disease transmission after a recent hurricane hit the Southeast. A commercial explains the latest food guide, and you start planning what breakfast you would like to eat tomorrow morning.

Source: Adapted from Lafayette County Health Department (2016).

Population Health Versus Public Health

Population health is a relatively new term related to public health. The term originated in Canada, and the Canadian Federal, Provincial, and Territorial Advisory Committee on Population Health defined it in 1997 as "the health of a population as measured by health status indicators and as influenced by social, economic, and physical environments, personal health practices, individual capacity and coping skills, human biology, early childhood development, and health services. As an approach, population health focuses on interrelated conditions and factors that influence the health of populations over the life course, identifies systematic variations in their patterns of occurrence, and applies the resulting knowledge to develop and implement policies and actions to improve the health and well-being of those populations" (Public Health Agency of Canada 2013).

Kindig and Stoddart (2003, 381) propose that "*population health as a concept of health* be defined as 'the health outcomes of a group of individuals, including the distribution of such outcomes within the group.'" Such populations can be geographic regions, such as nations or communities, or other groups, such as employees, ethnic groups, people with disabilities, or prisoners. "Many determinants of health, such as medical care systems, the social environment, and the physical environment, have their biological impact on individuals in part at a population level" (Kindig and Stoddart 2003, 381).

population health
Health as measured by health status indicators within populations and influenced by social, economic, and physical environments; personal health practices; health services; and various other factors. A population health approach focuses on interrelated conditions that influence the health of populations, identifies variations in observed patterns, and uses the resulting knowledge to inform policies to improve the health and well-being of populations.

Population health should not be viewed as separate from public health but rather as a complement to public health. Population health addresses the diverse range of social, cultural, environmental, and physical conditions that populations are born into and live with, and it considers the outcomes these determinants have on the health of populations.

Exhibit 1.7 lists a number of public health and population health professional associations.

Exhibit 1.7
Some Professional Associations for Public Health and Population Health

American Hospital Association (AHA)
Website: www.aha.org
Mission: "To advance the health of individuals and communities. The AHA leads, represents, and serves hospitals, health systems, and other related organizations that are accountable to the community and committed to health improvement."

American Public Health Association (APHA)
Website: www.apha.org
Mission: "Improve the health of the public and achieve equity in health status"

Association for Community Health Improvement (ACHI)
Website: www.healthycommunities.org
Mission: "To advance healthy communities by providing our members education, professional development, resources, and engagement opportunities in the fields of community health, population health, and community benefit"

Health Research & Educational Trust (HRET)
Website: www.hret.org
Mission: "Transforming health care through research and education"

National Association of County and City Health Officials (NACCHO)
Website: www.naccho.org
Mission: "To improve the public's health while adhering to a set of core values: equity, excellence, participation, respect, integrity, leadership, science, and innovation"

National Association of Local Boards of Health (NALBOH)
Website: www.nalboh.org
Mission: "To strengthen and improve public health governance"

Public Health Institute (PHI)
Website: www.phi.org
Mission: "PHI generates and promotes research, leadership, and partnerships to build capacity for strong public health policy, programs, systems, and practices."

Sources: AHA 2016; APHA 2016; ACHI 2016; HRET 2016; NACCHO 2016; NALBOH 2017; PHI 2016.

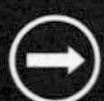

FOR DISCUSSION: PUBLIC HEALTH IN THE MEDIA

Explore the following links, and read about public health issues in the news. You may be surprised to see that public health is all around us! Discuss the stories that you find most surprising, whether because public health is the main issue or the public health system is involved in responding to a particular problem.

- *Environmental Health News* (www.environmentalhealthnews.org)
- *Food Safety News* (www.foodsafetynews.com/sections/nutrition-public-health)
- *Kaiser Health News* (http://khn.org)
- *The Nation's Health* (http://thenationshealth.aphapublications.org)
- *Public Health Newswire* (www.publichealthnewswire.org)
- *Science Daily* (www.sciencedaily.com/news/science_society/public_health)

Also check the *New York Times*, *Washington Post*, *Wall Street Journal*, and other major newspapers.

Key Chapter Points

- Public health is "the science and art of preventing disease, prolonging life, and promoting health and efficiency through organized community efforts" (Winslow 1920, 30).
- The mission of public health is to promote health, prevent disease, and protect populations so that they live a healthy life.
- The three *P*s of public health are *promotion*, *prevention*, and *protection*.
- The core functions of public health are assessment, policy development, and assurance.
- The public health system is defined as "all public, private, and voluntary entities that contribute to the delivery of essential public health services within a jurisdiction" (CDC 2014).
- The ten essential public health services (EPHS) are the functions that the public health system should undertake to prevent disease and promote health in all communities. They are based on the core functions of public health.

- Public health differs from healthcare in that public health focuses efforts on achieving and maintaining the health of populations. In contrast, healthcare uses diagnosis and treatment to achieve health in an individual.
- Disease prevention is the cornerstone of public health. There are three types of prevention: (1) primary, concerned with eliminating risk factors for a disease; (2) secondary, focused on early detection and treatment of a disease; and (3) tertiary, aimed at eliminating or moderating disability associated with an advanced disease (Fos and Fine 2000).
- We enjoy an increased life expectancy and improved quality of life as a result of the public health achievements of the twentieth century.
- Initiatives at the national, state, and local community levels aim to improve the health of populations. These initiatives require community members and public health–oriented stakeholders to work collaboratively.
- Collective impact initiatives "typically have five conditions that together produce true alignment and lead to powerful results: a common agenda, shared measurement systems, mutually reinforcing activities, continuous communication, and backbone support organizations" (MHD 2014, 56).
- Kindig and Stoddart (2003, 381) "propose that *population health* as a concept of health be defined as 'the health outcomes of a group of individuals, including the distribution of such outcomes within the group.' These populations are often geographic regions, such as nations or communities, but they can also be other groups, such as employees, ethnic groups, disabled persons, or prisoners. . . . [M]any determinants of health, such as medical care systems, the social environment, and the physical environment, have their biological impact on individuals in part at a population level."

Discussion Questions

1. Define *public health* and describe its mission.
2. What are the core functions of public health?
3. Describe the public health system, and provide two examples of representative stakeholders in this system.
4. Describe two of the essential public health services, and explain why they are important.
5. What are the three types of prevention? Provide an example of each.
6. Describe one public health initiative, and explain why it is relevant to achieving the public health mission.
7. Provide two examples of how public health achievements have influenced your daily life.

References

Advancing a Healthier Wisconsin Endowment. 2016. "HWPP Funded Partnership Awards." Medical College of Wisconsin. Updated March 28. www.mcw.edu/Advancing-Healthier-WI-Endowment/Funded-Awards/HWPP-Funded-Awards.htm.

American Hospital Association (AHA). 2016. "Vision & Mission." Accessed August 29. www.aha.org/about/mission.shtml.

American Public Health Association (APHA). 2016. "Our Mission." Accessed August 29. www.apha.org/about-apha/our-mission.

Arias, E. 2012. "United States Life Tables, 2008." *National Vital Statistics Reports* 61 (3): 1–63.

Association for Community Health Improvement (ACHI). 2016. "About ACHI." Accessed August 29. www.healthycommunities.org/About/.

Centers for Disease Control and Prevention (CDC). 2016. "Yellow Fever." Updated July 12. www.cdc.gov/yellowfever.

———. 2015. "National Health Initiatives, Strategies, and Action Plans." Updated November 9. www.cdc.gov/stltpublichealth/strategy/index.html.

———. 2014. "National Public Health Performance Standards." Updated May 29. www.cdc.gov/nphpsp/essentialservices.html.

———. 2013. "Ten Great Public Health Achievements in the 20th Century." Updated April 26. www.cdc.gov/about/history/tengpha.htm.

Collective Impact Forum. 2013. "Case Study: Shape Up Somerville." Published December 30. https://collectiveimpactforum.org/resources/case-study-shape-somerville.

Community Tool Box. 2016. "Ten Essential Public Health Services." Work Group for Community Health and Development, University of Kansas. Accessed May 19. http://ctb.ku.edu/en/table-of-contents/overview/models-for-community-health-and-development/ten-essential-public-health-services/main.

County Health Rankings & Roadmaps Program. 2016. "About." Accessed August 29. www.countyhealthrankings.org/about-project.

Fos, P. J., and D. J. Fine. 2000. *Designing Healthcare for Populations: Applied Epidemiology in Healthcare Administration.* San Francisco: Jossey-Bass.

Goldsteen, R. L., K. Goldsteen, and D. G. Graham. 2011. *Introduction to Public Health.* New York: Springer Publishing.

Health Research & Educational Trust (HRET). 2016. "About Us." Accessed August 29. www.hret.org/about/index.shtml.

Healthy People. 2016a. "About Healthy People." Updated August 25. www.healthypeople.gov/2020/About-Healthy-People.

——. 2016b. "Leading Health Indicators." Updated August 25. www.healthypeople.gov/2020/Leading-Health-Indicators.

Institute of Medicine (IOM). 2003. *Who Will Keep the Public Healthy? Educating Public Health Professionals for the 21st Century.* Washington, DC: National Academies Press.

——. 1988. *The Future of Public Health.* Washington, DC: National Academies Press.

Kania, J., and M. Kramer. 2013. "Embracing Emergence: How Collective Impact Addresses Complexity." *Stanford Social Innovation Review.* Published January 21. http://ssir.org/articles/entry/embracing_emergence_how_collective_impact_addresses_complexity.

——. 2011. "Collective Impact." *Stanford Social Innovation Review.* Accessed August 29, 2016. http://ssir.org/articles/entry/collective_impact.

Kerschner, J. E., and C. A. Maurana. 2012. "Community Medical Education Program" (online presentation). Wisconsin Office of Rural Health. Presented January 12. http://worh.org/files/MCW_CommMedEdu01-12-12.pdf.

Kindig, D., and G. Stoddart. 2003. "What Is Population Health?" *American Journal of Public Health* 93 (3): 380–83.

Lafayette County Health Department. 2016. "Day in the Life." Accessed August 29. www.lafayettecountyhealth.org/DayInTheLife.html.

Manchester Health Department (MHD). 2014. *Manchester Neighborhood Health Improvement Strategy.* Accessed December 15. www.manchesternh.gov/health/NeighborhoodHealthImprovementStrategy.pdf.

Murphy, S. L., J. Xu, and K. D. Kochanek. 2013. "Deaths: Final Data for 2010." *National Vital Statistics Reports* 61 (4): 1–117.

National Association of County and City Health Officials (NACCHO). 2016. "About." Accessed August 29. www.naccho.org/about.

National Association of Local Boards of Health (NALBOH). 2017. "About NALBOH." Accessed January 11. www.nalboh.org/?page=About.

Pfizer Global Pharmaceuticals. 2006. *Milestones in Public Health: Accomplishments in Public Health Over the Last 100 Years.* New York: Pfizer.

Public Health Agency of Canada. 2013. "What Is the Population Health Approach?" Updated January 15. www.phac-aspc.gc.ca/ph-sp/approach-approche/appr-eng.php.

Public Health Institute (PHI). 2016. "About PHI." Accessed August 29. www.phi.org/about-phi/.

Rosen, G. 1993. *A History of Public Health*, expanded ed. Baltimore, MD: Johns Hopkins University Press.

What Is Public Health? 2014. "Impact." Accessed December 15. www.whatispublichealth.org/impact/.

Winslow, C. E. A. 1920. "The Untilled Field of Public Health." *Science* 51 (1306): 23–33.

World Health Organization (WHO). 1946. *Constitution of the World Health Organization.* Accessed August 30, 2016. http://apps.who.int/gb/bd/PDF/bd47/EN/constitution-en.pdf.

CHAPTER 2

EPIDEMIOLOGY: THE BASIC SCIENCE OF PUBLIC HEALTH

"The science on which public health decisions are based is epidemiology, or the study of the distribution of diseases, health problems, or risk factors in the population and action taken to alleviate those problems."

—William Foege (2011)

Learning Objectives

After completing this chapter, you should be able to

- define *epidemiology* and describe its key components;
- describe the kinds of questions that epidemiology can answer;
- discuss the goals of epidemiology;
- explain the significance of the frequency of disease in populations;
- describe the tools used to study and control epidemics;
- discuss surveillance and provide an example; and
- explain the differences between endemics, epidemics, pandemics, and outbreaks and describe their significance when disseminating information to the community.

Introduction

This chapter highlights **epidemiology**, the science of public health. Epidemiology uses both quantitative and qualitative skills from various disciplines to help determine the extent to which a health condition is present in a community. Understanding the normal level of disease in a community is extremely important because it allows for public health interventions to be implemented when higher-than-expected levels of disease are detected. Epidemiology is an instrumental tool in helping to keep populations healthy.

epidemiology
The science of public health, which studies the distribution and determinants of health-related events in a population and applies the findings to help control health problems.

Epidemiology Defined

Fraser (1987, 309) defines *epidemiology* as follows:

> Epidemiology has features that resemble those of the traditional liberal arts. This makes it fit both for inclusion in an undergraduate curriculum and as an example in medical school of the continuing value of a liberal education. As a "low-technology" science, epidemiology is readily accessible to nonspecialists. Because it is useful for taking a first look at a new problem, it is applicable to a broad range of interesting phenomena. Furthermore, it emphasizes method rather than arcane knowledge and illustrates the approaches to problems and the kinds of thinking that a liberal education should cultivate: the scientific method, analogic thinking, deductive reasoning, problem solving within constraints, and concern for aesthetic values.

The word *epidemiology* has origins in the Greek words *epi*, meaning *on* or *upon*; *demos*, meaning *people*; and *logos*, meaning *study of* (Centers for Disease Control and Prevention 2012). Although many definitions have been proposed, the following definition, by Last (2001, 62), expresses the field's underlying principles and public health utility:

> Epidemiology is the study of the distribution and determinants of health-related states or events in specified populations, and the application of this study to the control of health problems.

Let's take a closer look at the key words and phrases of this definition. *Study* includes "surveillance, observation, hypothesis testing, analytic research, and experiments." *Distribution* refers to "analysis by time, place, and classes of persons affected" (Last 2001, 62). A study of distribution might show, for instance, that incidence rates for Kaposi sarcoma, stomach cancer, and multiple myeloma are about twice as high for African Americans as they are for the white population (American Cancer Society 2013). *Determinants* are "the physical, biological, social, cultural, and behavioral factors that influence health" (Last 2001, 62). Friis and Sellers (2014, 8) further describe determinants as those "factors or events that are capable of bringing about a change in health."

Examples might include climate change and infectious diseases such as Lyme disease, avian flu, or West Nile virus (New York Academy of Sciences 2010). *Health-related states or events* include "diseases, causes of death, behaviors such as use of tobacco, reactions to preventive regimens, and provision and use of health services" (Last 2001, 62)—for instance, chronic diseases, communicable diseases, disability, or mental illness. *Specified populations* are groups with "identifiable characteristics" (Last 2001, 62), such as people of a certain age, living in a certain geographic region, of a certain race or ethnicity, and so on. *Application to control* "makes explicit the aim of epidemiology to promote, protect, and restore health" (Last 2001, 62). Examples of such applications may include education programs about sexually transmitted diseases in schools, immunization programs at community health centers, and restaurant inspections. Two terms that are key to studying epidemiology are **morbidity**, which refers to sickness or illness, and **mortality**, which refers to death (Friis and Sellers 2014).

morbidity
Sickness or illness within a population group.

mortality
Death within a population group.

MORBIDITY AND MORTALITY WEEKLY REPORT

The Centers for Disease Control and Prevention (CDC) prepares the ***Morbidity and Mortality Weekly Report* (*MMWR*)** series, which has been called "the voice of CDC." The series is the CDC's "primary vehicle for scientific publication of timely, reliable, authoritative, accurate, objective, and useful public health information and recommendations." The data in the series are based on weekly reports to the CDC by state health departments. Readership of the series consists largely of "physicians, nurses, public health practitioners, epidemiologists and other scientists, researchers, educators, and laboratorians" (CDC 2016a).

Morbidity and Mortality Weekly Report (MMWR)
A series prepared by the Centers for Disease Control and Prevention to provide timely and reliable public health information and recommendations.

Epidemiology is often considered *population medicine* because, as the basic science of public health, it focuses on the population as the patient. This approach differs from that of clinical medicine, which focuses on the individual as the patient.

To illustrate this distinction, consider, for example, chronic obstructive pulmonary disease (COPD), a group of diseases—including emphysema, chronic bronchitis, and, in some cases, asthma—associated with airflow blockage and breathing-related problems (CDC 2015b). The clinical examination for COPD would focus on signs and symptoms, such as shortness of breath, persistent cough, and wheezing. The epidemiologic description, on the other hand, would focus on the gender, age group, race, and ethnicity of the people most affected by this disease; additional factors such as employment status and type, education level, and tobacco use and exposure; and geographic variations in the frequency of the disease (CDC 2015b).

Thus, epidemiology is related to **demography**, which is "the study of populations, especially with reference to size and density, fertility, mortality, growth, age distribution, migration, and vital statistics, and the interaction of all these with social and economic conditions" (Porta 2014, 71).

demography
The study of populations in terms of various factors (e.g., numbers, fertility, mortality, growth, vital statistics) and the interaction of these factors with the social and economic environments.

Questions and Goals

Friis and Sellers (2014) describe the types of questions that epidemiology can be used to address:

1. When should a factor be considered a cause of disease?
2. How does the occurrence of disease vary across populations in relation to demographic descriptors and location?
3. What are the appropriate public health, healthcare, and individual responses to the presence of disease in a community?
4. To what extent are the findings from one epidemiologic investigation applicable to other communities?

Epidemiology is interdisciplinary, in that it utilizes expertise from clinical, social, and behavioral sciences and such fields as biostatistics to promote health and control the spread of disease. Friis and Sellers (2014, 14) state that "epidemiology is concerned with efforts to describe, explain, predict, and control." Describing involves counting cases of a disease, determining the frequency of the disease in populations, and identifying trends in disease occurrence. Explaining involves communication about the cause of disease, including risk factors and information about how the disease spreads. Predicting involves estimating the number of cases of disease that could occur given the information known about the disease (e.g., mode of transmission, susceptible populations). Finally, controlling involves efforts to prevent the spread or distribution of the disease to unaffected individuals and to treat existing cases of the disease.

Following from these epidemiologic aims, Friis and Sellers (2014, 15) identify two main goals of epidemiology: "an improved understanding of the natural history of disease and the factors that influence its distribution" and "control of disease via carefully designed interventions."

Quantitative and Qualitative Data

To achieve its goals, epidemiology makes use of quantitative and qualitative data types. Examples of quantitative data types include categorical data (i.e., data distributed across nonoverlapping categories, such as race or gender) or continuum data (i.e., data on a scale, such as weight or test scores). Quantitative data are represented by numbers and can be illustrated in various forms, including tables, pie charts, line graphs, bar graphs, histograms, and maps (CDC 2008b). Exhibits 2.1, 2.2, and 2.3 provide representative examples of how quantitative epidemiologic data can be illustrated. Qualitative data, on the other hand, is represented by narrative, not numbers. The narrative is coded, and the codes provide "building blocks for theory or model building and the foundation on which the analyst's arguments rest" (MacQueen et al. 1998, 31).

Exhibit 2.1
Example of a Bar Graph Presenting Epidemiologic Data

Number of confirmed cases (N=58) of occupationally acquired HIV infection among health care workers reported to CDC—United States, 1985–2013

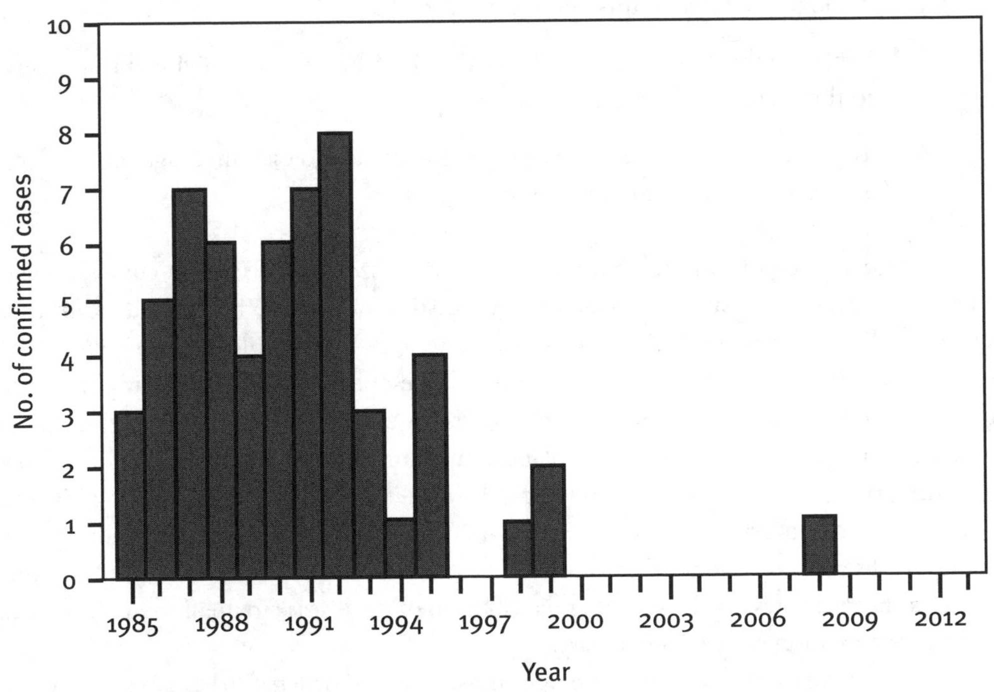

Note: HIV=human immunodeficiency virus.

Source: Reprinted from CDC (2015h).

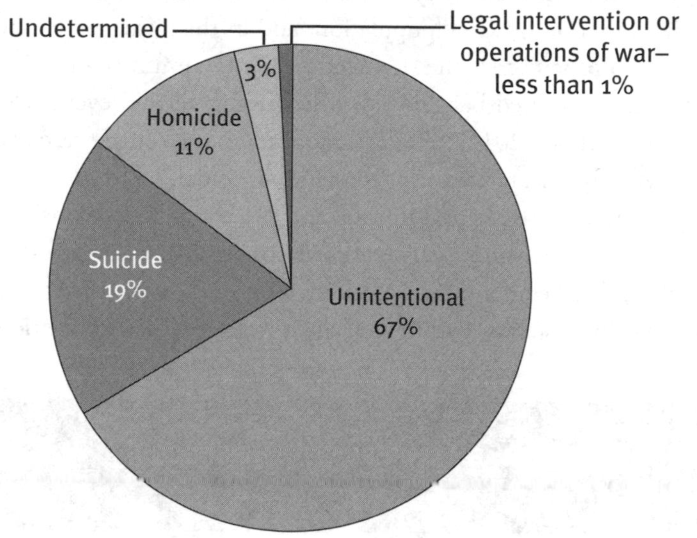

Source: Reprinted from CDC (2008a).

Exhibit 2.2 Example of a Pie Chart Presenting Epidemiologic Data

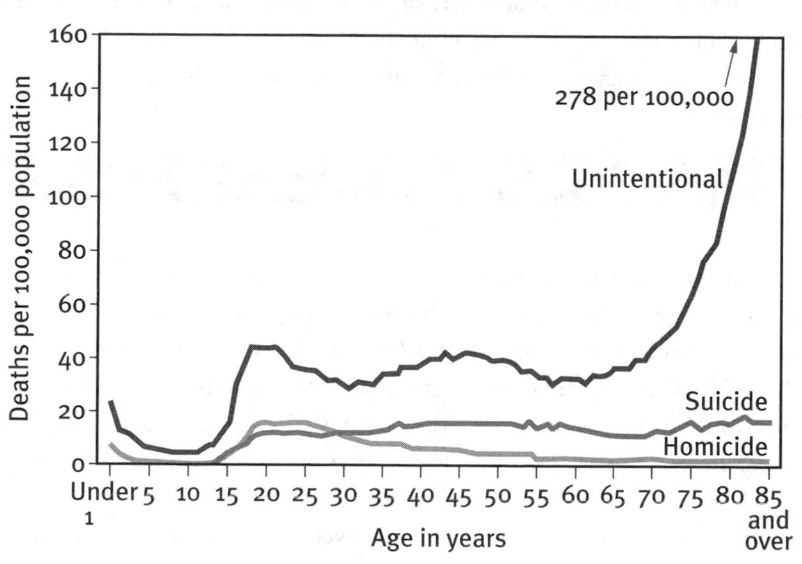

Source: Reprinted from CDC (2008a).

Exhibit 2.3 Example of a Line Graph Presenting Epidemiologic Data

Frequency of Disease

frequency
The rate of occurrence for a disease.

epidemic
The occurrence of an illness or other health-related event clearly in excess of normal expectancy.

outbreak
A localized epidemic, with an increase in the incidence of a disease within a limited area.

Epidemiology assesses the **frequency** of a disease relative to the disease's usual occurrence at the same time, within the same population, and in the same geographic area (Friis and Sellers 2014). An **epidemic** is "the occurrence in a community or region of cases of an illness, specific health-related behavior, or other health-related events clearly in excess of normal expectancy" (Porta 2014, 93). The reappearance of a single case of a communicable disease that previously disappeared also represents an epidemic. In addition, "the occurrence of two cases of a new disease linked in time and place" might be considered to be an epidemic, because the circumstances suggest disease transmission (Friis and Sellers 2014, 20). **Outbreaks** are localized epidemics in which increase in the incidence of a disease is limited to a certain area—for instance, within a village, town, or closed institution (Porta 2014).

FOR DISCUSSION: EXAMPLES OF EPIDEMICS

Epidemics include not only communicable or infectious diseases exceeding normal expectations but also conditions linked to occupational settings, environmental exposures, and lifestyle choices. Examples from these latter categories have included pneumoconiosis and advanced occupational lung disease among surface coal miners; carpal tunnel syndrome and traumatic injury risk factors among poultry-processing employees; childhood lead poisoning in areas surrounding a former lead paint production facility; complications related to chemical spills; and chronic diseases such as heart disease and cancer for which lifestyle choices are a contributing factor (CDC 2015c, 2016b).

Can you identify any epidemics or outbreaks that have made the local or national news recently?

endemic
Having a constant presence within a given area or population group.

pandemic
An epidemic occurring worldwide, or over a very wide area, usually affecting large numbers of people.

The term ***endemic*** describes "the constant occurrence of a disease, disorder, or noxious infectious agent within a geographic area or population group" (Porta 2014, 92). One example of an endemic condition is malaria in Africa, where temperature, humidity, and rainfall are conducive to the viability and reproduction of the *Anopheles* mosquito, the vector responsible for transmitting the disease (CDC 2010). Another example is cholera, which may persist in Haiti at endemic levels in part because of poor sanitation infrastructure (CDC 2015f).

A **pandemic** is "an epidemic occurring over a very wide area, crossing international boundaries, and usually affecting a large number of people" (Porta 2014, 209). A

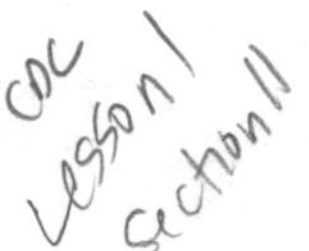

well-known pandemic was the influenza pandemic of 1918 and 1919, which killed an estimated 20 to 50 million people worldwide (CDC 2014c). According to the CDC (2015a), influenza viruses with pandemic potential include two "bird flu" viruses, avian influenza A (H5N1) and avian influenza H7N9. These viruses circulate among birds in parts of the world and are novel among humans, so people have little to no immunity against them. "Human infections with these viruses have occurred rarely, but if either of these viruses was to change in such a way that it was able to infect humans and spread easily from person to person, an influenza pandemic could result" (CDC 2015a).

The minimum number of cases or deaths required for an event to be considered an epidemic is called the **epidemic threshold** (Porta 2014). Exhibit 2.4 provides an example of the epidemic threshold for mortality due to pneumonia and influenza. It shows the seasonal pattern for pneumonia and influenza deaths from 2010 to January 2015. Note the seasonal baseline (the lower line), which reflects the "flu season" trends, and the threshold line above it. In Week 3 of 2015, for instance, the percentage of deaths resulting from pneumonia and influenza was 9.1 percent, well above that week's epidemic threshold of 7.1 percent (CDC 2015d).

epidemic threshold
The minimum number of cases or deaths required for an event to be considered an epidemic.

EXHIBIT 2.4
Epidemic Threshold for Pneumonia and Influenza, 2010–2015

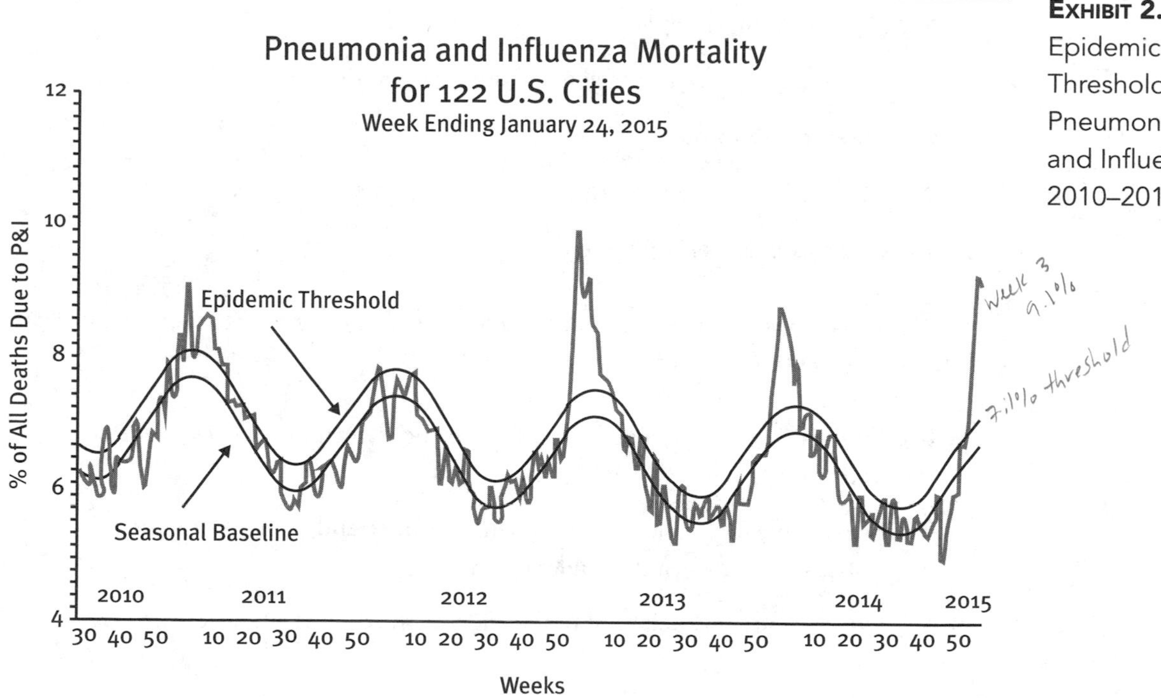

Source: Reprinted from CDC (2015d).

Epidemiologic Tools

This section examines some of the key tools used in epidemiology: surveillance, the control measures of quarantine and isolation, and the use of police power for public health.

Surveillance

surveillance
The ongoing systematic collection, analysis, and interpretation of health data. Surveillance is essential to the planning, implementation, and evaluation of public health practice.

Surveillance, as defined by the CDC (1986), is "the ongoing systematic collection, analysis, and interpretation of health data, essential to the planning, implementation, and evaluation of public health practice, closely integrated with the timely dissemination of these data to those who need to know. The final link in the surveillance chain is the application of these data to prevention and control. A surveillance system includes a functional capacity for data collection, analysis, and dissemination linked to public health programs." The CDC (1986) further states that sources of data may relate directly to disease or to factors that influence disease. Thus, they may include the following:

- Mortality and morbidity reports
- Diagnoses from laboratory reports
- Disease outbreak reports
- Reports of vaccine utilization and adverse reactions
- Absenteeism records
- Changes in disease determinants (agent, vectors, reservoirs)
- Changes in susceptibility to disease

Surveillance is an important epidemiologic and clinical tool because it can assist with the following (CDC 2013):

- Establishing the baseline rate of disease and detecting changes in the rate of disease
- Estimating the magnitude (prevalence), time trend, and geographic distribution of a health problem
- Understanding the natural progression of the disease and associated risk factors
- Generating hypotheses as to the cause and spread of the disease
- Generating research initiatives into the cause, prevention, and control of the disease

Exhibit 2.5
Components of a Generic Surveillance System

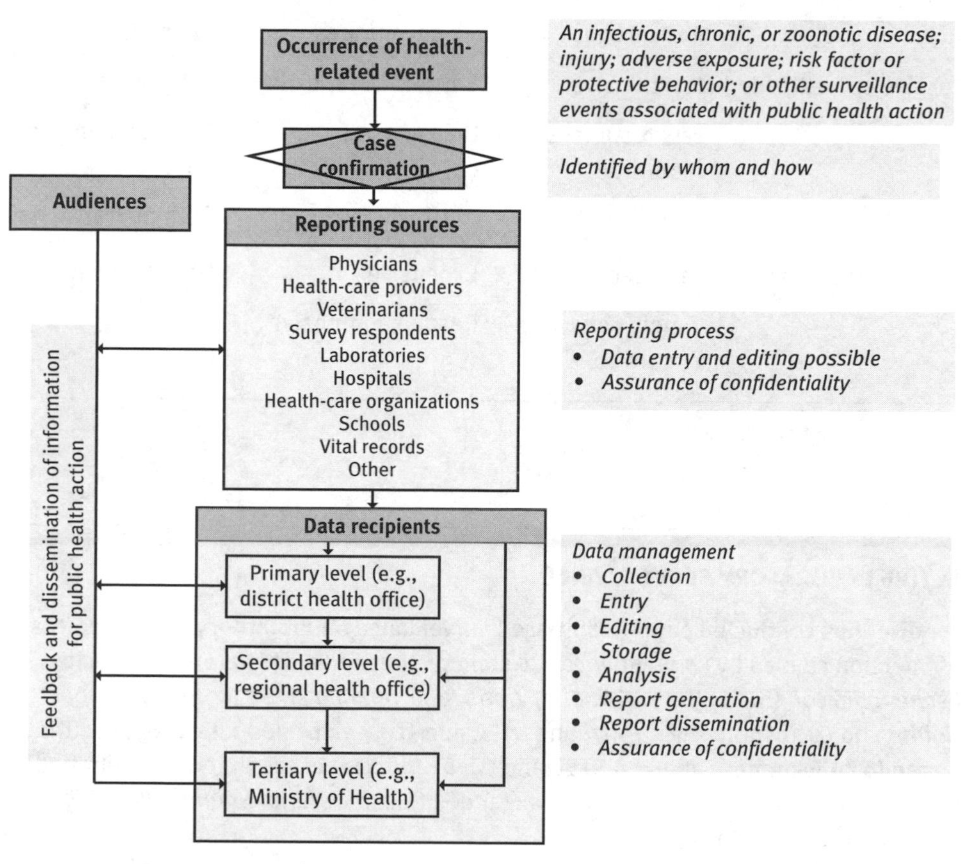

Source: Adapted from CDC (2001).

Surveillance can inform public health efforts by evaluating control measures, monitoring changes in the presentation of communicable and chronic diseases, detecting changes in the practice of healthcare, and facilitating planning among the partners in the public health system (CDC 2013). Exhibit 2.5 illustrates the components of a basic surveillance system.

The collection of surveillance data can be categorized as either passive or active. **Passive surveillance**, the more common of the two types, comes from standardized reporting forms submitted by healthcare providers and laboratories. It can also include existing health data that have been collected for other reasons. **Active surveillance** involves the collection of data by local public health practitioners via in-person interviews, phone calls, and other methods. Active surveillance therefore requires more resources than passive surveillance (CDC 2013). Exhibit 2.6 highlights the advantages, disadvantages, and select examples of passive and active surveillance. Exhibit 2.7 provides a more detailed example of active surveillance from the CDC's Foodborne Diseases Active Surveillance Network (FoodNet).

passive surveillance
Surveillance efforts that largely depend on the submission of standardized reporting forms from healthcare providers and laboratories.

active surveillance
Surveillance efforts that involve local public health practitioners collecting information via in-person interviews, phone calls, and other methods.

EXHIBIT 2.6
Passive and Active Surveillance

	Advantages	Disadvantages	Examples
Passive surveillance	Inexpensive Few resources required	Barriers to reporting Delays in reporting Missing data	Lab reports Hospital discharge data Administrative data
Active surveillance	Targeted data Timely collection of data	Expensive Resource intensive	Health behavior surveys

Source: Adapted from CDC (2013).

EXHIBIT 2.7
Foodborne Diseases Active Surveillance Network (FoodNet)

ACTIVE LABORATORY SURVEILLANCE

FoodNet has conducted population-based surveillance for laboratory-confirmed cases of infection caused by *Campylobacter*, *Listeria*, *Salmonella*, *Shiga* toxin-producing *Escherichia coli* (STEC) O157, *Shigella*, *Vibrio*, and *Yersinia* since 1996; *Cryptosporidium* and *Cyclospora* since 1997; and STEC non-O157 since 2000. In 2009, FoodNet began to collect information on STEC and *Campylobacter* cases that were identified by culture-independent methods and expanded this to *Listeria*, *Salmonella*, *Shigella*, *Yersinia*, and *Vibrio* in 2011.

FoodNet is an active surveillance system, meaning that public health officials routinely communicate with more than 650 clinical laboratories serving the surveillance area to identify new cases and conduct periodic audits to ensure that all cases are reported.

FoodNet collects information on laboratory-confirmed cases (defined as isolation for bacteria or identification for parasites of an organism from a clinical specimen) and cases diagnosed using culture-independent methods. Once a case is identified, FoodNet personnel at each site collect information about core variables and enter this information into a database, and transmit data to CDC. The data include:

- Hospitalizations occurring within 7 days of the specimen collection date
- The patient's status (alive or dead) at hospital discharge (or at 7 days after the specimen collection date if the patient is not hospitalized)
- Whether the patient traveled abroad in the 7 days before illness began, and selected food and environmental exposures for select pathogens

FoodNet also conducts surveillance for cases of hemolytic uremic syndrome (HUS) through a network of pediatric nephrologists and infection-control practitioners who

(continued)

Exhibit 2.7 Foodborne Diseases Active Surveillance Network (FoodNet) *(continued)*

report all illnesses diagnosed as HUS on the basis of physician diagnosis. FoodNet staff review hospital discharge data for pediatric HUS cases to validate surveillance reports and identify additional cases by using ICD-9-CM/ICD-10 codes specifying HUS, acute renal failure with the hemolytic anemia and thrombocytopenia, or thrombotic thrombocytopenic purpura with diarrhea caused by an unknown pathogen or *E. coli.*

In addition to routine surveillance, FoodNet also conducts special surveillance projects. In 2002, two sites conducted population-based surveillance for reactive arthritis associated with *Campylobacter*, *Salmonella*, *Shigella*, *Yersinia*, and STEC infections. In 2009, FoodNet conducted a pilot surveillance program for community-acquired *Clostridium difficile* infections in Connecticut and New York. In 2010, FoodNet conducted a pilot surveillance program for *Cronobacter sakazakii* infections in selected sites.

BURDEN OF ILLNESS

The burden of illness pyramid is a model for understanding foodborne disease reporting and illustrates steps that must occur for an episode of illness in the population to be registered in surveillance.

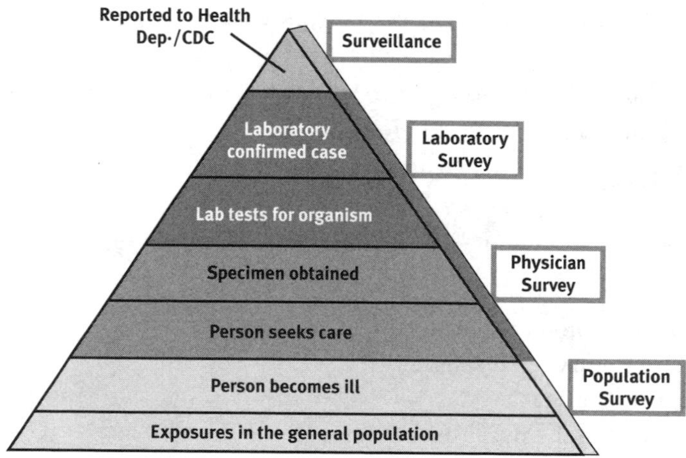

Starting from the bottom of the pyramid:

- Some members of the general population are exposed to an organism.
- Some of these exposed people become ill.
- Some of these ill people seek medical care.
- A specimen is obtained from some of these people and submitted to a clinical laboratory.
- A laboratory tests some of these specimens for a given pathogen.

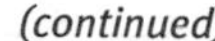
(continued)

Exhibit 2.7 Foodborne Diseases Active Surveillance Network (FoodNet) *(continued)*

- The laboratory identifies the causative organism in some of these tested specimens and thereby confirms the case.
- The laboratory-confirmed case is reported to a local or state health department.

FoodNet conducts laboratory surveys, physician surveys, and population surveys to collect information about each of these steps. This information is used to calculate estimates of the actual number of people who become ill. Other information is used to estimate the proportion of these illnesses transmitted by food.

Source: Reprinted from CDC (2015e).

population-based surveillance Surveillance that involves the reporting of information from healthcare providers and laboratories about unusual diseases or diseases that are required by law to be reported.

Surveillance systems can be either population based or sentinel. A **population-based surveillance** system relies on information reported by healthcare providers and laboratories, usually on standardized forms, about unusual diseases or diseases that are deemed notifiable or reportable (CDC 2013). A **notifiable disease** is one for which "regular, frequent, and timely information on individual cases is considered necessary" for the control of the disease; a **reportable disease** is one that, by law, must be reported to state and territorial authorities (CDC 2015g). In the reporting process for population-based surveillance, the healthcare provider or laboratory goes to the local health department, which discusses the information with the state or county health department, which then reports to the CDC at the national level. Depending on the severity of the disease and the risk for human transmission and mortality, the World Health Organization may be notified. Exhibit 2.8 lists the diseases that were designated as notifiable in the United States for 2016.

Exhibit 2.8 Infectious Diseases Designated as Notifiable for the United States, 2016

- Anthrax
- Arboviral diseases, neuroinvasive and non-neuroinvasive
  - California Serogroup virus diseases
  - Chikungunya virus disease
  - Eastern Equine Encephalitis virus disease
  - Powassan virus disease
  - St. Louis Encephalitis virus disease
  - West Nile virus disease
  - Western Equine Encephalitis virus disease
- Babesiosis
- Botulism
  - Botulism, foodborne
  - Botulism, infant
  - Botulism, other
  - Botulism, wound

(continued)

Exhibit 2.8
Infectious Diseases Designated as Notifiable for the United States, 2016
(continued)

Brucellosis
Campylobacteriosis
Chancroid
Chlamydia trachomatis infection
Cholera
Coccidioidomycosis / valley fever
Congenital Syphilis
Cryptosporidiosis
Cyclosporiasis
Dengue virus infections
    Dengue
    Dengue-like illness
    Severe dengue
Diphtheria
Ehrlichiosis and Anaplasmosis
    Anaplasma phagocytophilum infection
    Ehrlichia chaffeensis infection
    Ehrlichia ewingii infection
    Undetermined Human Ehrlichiosis / Anaplasmosis
Giardiasis
Gonorrhea
Haemophilus influenzae, invasive disease
Hansen's disease / leprosy
Hantavirus infection, non-Hantavirus pulmonary syndrome
Hantavirus pulmonary syndrome (HPS)
Hemolytic uremic syndrome, postdiarrheal (HUS)
Hepatitis A, acute
Hepatitis B, acute
Hepatitis B, chronic
Hepatitis B, perinatal infection
Hepatitis C, acute
Hepatitis C, chronic
HIV infection (AIDS has been reclassified as HIV Stage III) (AIDS/HIV)
Influenza-associated pediatric mortality
Invasive Pneumococcal Disease (IPD) / *Streptococcus pneumoniae*, invasive disease
Legionellosis / Legionnaire's disease or Pontiac fever
Leptospirosis
Listeriosis
Lyme disease
Malaria
Measles/Rubeola

(continued)

notifiable disease
A disease for which frequent and timely information about individual cases is considered necessary for public health.

reportable disease
A disease for which an occurrence must, by law, be reported to authorities.

EXHIBIT 2.8
Infectious Diseases Designated as Notifiable for the United States, 2016 *(continued)*

Meningococcal disease
Mumps
Novel influenza A virus infections
Pertussis / whooping cough
Plague
Poliomyelitis, paralytic
Poliovirus infection, nonparalytic
Psittacosis/Ornithosis
Q fever
  Q fever, acute
  Q fever, chronic
Rabies, animal
Rabies, human
Rubella / German measles
Rubella, congenital syndrome (CRS)
Salmonellosis
Severe acute respiratory syndrome–associated coronavirus disease (SARS)
Shiga toxin-producing *Escherichia coli* (STEC)
Shigellosis
Smallpox/Variola
Spotted Fever Rickettsiosis
Streptococcal toxic shock syndrome (STSS)
Syphilis
  Syphilis, early latent
  Syphilis, late latent
  Syphilis, late with clinical manifestations (including late benign syphilis and cardiovascular syphilis)
  Syphilis, primary
  Syphilis, secondary
  Syphilitic stillbirth
Tetanus
Toxic shock syndrome (other than Streptococcal) (TSS)
Trichinellosis/Trichinosis
Tuberculosis (TB)
Tularemia
Typhoid fever
Vancomycin-intermediate *Staphylococcus aureus* and Vancomycin-resistant *Staphylococcus aureus* (VISA/VRSA)
Varicella/chickenpox
Varicella deaths

(continued)

Exhibit 2.8
Infectious Diseases Designated as Notifiable for the United States, 2016
(continued)

Vibriosis
Viral hemorrhagic fever (VHF)
  Crimean-Congo hemorrhagic fever virus
  Ebola virus
  Lassa virus
  Lujo virus
  Marburg virus
  New World Arenavirus—Guanarito virus
  New World Arenavirus—Junin virus
  New World Arenavirus—Machupo virus
  New World Arenavirus—Sabia virus
Yellow fever
Zika virus disease and Zika virus, congenital infection
  Zika virus disease
  Zika virus, congenital infection

Source: Reprinted from CDC (2016c).

Sentinel surveillance systems focus on "selected population samples chosen to represent the relevant experience of particular groups" (Porta 2014, 260). For example, colleges or family physician networks might serve as representative subsets of larger populations in cooperative efforts for the early detection of influenza epidemics. The use of animals as sentinels can help detect the circulation of arboviruses (viruses that are transmitted to humans primarily through the bites of infected mosquitoes, ticks, sand flies, or midges). Examples of arboviruses include West Nile virus and Eastern Equine Encephalitis, both mosquito-borne diseases (CDC 2011). Sentinel surveillance can use both passive and active surveillance methods (CDC 2013).

sentinel surveillance
Surveillance conducted on population samples that have been selected to represent the experience of larger groups.

The **stakeholders** in a surveillance system may include the following:

stakeholder
An individual or organization that has an interest in a particular issue.

- Users of the data and results
- Public health practitioners
- Healthcare practitioners
- Community representatives and the population under surveillance
- Local, state, and national governments
- Nonprofit organizations

The people who maintain surveillance systems should be engaged stakeholders to ensure that the information being collected, analyzed, and reported is useful (CDC 2013). The

Exhibit 2.9 Representative Dissemination Methods for Stakeholders

Stakeholder Type	Dissemination Method
Decision makers	Reports
	Staff meetings
	Conferences
Healthcare community	Bulletins (for an example, see the *MMWR* presented in the case study later in the chapter)
	Meetings
	Electronic communication
The public	Press releases
	Community meetings
	Media announcements

Source: Adapted from CDC (2013).

quarantine Restriction of the activities of people who have been exposed to a communicable disease.

findings from surveillance must be disseminated to the decision makers, the reporting healthcare community, and the public (see exhibit 2.9).

isolation Separation of infected people from other individuals with the aim of preventing the transmission of an infectious agent.

Control Measures

Two control measures that can help prevent the spread of communicable disease are **quarantine** and **isolation**. Additional measures include early detection, rapid diagnosis, and the use of antibiotics and antivirals.

Quarantine separates people who have been exposed to a specific illness—even if they are not yet sick and do not have symptoms—from others in the population (MOHAKCA 2016). The reason people may be quarantined even when they are not ill is that, depending on the illness, people can often spread a disease before they develop symptoms. People under quarantine are often confined in their homes until the risk of the disease developing has passed; the time frame depends upon the disease and its **incubation period** (MOHAKCA 2016).

incubation period The length of time between invasion by an infectious agent and the appearance of the first sign of disease.

Isolation applies to people who are known to be ill with a contagious disease. It separates those people who are ill or infected from those who are not, with the aim of preventing the spread or transmission of disease (MOHAKCA 2016). Where people are isolated and for how long will depend on the severity of the disease. Some people may be placed in isolation at home, whereas others may be hospitalized (MOHAKCA 2016).

These control measures were used in 2014, for instance, when several healthcare workers who had traveled to Africa to help with the Ebola outbreak were quarantined upon their return to the United States. Quarantine lasted for 21 days, which is the incubation period for Ebola. People who did not develop signs and symptoms of an Ebola infection during this period were released from quarantine. People in quarantine who did develop the signs and symptoms were placed in isolation; in addition, health officials observed other individuals who may have had contact with those people for the incubation period of the disease (Hartocollis 2014). Only four hospitals in the United States had appropriate units to contain a highly infectious disease such as Ebola. These hospitals were the National Institutes of Health in Bethesda, Maryland; Emory University Hospital in Atlanta, Georgia; University of Nebraska Medical Center; and Saint Patrick Hospital in Missoula, Montana (Courage 2014).

Public Health Police Power

Sometimes, a governmental public health organization must have the authority of police power to protect the population from individuals who might put the general population at harm. The CDC (2014a) states, "In addition to serving as medical functions, isolation and quarantine are also 'police power' functions, derived from the right of the state to take action affecting individuals for the benefit of society." "By definition, both isolation and quarantine restrict the movement of individuals. While voluntary isolation and quarantine may be successful, involuntary restriction may be necessary in certain circumstances" (MOHAKCA 2016).

In the United States, police power at the state level aims to protect the health, safety, and welfare of the people within each state's borders. State laws to enforce the use of isolation and quarantine vary from one state to another. In some states, local health authorities implement state law. Breaking a quarantine order is usually a criminal misdemeanor (CDC 2014a). At the federal level, the government uses quarantine and isolation measures to prevent the introduction of communicable diseases into the United States (CDC 2014a). The following communicable diseases are authorized for federal quarantine and isolation by executive order of the US president (CDC 2014a):

- Cholera
- Diphtheria
- Infectious tuberculosis
- Plague
- Smallpox
- Yellow fever
- Viral hemorrhagic fevers

- Severe acute respiratory syndromes
- Flu that can cause a pandemic

When implementing such public health orders, authorities should support and compensate—via shelter, food, and compensation for lost wages—the people who have sacrificed their individual freedoms for the public good. Considerations must also be in place to protect the individuals' dignity and privacy.

Case Study

Ebola Viral Disease Outbreak

The following case has been reproduced from the CDC (2014b). The report, prepared by Meredith G. Dixon, MD, and Ilana J. Schafer, DVM, was posted on the CDC's MMWR *website (www.cdc.gov/mmwr) on June 24, 2014.*

EBOLA VIRAL DISEASE OUTBREAK—WEST AFRICA, 2014

On March 21, 2014, the Guinea Ministry of Health reported the outbreak of an illness characterized by fever, severe diarrhea, vomiting, and a high case-fatality rate (59%) among 49 persons (1). Specimens from 15 of 20 persons tested at Institut Pasteur in Lyon, France, were positive for an Ebola virus by polymerase chain reaction (2). Viral sequencing identified Ebola virus (species Zaïre ebolavirus), one of five viruses in the genus Ebolavirus, as the cause (2). Cases of Ebola viral disease (EVD) were initially reported in three southeastern districts (Gueckedou, Macenta, and Kissidougou) of Guinea and in the capital city of Conakry. By March 30, cases had been reported in Foya district in neighboring Liberia (1), and in May, the first cases identified in Sierra Leone were reported. As of June 18, the outbreak was the largest EVD outbreak ever documented, with a combined total of 528 cases (including laboratory-confirmed, probable, and suspected cases) and 337 deaths (case-fatality rate=64%) reported in the three countries. The largest previous outbreak occurred in Uganda during 2000–2001, when 425 cases were reported with 224 deaths (case-fatality rate=53%) (3). The current outbreak also represents the first outbreak of EVD in West Africa (a single case caused by Taï Forest virus was reported in Côte d'Ivoire in 1994 [3]) and marks the first time that Ebola virus transmission has been reported in a capital city.

(continued)

CHARACTERISTICS OF EVD

EVD is characterized by the sudden onset of fever and malaise, accompanied by other nonspecific signs and symptoms such as myalgia, headache, vomiting, and diarrhea. Among EVD patients, 30%–50% experience hemorrhagic symptoms (4). In severe and fatal forms, multi-organ dysfunction, including hepatic damage, renal failure, and central nervous system involvement occur, leading to shock and death. The first two Ebolavirus species were initially recognized in 1976 during simultaneous outbreaks in Sudan (Sudan ebolavirus) and Zaïre (now Democratic Republic of the Congo) (Zaïre ebolavirus) (5). Since 1976, there have been more than 20 EVD outbreaks across Central Africa, with the majority caused by Ebola virus (species Zaïre ebolavirus), which historically has demonstrated the highest case-fatality rate (up to 90%) (3).

The wildlife reservoir has not been definitively ascertained; however, evidence supports fruit bats as one reservoir (6). The virus initially is spread to the human population after contact with infected wildlife and is then spread person-to-person through direct contact with body fluids such as, but not limited to, blood, urine, sweat, semen, and breast milk. The incubation period is 2–21 days. Patients can transmit the virus while febrile and through later stages of disease, as well as postmortem, when persons contact the body during funeral preparations. Additionally, the virus has been isolated in semen for as many as 61 days after illness onset.

Diagnosis is made most commonly through detection of Ebola virus RNA or Ebola virus antibodies in blood (5). Testing in this outbreak is being performed by Institut Pasteur, the European Mobile Laboratory, and CDC in Guinea; by the Kenema Government Hospital Viral Hemorrhagic Fever Laboratory in Sierra Leone; and by the Liberia Institute of Biomedical Research. Patient care is supportive; there is no approved treatment known to be effective against Ebola virus. Clinical support consists of aggressive volume and electrolyte management, oral and intravenous nutrition, and medications to control fever and gastrointestinal distress, as well as to treat pain, anxiety, and agitation (4,5). Diagnosis and treatment of concomitant infections and superinfections, including malaria and typhoid, also are important aspects of patient care (4).

Keys to controlling EVD outbreaks include 1) active case identification and isolation of patients from the community to prevent continued virus spread; 2) identifying contacts of ill or deceased persons and tracking the contacts daily for the entire incubation period of 21 days; 3) investigation of retrospective and current cases to document all historic and ongoing chains of virus transmission; 4) identifying deaths in the community and using safe burial practices; and 5) daily reporting of cases (4,7,8). Education of health-care workers regarding safe infection-control practices, including appropriate use of personal protective equipment, is essential to protect them and their patients because health-care–associated transmission has played a part in transmission during previous outbreaks (4,9).

(continued)

EFFORTS TO CONTROL THE CURRENT OUTBREAK

To implement prevention and control measures in both Guinea and Liberia, ministries of health with assistance from Médecins Sans Frontières, the World Health Organization, and others, put in place Ebola treatment centers to provide better patient care and interrupt virus transmission. Teams from CDC traveled to Guinea and Liberia at the end of March as part of a response by the Global Outbreak Alert and Response Network to assist the respective ministries of health in characterizing and controlling the outbreak through collection of case reports, interviewing of patients and family members, coordination of contact tracing, and consolidation of data into centralized databases. Cases are categorized into one of three case definitions: suspected (alive or dead person with fever and at least three additional symptoms, or fever and a history of contact with a person with hemorrhagic fever or a dead or sick animal, or unexplained bleeding); probable (meets the suspected case definition and has an epidemiologic link to a confirmed or probable case); confirmed (suspected or probable case that also has laboratory confirmation).

In late April, it appeared that the outbreak was slowing when Liberia did not report new cases for several weeks after April 9, and the number of new reported cases in Guinea decreased to nine for the week of April 27 (Figure 1). Since then, however, the EVD outbreak has resurged, with neighboring Sierra Leone reporting its first laboratory-confirmed case on May 24, Liberia reporting a new case on May 29 that originated in Sierra Leone, and Guinea reporting a new high of 38 cases for the week of May 25.

As of June 18, the total EVD case count reported for all three countries combined was 528, including 364 laboratory-confirmed, 99 probable, and 65 suspected cases, with 337 deaths (case-fatality rate=64%). Guinea had reported 398 cases (254 laboratory-confirmed, 88 probable, and 56 suspected) with 264 deaths (case-fatality rate=66%) across nine districts (Figure 1). Sierra Leone had reported 97 cases (92 laboratory-confirmed, three probable, and two suspected) with 49 deaths (case-fatality rate=51%) across five districts and the capital, Freetown. Liberia had reported 33 cases (18 confirmed, eight probable, and seven suspected) with 24 deaths (case-fatality rate=73%) across four districts.

Major challenges faced by all partners in the efforts to control the outbreak include its wide geographic spread (Figure 2), weak health-care infrastructures, and community mistrust and resistance (10). Retrospective case investigation has indicated that the first case of EVD might have occurred as early as December 2013 (Figure 1) (2). To control the outbreak, additional strategies such as involving community leaders in response efforts are needed to alleviate concerns of hesitant and fearful populations so that health-care workers can care for patients in treatment centers and thorough contact tracing can be performed. Enhancing communication across borders with respect to disease surveillance will assist in the control and prevention of more cases in this EVD outbreak.

(continued)

Figure 1: Number of cases of Ebola viral disease (n=398*), by week of symptom onset—Guinea, 2014

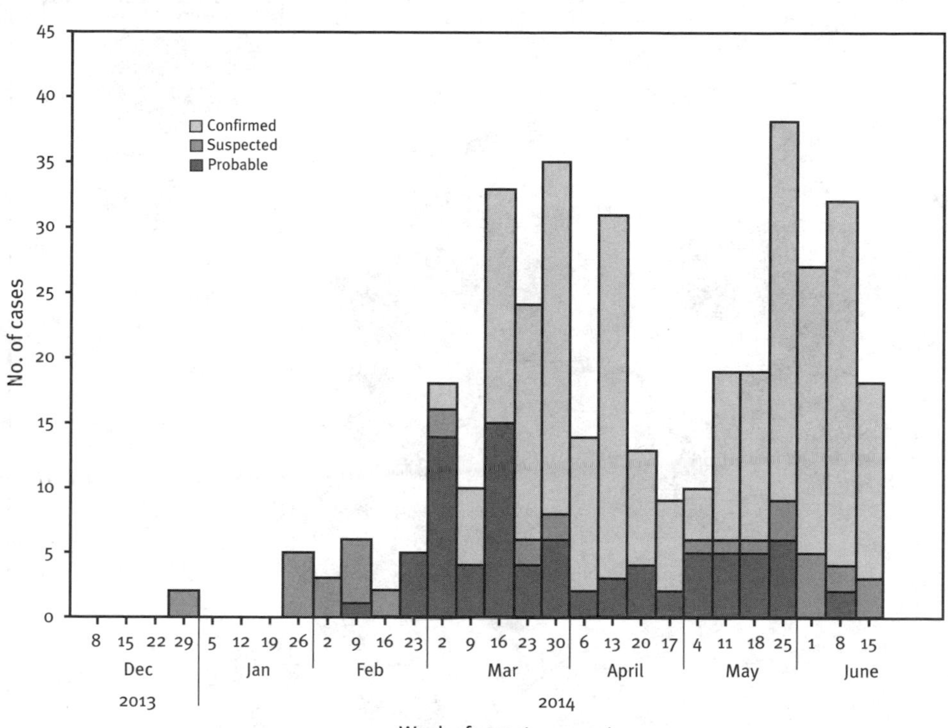

* Cases reported as of June 18, 2014.

The figure above is a bar chart showing the number of cases of Ebola viral disease (EVD) in the ongoing outbreak that were reported from Guinea, by week of symptom onset during 2014. Although cases also were reported from Liberia and Sierra Leone, as of June 18, 2014, the majority (398) of the 528 total EVD cases had been reported from Guinea.

In June 2014, the World Health Organization, via the Global Outbreak Alert and Response Network, requested additional support from CDC and other partners, necessitating the deployment of additional staff members to Guinea and Sierra Leone to further coordinate efforts aimed at halting and preventing virus transmission. Persistence of the outbreak necessitates high-level, regional and international coordination to bolster response efforts among involved and neighboring nations and other response partners in order to expeditiously end this outbreak.

(continued)

Figure 2: Location of cases of Ebola viral disease*—West Africa, 2014

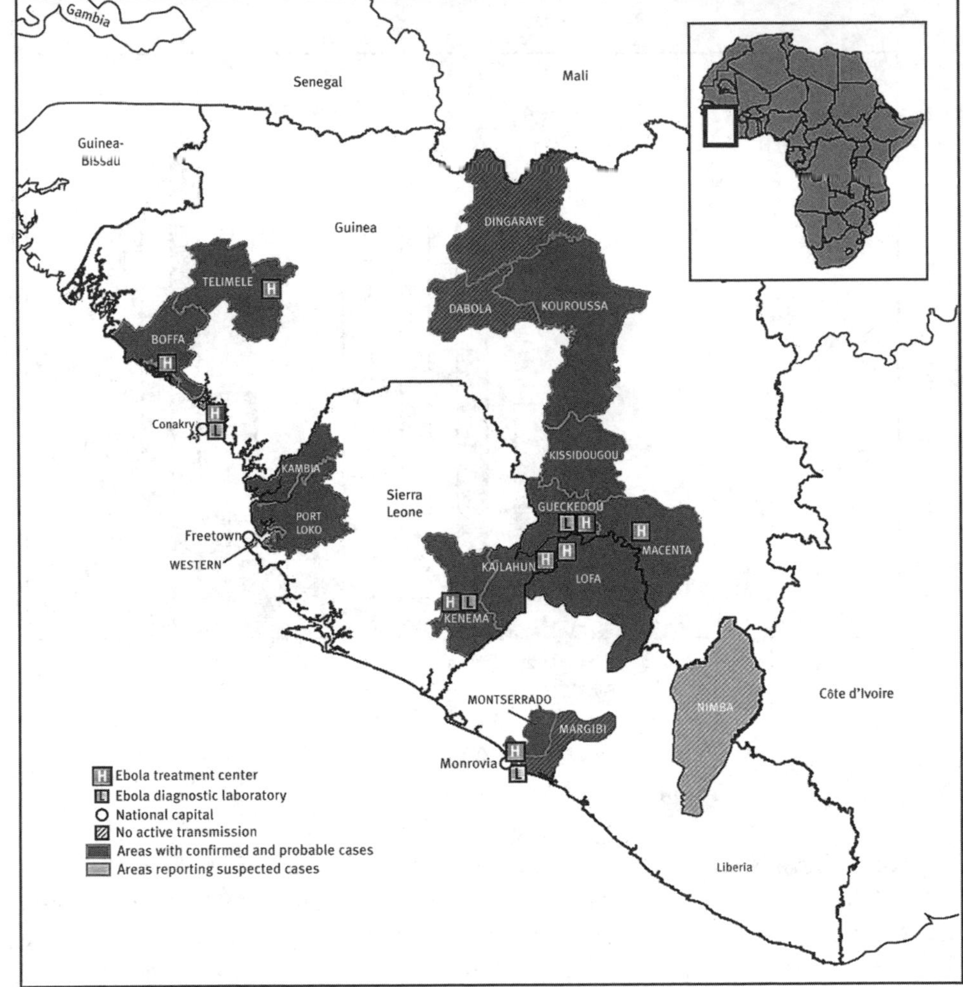

* Cases reported as of June 18, 2014.

The figure above is a map of West Africa, showing the wide geographic spread of cases of Ebola viral disease during the ongoing outbreak. As of June 18, 2014, a total of 528 cases, including 337 deaths, had been reported from Guinea, Liberia, and Sierra Leone.

ACKNOWLEDGMENTS

The West Africa Ebola national and international response teams, including the ministries of health of Guinea, Liberia, and Sierra Leone; the World Health Organization; Médecins Sans Frontières; CDC response teams; the United Nations Children's Fund; the International Federation of Red Cross; Institut Pasteur; the European Mobile

(continued)

Laboratory; the Kenema Government Hospital Viral Hemorrhagic Fever Laboratory; the Liberia Institute of Biomedical Research; African Field Epidemiology Network; Elizabeth Ervin, Viral Special Pathogens Branch, National Center for Emerging and Zoonotic Infectious Diseases, CDC.

REFERENCES

1. World Health Organization. Global alert and response: Ebola virus disease (EVD). Geneva, Switzerland: World Health Organization; 2014. Available at http://www.who.int/csr/don/archive/disease/ebola/en.
2. Baize S, Pannetier D, Oestereich L, et al. Emergence of Zaire Ebola virus disease in Guinea—preliminary report. N Engl J Med 2014; April 16 (e-pub ahead of print).
3. World Health Organization. Ebola viral disease: fact sheet. Geneva, Switzerland: World Health Organization; 2014. Available at http://www.who.int/mediacentre/factsheets/fs103/en.
4. Médecins Sans Frontières. Filovirus haemorrhagic fever guideline. Barcelona, Spain: Médecins Sans Frontières; 2008:39–48.
5. Formenty P. Ebola-Marburg viral diseases. In: Control of communicable diseases manual. Heymann DL, ed. Washington, DC: American Public Health Association; 2008:204–7.
6. Leroy EM, Kumulungui B, Pourrut X, et al. Fruit bats as reservoirs of Ebola virus. Nature 2005;438:575–6.
7. Rollin P, Roth C. Lassa fever. In: Control of communicable diseases manual. Heymann DL, ed. Washington, DC: American Public Health Association; 2008:335–7.
8. Nkoghe D, Formenty P, Leroy EM, et al. Multiple Ebola virus haemorrhagic fever outbreaks in Gabon, from October 2001 to April 2002 [French]. Bull Soc Pathol Exot 2005;98:224–9.
9. Pattyn SR, ed. Ebola virus haemorrhagic fever. Amsterdam, The Netherlands: Elsevier; 1978.
10. Ebola in West Africa: gaining community trust and confidence [Editorial]. Lancet 2014;383:1946.

CASE STUDY DISCUSSION QUESTIONS

1. What aspects of this case study exemplify the basic science of public health (e.g., population affected, distribution, determinants)?
2. Describe how we can use epidemiology to explain and predict the Ebola outbreak. What kind of questions should we attempt to answer?
3. Describe the clinical versus epidemiologic descriptions of the Ebola outbreak.

4. Propose a passive and active surveillance system for an Ebola outbreak. How should the findings be disseminated and to what stakeholders?
5. What type of control measures should be implemented and when?
6. Are there other data that should be collected, and how should they be presented?

Key Chapter Points

- Epidemiology is "the study of the distribution and determinants of health-related states or events in specified populations, and the application of this study to the control of health problems" (Last 2001, 62). It is the science of public health. Morbidity, which refers to sickness or illness, and mortality, which refers to death, are key to the study of epidemiology.
- Epidemiology is often referred to as *population medicine*, because it focuses on the population as the patient—rather than treating the individual as the patient, as is the case in clinical medicine.
- The aims of epidemiology are to describe, explain, predict, and control disease frequency in populations.
- An epidemic is the "occurrence in a community or region of cases of an illness, specific health-related behavior, or other health-related events clearly in excess of normal expectancy" (Porta 2014, 93). Epidemics include not only communicable or infectious diseases but also conditions associated with occupational settings, environmental exposures, and lifestyle choices.
- An endemic condition is a disease, disorder, or infectious agent that occurs constantly within a given geographic area or population group.
- A pandemic is an epidemic that occurs worldwide, or over a very wide area, and usually affects large numbers of people.
- Surveillance, as defined by the CDC (1986), is "the ongoing systematic collection, analysis, and interpretation of health data, essential to the planning, implementation, and evaluation of public health practice, closely integrated with the timely dissemination of these data to those who need to know."
- Surveillance data can be categorized as passive or active. Passive surveillance involves the submission of completed, standardized reporting forms from healthcare providers and laboratories; it may also use existing health data that have been collected for other reasons. Active surveillance involves local public health practitioners collecting information via in-person interviews, phone calls, and other methods.

- Population-based surveillance reports information, usually on standardized forms, from healthcare providers and laboratories for unusual diseases or diseases that are required by a legal mandate to be reported. Sentinel surveillance is conducted on population samples chosen to represent the experience of particular groups.
- Quarantine and isolation are control measures that can be implemented to help prevent the spread of communicable diseases. Quarantine separates people who have been exposed to a specific illness (but who may not be sick or have symptoms) from others. Isolation separates people who are already ill or infected from those who are not.
- Governments have police power authority to protect the health, safety, and welfare of their people. Examples of this kind of authority include state laws to enforce the use of isolation and quarantine.

Discussion Questions

1. Explain how epidemiology is the basic science of public health.
2. What are the key components of the definition of *epidemiology*?
3. What are the goals of epidemiology?
4. Describe how epidemics include not only communicable diseases but also other conditions that occur in excess of what is expected.
5. What is surveillance? Describe the types of data useful for surveillance; the types of surveillance and surveillance systems; the stakeholders in a surveillance system; and how the findings from surveillance should be disseminated.
6. Propose a surveillance system for influenza in the United States.
7. What is the epidemic threshold? Discuss potential reasons why it could be exceeded in the case of influenza.
8. Discuss control measures for communicable diseases.

References

American Cancer Society. 2013. *Cancer Facts & Figures for African Americans 2013–2014*. Atlanta, GA: American Cancer Society.

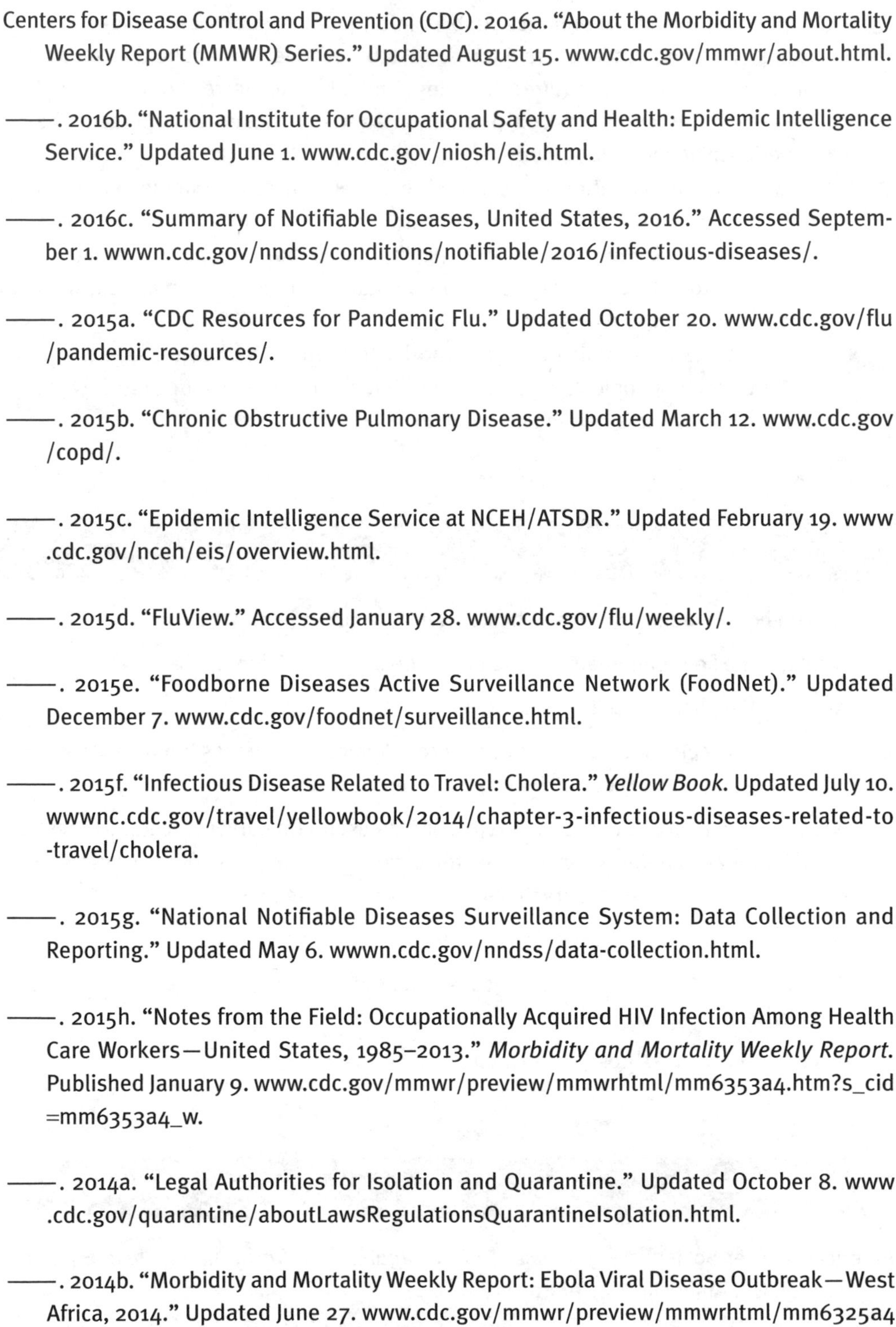

Centers for Disease Control and Prevention (CDC). 2016a. "About the Morbidity and Mortality Weekly Report (MMWR) Series." Updated August 15. www.cdc.gov/mmwr/about.html.

——. 2016b. "National Institute for Occupational Safety and Health: Epidemic Intelligence Service." Updated June 1. www.cdc.gov/niosh/eis.html.

——. 2016c. "Summary of Notifiable Diseases, United States, 2016." Accessed September 1. wwwn.cdc.gov/nndss/conditions/notifiable/2016/infectious-diseases/.

——. 2015a. "CDC Resources for Pandemic Flu." Updated October 20. www.cdc.gov/flu/pandemic-resources/.

——. 2015b. "Chronic Obstructive Pulmonary Disease." Updated March 12. www.cdc.gov/copd/.

——. 2015c. "Epidemic Intelligence Service at NCEH/ATSDR." Updated February 19. www.cdc.gov/nceh/eis/overview.html.

——. 2015d. "FluView." Accessed January 28. www.cdc.gov/flu/weekly/.

——. 2015e. "Foodborne Diseases Active Surveillance Network (FoodNet)." Updated December 7. www.cdc.gov/foodnet/surveillance.html.

——. 2015f. "Infectious Disease Related to Travel: Cholera." *Yellow Book*. Updated July 10. wwwnc.cdc.gov/travel/yellowbook/2014/chapter-3-infectious-diseases-related-to-travel/cholera.

——. 2015g. "National Notifiable Diseases Surveillance System: Data Collection and Reporting." Updated May 6. wwwn.cdc.gov/nndss/data-collection.html.

——. 2015h. "Notes from the Field: Occupationally Acquired HIV Infection Among Health Care Workers—United States, 1985–2013." *Morbidity and Mortality Weekly Report*. Published January 9. www.cdc.gov/mmwr/preview/mmwrhtml/mm6353a4.htm?s_cid=mm6353a4_w.

——. 2014a. "Legal Authorities for Isolation and Quarantine." Updated October 8. www.cdc.gov/quarantine/aboutLawsRegulationsQuarantineIsolation.html.

——. 2014b. "Morbidity and Mortality Weekly Report: Ebola Viral Disease Outbreak—West Africa, 2014." Updated June 27. www.cdc.gov/mmwr/preview/mmwrhtml/mm6325a4.htm.

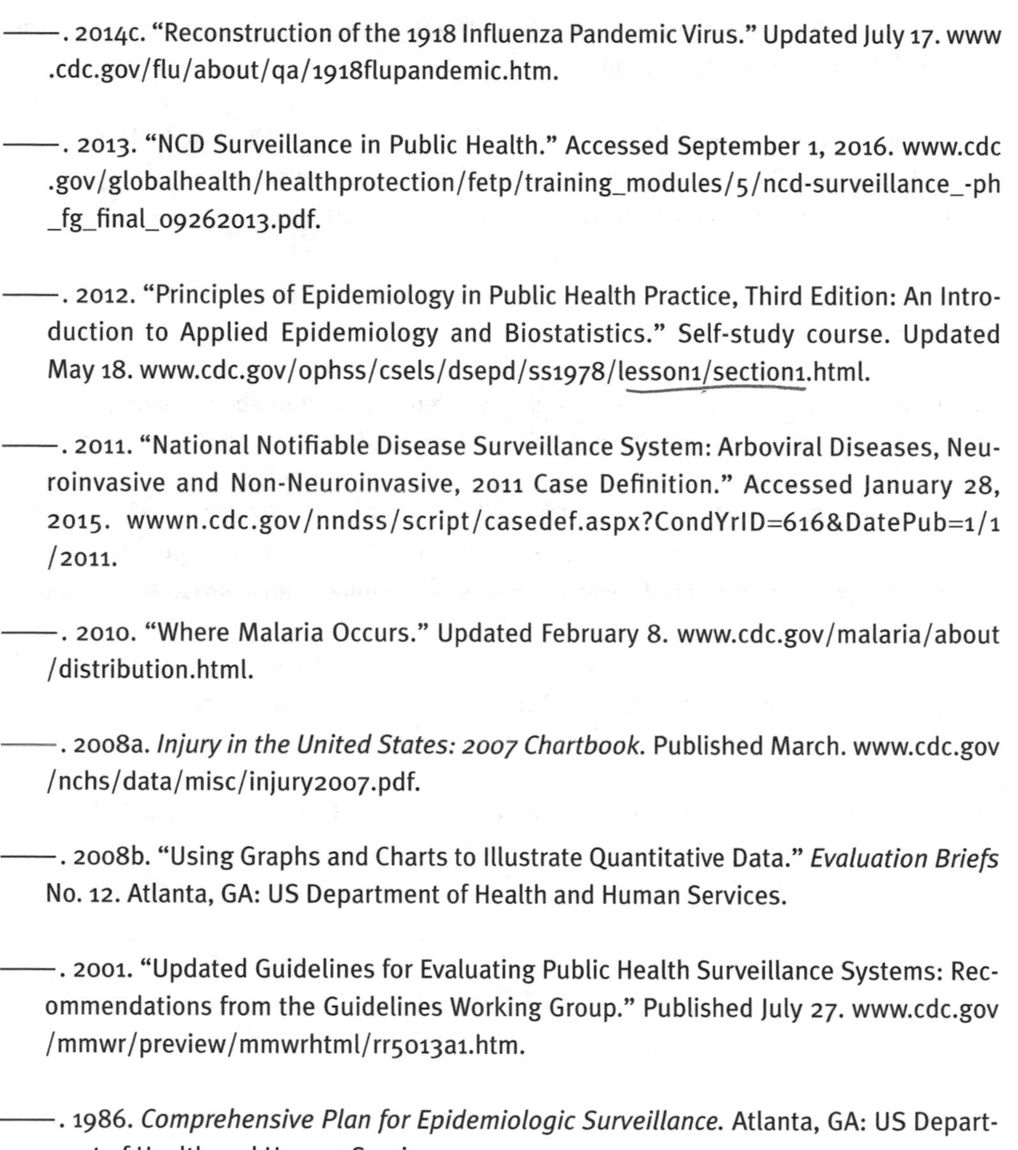

——. 2014c. "Reconstruction of the 1918 Influenza Pandemic Virus." Updated July 17. www.cdc.gov/flu/about/qa/1918flupandemic.htm.

——. 2013. "NCD Surveillance in Public Health." Accessed September 1, 2016. www.cdc.gov/globalhealth/healthprotection/fetp/training_modules/5/ncd-surveillance_-ph_fg_final_09262013.pdf.

——. 2012. "Principles of Epidemiology in Public Health Practice, Third Edition: An Introduction to Applied Epidemiology and Biostatistics." Self-study course. Updated May 18. www.cdc.gov/ophss/csels/dsepd/ss1978/lesson1/section1.html.

——. 2011. "National Notifiable Disease Surveillance System: Arboviral Diseases, Neuroinvasive and Non-Neuroinvasive, 2011 Case Definition." Accessed January 28, 2015. wwwn.cdc.gov/nndss/script/casedef.aspx?CondYrID=616&DatePub=1/1/2011.

——. 2010. "Where Malaria Occurs." Updated February 8. www.cdc.gov/malaria/about/distribution.html.

——. 2008a. *Injury in the United States: 2007 Chartbook*. Published March. www.cdc.gov/nchs/data/misc/injury2007.pdf.

——. 2008b. "Using Graphs and Charts to Illustrate Quantitative Data." *Evaluation Briefs* No. 12. Atlanta, GA: US Department of Health and Human Services.

——. 2001. "Updated Guidelines for Evaluating Public Health Surveillance Systems: Recommendations from the Guidelines Working Group." Published July 27. www.cdc.gov/mmwr/preview/mmwrhtml/rr5013a1.htm.

——. 1986. *Comprehensive Plan for Epidemiologic Surveillance*. Atlanta, GA: US Department of Health and Human Services.

Courage, K. H. 2014. "Inside the 4 Biocontainment Hospitals That Are Stopping Ebola." *Scientific American*. Published October 24. www.scientificamerican.com/article/inside-the-4-u-s-biocontainment-hospitals-that-are-stopping-ebola-video/.

Foege, W. 2011. "Quotable Epidemiology Quotes." *Epimonitor*. Accessed August 30, 2016. www.epimonitor.net/Quotable_Quotes.htm.

Fraser, D. W. 1987. "Epidemiology as a Liberal Art." *New England Journal of Medicine* 316 (6): 309–14.

Friis, R. H., and T. A. Sellers. 2014. *Epidemiology for Public Health Practice*, 5th ed. Burlington, MA: Jones & Bartlett Learning.

Hartocollis, A. 2014. "Craig Spencer, New York Doctor with Ebola, Will Leave Bellevue Hospital." *New York Times*. Published November 10. www.nytimes.com/2014/11/11/nyregion/craig-spencer-new-york-doctor-with-ebola-will-leave-bellevue-hospital.html.

Last, J. M. (ed.). 2001. *A Dictionary of Epidemiology*, 4th ed. New York: Oxford University Press.

MacQueen, K. M., E. McLellan, K. Kay, and B. Milstein. 1998. "Codebook Development for Team-Based Qualitative Analysis." *Cultural Anthropology Methods* 10 (2): 31–36.

Metropolitan Official Health Agencies of the Kansas City Area (MOHAKCA). 2016. *What Physicians Need to Know about Isolation and Quarantine.* Accessed September 2. www.marc.org/Community/Public-Health/Assets/IandQ-physicians.aspx.

New York Academy of Sciences. 2010. "Emerging Infectious Diseases in Response to Climate Change" (webinar). Accessed February 1, 2015. www.nyas.org/Events/WebinarDetail.aspx?cid=90cad802-77a9-4c77-a441-85d8868ea555.

Porta, M. (ed.). 2014. *A Dictionary of Epidemiology*, 6th ed. New York: Oxford University Press.

CHAPTER 3

DESCRIPTIVE EPIDEMIOLOGY: THE SIGNIFICANCE OF PERSON, PLACE, AND TIME

"The only way to keep your health is to eat what you don't want, drink what you don't like, and do what you'd rather not."

—Mark Twain (1897)

LEARNING OBJECTIVES

After completing this chapter, you should be able to

- describe the epidemiologic contributions of John Snow,
- discuss a natural experiment and its utility,
- compare the two branches of epidemiology,
- discuss indicators useful in descriptive epidemiology, and
- explain the epidemiologic transition and its significance.

Introduction

descriptive epidemiology
The branch of epidemiology that helps answer questions of what (health issue of concern), who (person), where (place), when (time), and why/how (causes, risk factors, modes of transmission).

Epidemiology has two branches: **descriptive epidemiology** and analytic epidemiology. This chapter will focus on the first branch, exploring how descriptive epidemiology helps answer questions about person, place, and time for a given disease. Analytic epidemiology will be discussed later, in chapter 6. The descriptive epidemiology approach must precede the analytic approach because it helps frame the context of the health issue.

The Development of Epidemiology

The Father of Epidemiology

cholera
An acute illness caused by infection of the intestine with the bacterium *Vibrio cholerae*.

John Snow, a British physician, is widely regarded as the "father of epidemiology." His work investigating **cholera** demonstrates the value—and timeless utility—of descriptive epidemiology as a tool for the prevention of disease and promotion of health. Snow's approach to stopping the outbreak of a disease with a high mortality rate is still in use today (albeit with more sophisticated technology), and the basics of his approach have been discussed in classrooms across the world for more than a century.

Case Study

John Snow and the London Cholera Epidemic

This case study has been adapted from course materials provided by the Centers for Disease Control and Prevention (CDC 2012a).

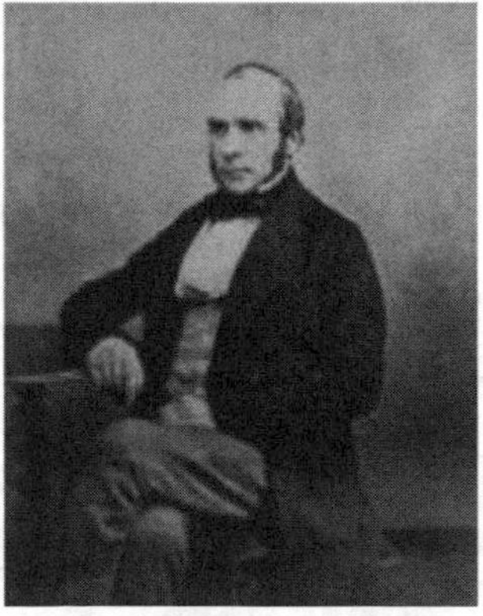

In the mid-1800s, an anesthesiologist named John Snow was conducting a series of investigations in London that warrant his being considered the "father of field epidemiology." Twenty years before the development of the microscope, Snow conducted

(continued)

studies of cholera outbreaks both to discover the cause of disease and to prevent its recurrence. Because his work illustrates the classic sequence from descriptive epidemiology to hypothesis generation to hypothesis testing (analytic epidemiology) to application, two of his investigations will be described in detail.

Snow conducted one of his now famous studies in 1854 when an epidemic of cholera erupted in the Golden Square of London (Snow 1936). He began his investigation by determining where in this area persons with cholera lived and worked. He marked each residence on a map of the area, as shown in Figure 1. Today, this type of map, showing the geographic distribution of cases, is called a **spot map**.

spot map
A map showing the geographic location of people with a specific disease or attribute. Spot maps have proved useful in the investigation of localized disease outbreaks.

Figure 1: Spot Map of Deaths from Cholera in Golden Square Area, London, 1854

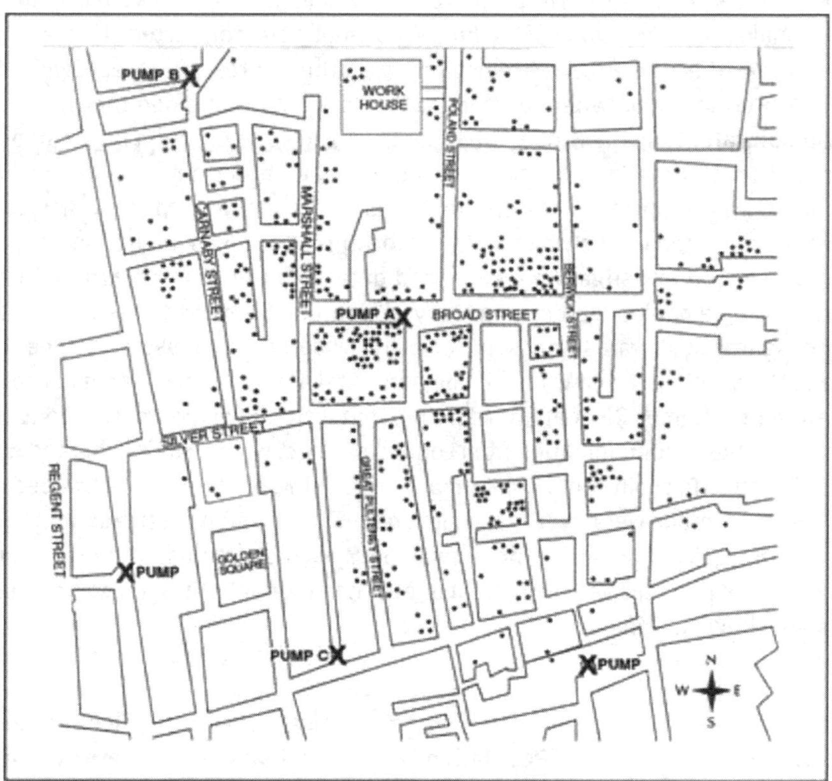

London street map. An *X* indicates the locations of various water pumps. Dots indicate the locations of cholera cases. A relationship between Pump A and cholera cases can be seen.

Source: Snow (1936).

(continued)

Because Snow believed that water was a source of infection for cholera, he marked the location of water pumps on his spot map, then looked for a relationship between the distribution of households with cases of cholera and the location of pumps. He noticed that more case households clustered around Pump A, the Broad Street pump, than around Pump B or C. When he questioned residents who lived in the Golden Square area, he was told that they avoided Pump B because it was grossly contaminated, and that Pump C was located too inconveniently for most of them. From this information, Snow concluded that the Broad Street pump (Pump A) was the primary source of water and the most likely source of infection for most persons with cholera in the Golden Square area. He noted with curiosity, however, that no cases of cholera had occurred in a two-block area just to the east of the Broad Street pump. Upon investigating, Snow found a brewery located there with a deep well on the premises. Brewery workers got their water from this well, and also received a daily portion of malt liquor. Access to these uncontaminated rations could explain why none of the brewery's employees contracted cholera.

To confirm that the Broad Street pump was the source of the epidemic, Snow gathered information on where persons with cholera had obtained their water. Consumption of water from the Broad Street pump was the one common factor among the cholera patients. After Snow presented his findings to municipal officials, the handle of the pump was removed and the outbreak ended. The site of the pump is now marked by a plaque mounted on the wall outside of the appropriately named John Snow Pub.

Snow's second investigation reexamined data from the 1854 cholera outbreak in London. During a cholera epidemic a few years earlier, Snow had noted that districts with the highest death rates were serviced by two water companies: the Lambeth Company and the Southwark and Vauxhall Company. At that time, both companies obtained water from the Thames River at intake points that were downstream from London and thus susceptible to contamination from London sewage, which was discharged directly into the Thames. To avoid contamination by London sewage, in 1852 the Lambeth Company moved its intake water works to a site on the Thames well upstream from London. Over a seven-week period during the summer of 1854, Snow compared cholera mortality among districts that received water from one or the other or both water companies. The results are shown in Table 1.

TABLE 1 Mortality from Cholera in the Districts of London Supplied by the Southwark and Vauxhall and the Lambeth Companies, July 9–August 26, 1854

Districts with Water Supplied by:	Population (1851 Census)	Number of Deaths from Cholera	Cholera Death Rate per 1,000 Population
Southwark and Vauxhall only	167,654	844	5.0
Lambeth only	19,133	18	0.9
Both companies	1,300,149	652	2.2

Source: Snow (1936).

(continued)

The data in Table 1 show that the cholera death rate was more than five times higher in districts served only by the Southwark and Vauxhall Company (intake downstream from London) than in those served only by the Lambeth Company (intake upstream from London). Interestingly, the mortality rate in districts supplied by both companies fell between the rates for districts served exclusively by either company. These data were consistent with the hypothesis that water obtained from the Thames below London was a source of cholera. Alternatively, the populations supplied by the two companies may have differed on other factors that affected their risk of cholera.

To test his water supply hypothesis, Snow focused on the districts served by both companies, because the households within a district were generally comparable except for the water supply company. In these districts, Snow identified the water supply company for every house in which a death from cholera had occurred during the seven-week period. Table 2 shows his findings.

TABLE 2
Mortality from Cholera in London Related to the Water Supply of Individual Houses in Districts Served by Both the Southwark and Vauxhall Company and the Lambeth Company, July 9–August 26, 1854

Water Supply of Individual House	Population (1851 Census)	Number of Deaths from Cholera	Cholera Death Rate per 1,000 Population
Southwark and Vauxhall only	98,862	419	4.2
Lambeth only	154,615	80	0.5

Source: Snow (1936).

This study, demonstrating a higher death rate from cholera among households served by the Southwark and Vauxhall Company in the mixed districts, added support to Snow's hypothesis. It also established the sequence of steps used by current-day epidemiologists to investigate outbreaks of disease. Based on a characterization of the cases and population at risk by time, place, and person, Snow developed a testable hypothesis. He then tested his hypothesis with a more rigorously designed study, ensuring that the groups to be compared were comparable. After this study, efforts to control the epidemic were directed at changing the location of the water intake of the Southwark and Vauxhall Company to avoid sources of contamination. Thus, with no knowledge of the existence of microorganisms, Snow demonstrated through epidemiologic studies that water could serve as a vehicle for transmitting cholera and that epidemiologic information could be used to direct prompt and appropriate public health action.

REFERENCE

1. Snow J. 1936. *Snow on Cholera.* London: Oxford University Press.

In addition to Snow, a number of other thinkers made significant contributions to the early development of epidemiology. John Graunt, for instance, was a British biostatistician from the mid-1600s who compiled **vital statistics**. In the 1800s, William Farr, also British, developed a system for classifying medical conditions; his system became the foundation for the International Classification of Diseases system we use today. The Hungarian physician Ignaz Semmelweis determined that the practice of hand-washing was essential to reducing the transmission of disease to women during childbirth (Friis and Sellers 2014).

vital statistics
Systematically tabulated data concerning births, marriages, separations, divorces, and deaths.

Expansion and Evolution

The field of epidemiology has grown significantly since the time of John Snow, largely in response to advances in technology and improved understanding of not only what makes people sick but also what keeps people healthy.

In the middle and late 1800s, epidemiologic methods were applied to the investigation of disease occurrence, first with a focus on acute infectious diseases. In the 1930s and 1940s, epidemiologists extended their focus to noninfectious diseases. The CDC (2012a) states: "The period since World War II has seen an explosion in the development of research methods and the theoretical underpinnings of epidemiology. Epidemiology has been applied to the entire range of health-related outcomes, behaviors, and even knowledge and attitudes." Pioneering work from this era included research by Doll and Hill (1950) that linked lung cancer to smoking and the 1948 study of cardiovascular disease among residents of Framingham, Massachusetts (Kannel 2000). In the 1960s and early 1970s, health workers applied epidemiologic methods to eradicate naturally occurring smallpox (Fenner et al. 1988)—an unprecedented achievement in applied epidemiology (CDC 2012a).

During the 1980s, the field of epidemiology was extended to studies of injuries and violence. In the 1990s, the new fields of molecular and genetic epidemiology started looking at specific pathways, molecules, and genes that influence risk for disease. Meanwhile, epidemiologists were constantly challenged as new infectious agents emerged, were identified, or changed. The concerns of epidemiologists expanded further in the 1990s and 2000s—particularly after the September 11 attacks of 2001—to include the possible deliberate spread of infectious organisms through biological warfare and bioterrorism (CDC 2012a).

The CDC (2012a) states: "Today, public health workers throughout the world accept and use epidemiology regularly to characterize the health of their communities and to solve day-to-day problems, large and small."

natural experiment
An experiment in which the manipulation of a study factor is not under the experimenter's control but rather is a result of natural phenomena or policies.

Natural Experiments

Some of the health policies in place today, such as laws concerning seatbelt and helmet use, have come from **natural experiments**. A natural experiment is one in which the manipulation of a study factor is not under the experimenter's control but rather is a result of natural phenomena or policies that influence health (Friis and Sellers 2014). Natural experiments make use of "naturally occurring circumstances in which subsets of the population have different levels of exposure to a supposed causal factor in a situation resembling an actual experiment" (Porta 2014, 193). The presence of people in particular subsets is typically not random, as it would be in a true experiment, but "it suffices that their presence is independent of (unrelated to) potential confounders" (Porta 2014, 193).

John Snow's work on the cholera epidemic in London is an example of a natural experiment. Residents received their water from either the Southwark and Vauxhall or Lambeth water company, and Snow demonstrated that those who contracted cholera had generally received their water from the polluted Southwark and Vauxhall source (Friis and Sellers 2014). A true experiment in which Snow assigned subjects to groups exposed to a lethal infection would have been unethical; however, tracing the existing sources of people's drinking water, using what has been called **"shoe-leather" epidemiology**, enabled him to make crucially important observations (Porta 2014).

"shoe-leather" epidemiology
Epidemiologic studies conducted by asking questions directly to the people. The name comes from the idea of walking from door to door and wearing out shoe leather in the process.

In the example of seatbelt and helmet laws, natural experiments indicated that more deaths occurred among people who did not wear their seatbelt or helmet when driving than among people who did, so authorities implemented laws to protect the population. Additional natural experiment examples have involved efforts to discourage smoking. A natural experiment with a tobacco tax examined whether increasing the price of tobacco resulted in decreased sales (Friis and Sellers 2014). In another example, the city of Helena, Montana, implemented a smoking ban in all public places, including restaurants and bars, for a period of six months. As a result of this policy, the heart attack rate declined by 60 percent. After the smoking ban was later reversed, the heart attack rate increased (Sargent, Shepard, and Glantz 2004).

Person, Place, and Time

Descriptive epidemiology—the first of epidemiology's two branches—can identify patterns among cases and in populations by person, place, and time. Based on these observations, epidemiologists reach hypotheses about the causes of these patterns and about the factors that affect the risk of disease (CDC 2012d).

A descriptive epidemiology approach allows us to examine a health issue from varied perspectives, answering questions of what (health issue of concern), who (person), where (place), when (time), and why/how (causes, risk factors, modes of transmission). An epidemiologist studies the available data and determines what information is provided. Just as important, the epidemiologist notes the limitations of existing data. The epidemiologist also notes the patterns exhibited by the data. For example, in what time of year, in which geographic area, and among which demographic groups is the disease occurring? The epidemiologist can visually present the information using maps, tables, and graphs.

Finally, the epidemiologist will identify those segments of the population that are primarily affected by the health issue. This descriptive epidemiologic information, in total, helps the epidemiologist hypothesize about the cause of the disease (CDC 2012c). To test those hypotheses, the epidemiologist usually must turn to the second branch, analytic epidemiology (CDC 2012d), discussed in chapter 6.

The following sections will look more closely at the attributes of person, place, and time.

Person

The CDC (2012c) categorizes age, sex, ethnicity/race, and socioeconomic status as "person" attributes, and they represent one type of determinant for which information is gathered for descriptive epidemiologic purposes. "Because personal characteristics may affect illness, organization and analysis of data by 'person' may use inherent characteristics of people (for example, age, sex, race), biologic characteristics (immune status), acquired characteristics (marital status), activities (occupation, leisure activities, use of medications/tobacco/drugs), or the conditions under which they live (socioeconomic status, access to medical care)" (CDC 2012c). Exhibit 3.1 shows a presentation of data focusing on person attributes.

FOR DISCUSSION: PERSON ATTRIBUTES AND HOSPITALIZATION FOR LABORATORY-CONFIRMED INFLUENZA

Review the chart in exhibit 3.1. Can you identify the age groups at the greatest risk for hospitalization from laboratory-confirmed influenza? Why do you think these groups are the most susceptible?

Example: The Latino Paradox

Past research has shown that outcomes related to poor health and mortality among the non-Hispanic white and black populations in the United States are related to low socioeconomic status (Sorlie, Backlund, and Keller 1995). However, research has also suggested that Hispanics in the United States have lower mortality rates in adulthood than non-Hispanic whites do. This phenomenon has been called a paradox because Hispanics, on average, have lower socioeconomic status than non-Hispanic whites do (Palloni and Arias 2004).

Exhibit 3.2 provides a comparison of life expectancy at birth among various groups. Among the six groups shown, "Hispanic females have the highest life expectancy

Exhibit 3.1
Rates of Hospitalization for Laboratory-Confirmed Influenza, by Age Group and Surveillance Week

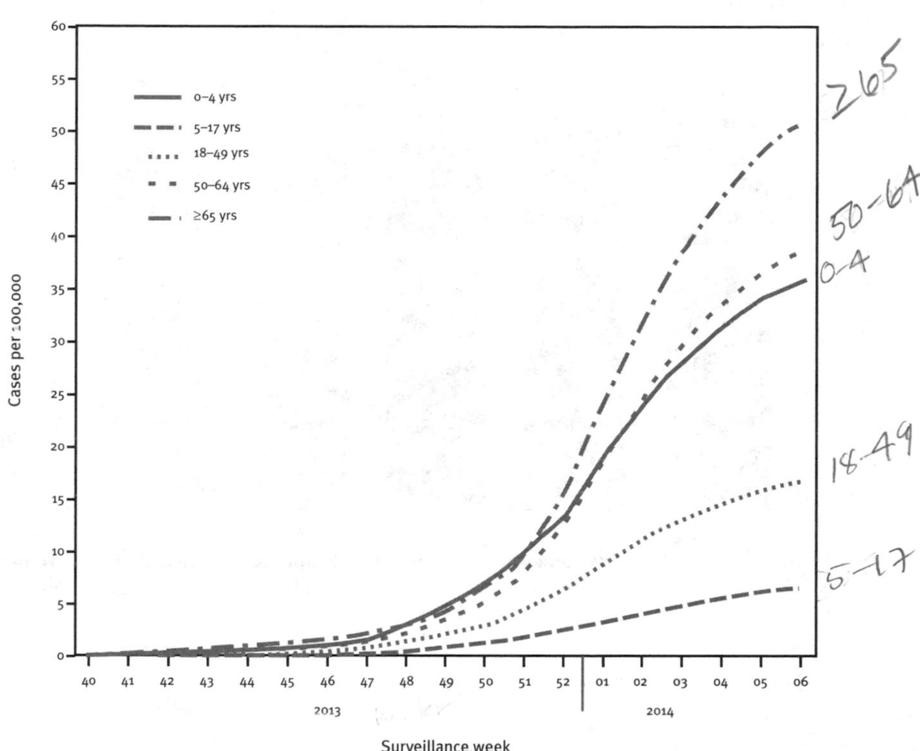

The figure above shows rates of hospitalization for laboratory-confirmed influenza, by age group and surveillance week during 2013–14. CDC monitors hospitalizations associated with laboratory-confirmed influenza in adults and children through the Influenza Hospitalization Surveillance Network (FluSurv-Net), which covers approximately 27 million persons, 8.5 percent of the US population. From October 1, 2013, through February 8, 2014 (week 6), a total of 6,655 laboratory-confirmed influenza-associated hospitalizations were reported. This yields a rate of 24.6 hospitalizations per 100,000 population.

Source: Reprinted from CDC (2014b).

at birth (83.1 years), followed by non-Hispanic white females (80.5 years), Hispanic males (77.9 years), non-Hispanic black females (76.3 years), non-Hispanic white males (75.6 years), and non-Hispanic black males (69.3 years). The smallest differential is between Hispanic and non-Hispanic white females, with Hispanic females having an advantage of 2.6 years. The largest differential is between Hispanic females and non-Hispanic black males, with Hispanic females having a life expectancy at birth 13.8 years greater" (Arias 2010, 11).

Exhibit 3.2
Life Expectancy at Birth, by Hispanic Origin, Race, and Sex, United States, 2006

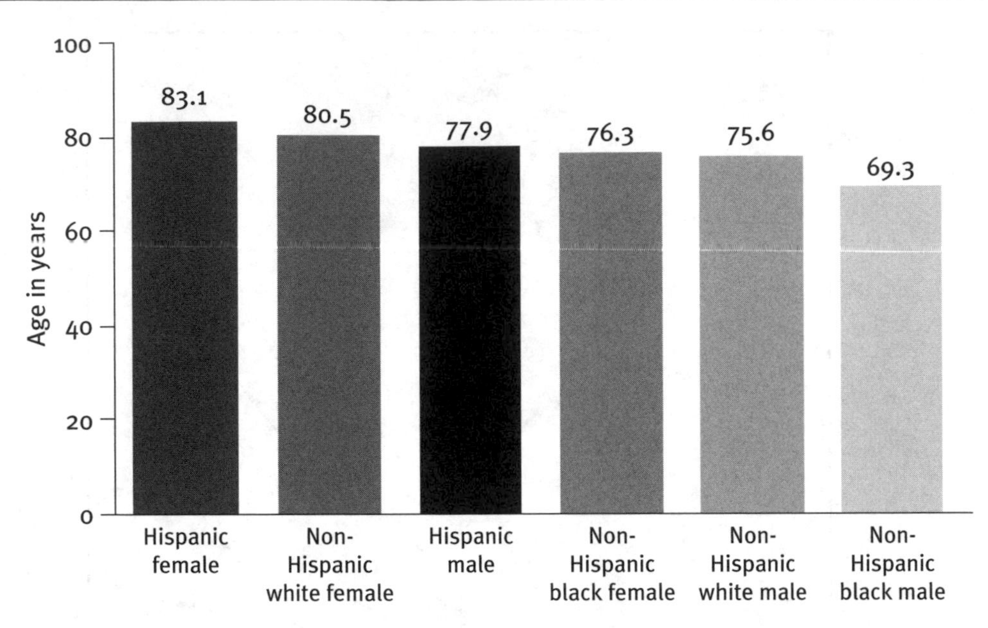

Source: Reprinted from Arias (2010).

Palloni and Arias (2004) have proposed several explanations for the "Latino paradox," involving both issues with the data analyzed and effects of migration and culture. Data issues include possible misclassification of ethnicity between **vital records** and US Census data, misstatement of ages, and incorrect linkage between data sets, leading to a low estimate of Hispanic deaths (Palloni and Arias 2004). Another possible explanation, the "healthy migrant effect," proposes that only migrants who are healthy enough to travel actually migrate. At the same time, the "salmon bias effect" proposes that migrants who become ill travel back home. Both those proposals could contribute to the relatively low number of recorded deaths among the Hispanic population. In general, however, the relatively low mortality rate among the Hispanic population appears to be related to the role of family structure, social networks, and lifestyle practices. Such cultural factors could provide a "protective barrier" to the low socioeconomic status and related challenges (Arias 2010; Palloni and Arias 2004).

vital records
Legal certificates of births, marriages, divorces, and deaths.

We will discuss public health data sets, such as vital records and US Census data, and their utility, advantages, and disadvantages in chapter 4.

Place

"Place" attributes represent a second category of determinants for which information is collected for descriptive epidemiologic purposes. "Describing the occurrence of disease by place provides insight into the geographic extent of the problem and its geographic variation. Characterization by place refers not only to place of residence but to any geographic location relevant to disease occurrence. Such locations include place of diagnosis or report, birthplace, site of employment, school district, hospital unit, or recent travel destinations. The unit may be as large as a continent or country or as small as a street address, hospital wing, or operating room. Sometimes place refers not to a specific location at all but to a place category, such as urban or rural, domestic or foreign, and institutional or noninstitutional" (CDC 2012c).

Variation in disease according to place can be attributed to a number of factors, including differences in how disease is detected and how information about disease is collected and reported in dissimilar places. Other factors may include the social, genetic, and demographic characteristics of a place's population, as well as local environmental conditions such as climate, pollution, and naturally occurring **carcinogens** and other elements (Friis and Sellers 2014).

carcinogen
An agent that can cause cancer.

Example: Lyme Disease

One example that demonstrates the distribution of disease by place involves Lyme disease, which is caused by the *Borrelia burgdorferi* bacterium and is transmitted to humans through the bites of infected ticks. The CDC (2016b) explains: "Typical symptoms include fever, headache, fatigue, and a characteristic skin rash. . . . If left untreated, infection can spread to joints, the heart, and the nervous system. Lyme disease is diagnosed based on symptoms, physical findings (e.g., rash), and the possibility of exposure to infected ticks; laboratory testing is helpful if used correctly and performed with validated methods. Most cases of Lyme disease can be treated successfully with a few weeks of antibiotics. Steps to prevent Lyme disease include using insect repellent, removing ticks promptly, applying pesticides, and reducing tick habitat."

Lyme disease is the most commonly reported vector-borne illness and one of the most common notifiable diseases in the United States; however, it is heavily concentrated in certain parts of the country. More than 95 percent of confirmed Lyme disease cases from 2014 were from Connecticut, Delaware, Maine, Maryland, Massachusetts, Minnesota, New Hampshire, New Jersey, New York, Pennsylvania, Rhode Island, Vermont, Virginia, and Wisconsin (CDC 2015c). Exhibit 3.3 shows the distribution of reported Lyme disease cases, both in 2001 and 2013.

Exhibit 3.3
Reported Cases of Lyme Disease in the United States, 2001 and 2013

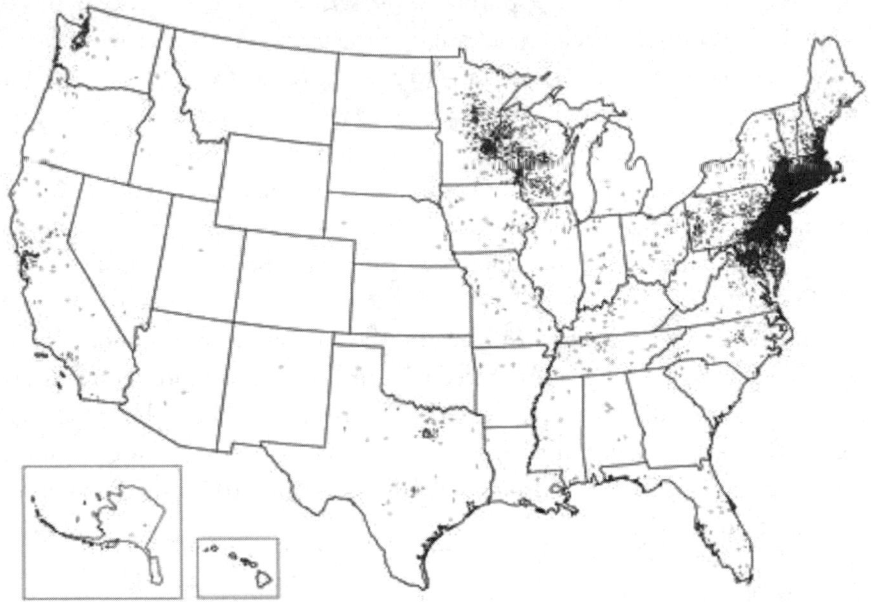

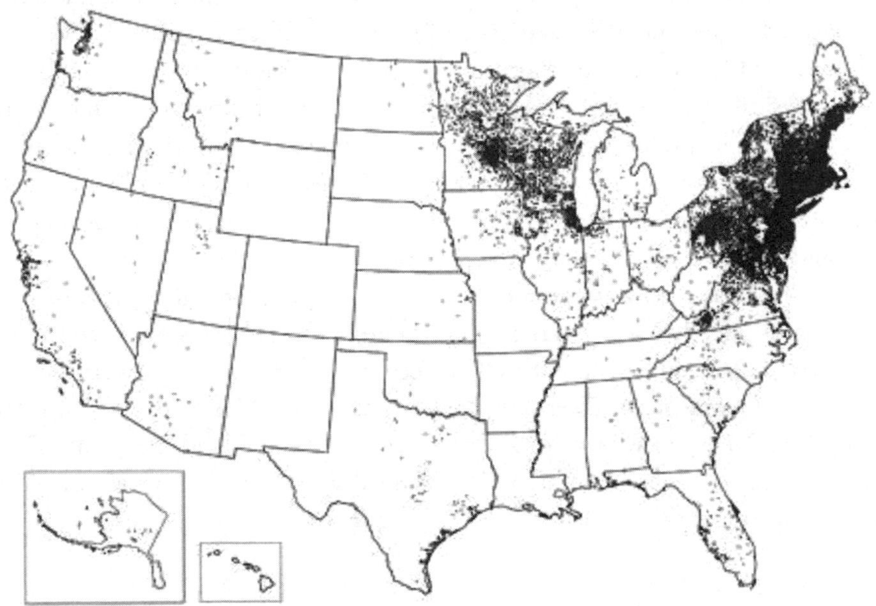

Source: Reprinted from CDC (2015c).

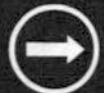

FOR DISCUSSION: THE DISTRIBUTION OF LYME DISEASE

Describe the change in the distribution of reported Lyme disease cases shown in exhibit 3.3. Why do you think Lyme disease cases are generally limited to the Northeast and the Midwest?

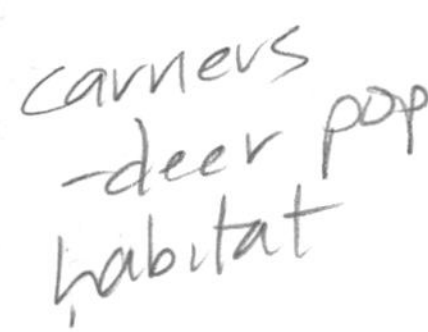

TIME

"Time" characteristics represent a third type of determinant for which information is collected for descriptive epidemiology. The CDC (2012c) states, "Displaying the patterns of disease occurrence by time is critical for monitoring disease occurrence in the community and for assessing whether the public health interventions made a difference."

Diseases may show a variety of patterns in relation to time. A **secular trend**, often called a temporal trend, represents change over a long period of time—usually years or decades. For instance, the long-term decline of tuberculosis mortality would be an example of a secular trend. So, too, would be the rise and subsequent decline in coronary heart disease mortality experienced by many industrialized countries over the last 50 years (Porta 2014). Some diseases occur in a cyclic or seasonal pattern. Certain acute infectious diseases, for instance, peak in one season and reach a low point in the opposite season (Porta 2014). Diseases may also happen in clusters of cases. **Clusters** can be defined as "aggregations of relatively uncommon events or diseases in space and/or time in amounts that are believed or perceived to be greater than could be expected by chance" (Porta 2014, 47). Detailed examples of each of these types of patterns follow.

secular trend
A pattern reflecting change over an extended period, usually years or decades; also called a *temporal trend.*

cluster
An aggregation of an event or disease in a place or time in an amount greater than would be expected by chance.

Example: Secular Trends for Varicella and Polio

Secular trends can be clearly demonstrated for two well-known communicable diseases: varicella, or chickenpox, and poliomyelitis, or polio.

The incidence of varicella, as well as the number of varicella-related hospitalizations, decreased significantly after a vaccine was licensed for use in 1995. Between that year and 2010, the number of cases declined by 97 percent. Cases declined most among children from 5 to 9 years of age, though the decline occurred in all age groups, including infants and adults. Varicella vaccine coverage among children 19 to 35 months old was estimated by the National Immunization Survey to be 90.8 percent in 2011 (CDC 2015b). Exhibit 3.4 charts varicella cases in one California county in the years following the licensure of the vaccine.

EXHIBIT 3.4
Varicella Cases in Antelope Valley, CA, 1995–2004

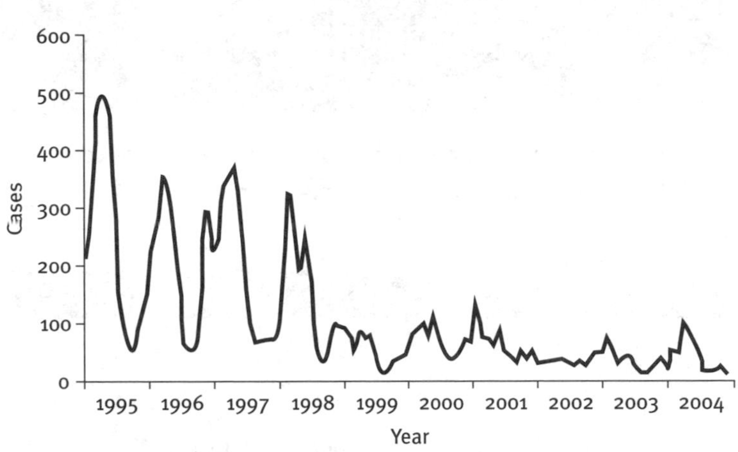

Source: Reprinted from CDC (2012f).

The second example of a secular trend is the decline of polio cases in the decades after the development of the polio vaccine. The CDC (2015a) reports: "From 1980 through 1999, a total of 162 confirmed cases of paralytic poliomyelitis were reported, an average of eight cases per year. Six cases were acquired outside the United States and imported. The last imported case was reported in 1993. Two cases were classified as indeterminant (no poliovirus isolated from samples obtained from the patients, and patients had no history of recent vaccination or direct contact with a vaccine recipient). The remaining 154 (95 percent) cases were vaccine-associated paralytic polio (VAPP) caused by live oral polio vaccine." In an effort to eliminate VAPP from the United States, the Advisory Committee on Immunization Practices recommended in 2000 that the United States exclusively use inactivated polio vaccine. "The last case of VAPP acquired in the United States was reported in 1999. In 2005, an unvaccinated US resident was infected with polio vaccine virus in Costa Rica and subsequently developed VAPP. A second case of VAPP from vaccine-derived poliovirus in a person with long-standing combined immunodeficiency was reported in 2009. Also in 2005, several asymptomatic infections with a vaccine-derived poliovirus were detected in unvaccinated children in Minnesota" (CDC 2015a). Exhibit 3.5 shows the secular trend of VAPP and imported polio during these years.

Example: The Cyclic Pattern of Influenza

Influenza is an excellent example of an illness that exhibits a cyclical or seasonal pattern. In the Northern hemisphere, the flu is most common in fall and winter, though the exact timing and duration of flu seasons vary (CDC 2016a). Most often, flu activity peaks

Exhibit 3.5
Poliomyelitis in the United States, 1980–2009

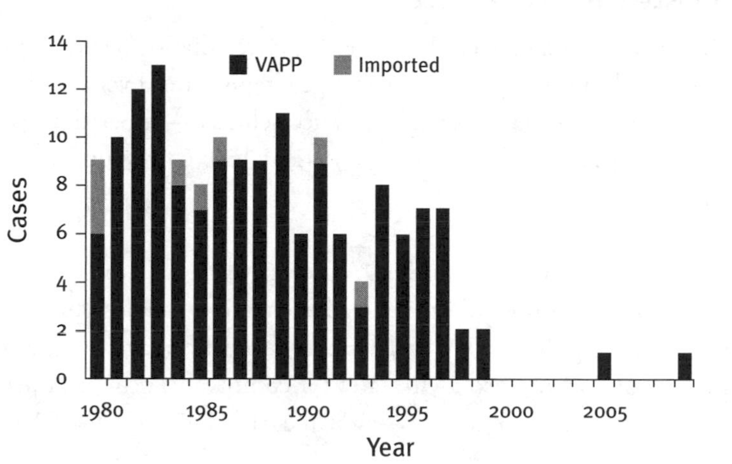

Source: Reprinted from CDC (2015a).

between December and February. Exhibit 3.6 shows how often each month was the peak month of flu activity in the United States between the 1982–1983 and 2015–2016 flu seasons. The peak month is the month with the highest percentage of respiratory specimens testing positive for influenza virus infection. During this period of 34 years, the most common peak month was February (14 seasons), followed by December (7 seasons), March (6 seasons), and January (5 seasons) (CDC 2016a).

Exhibit 3.6
Peak Month of Flu Activity, 1982–1983 through 2015–2016

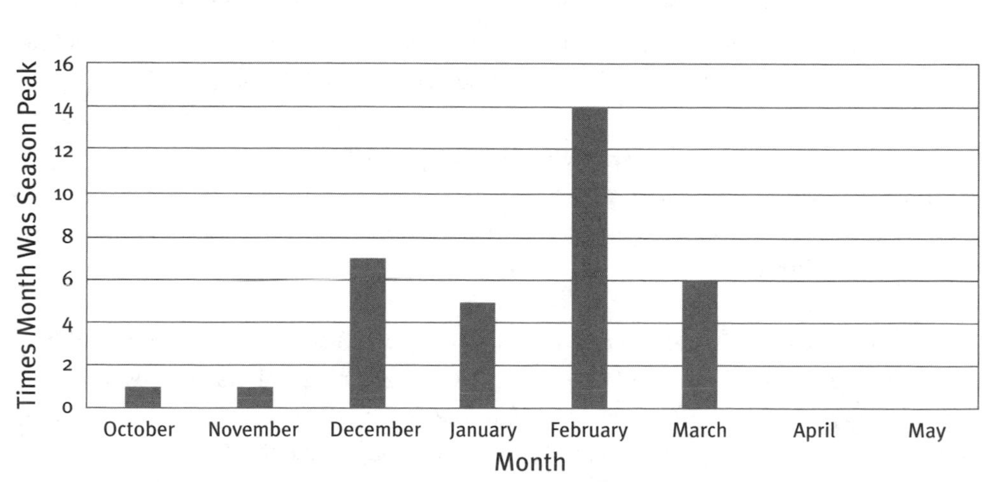

Source: Reprinted from CDC (2016a).

Example: Clusters of Cancer Cases

cancer cluster
Occurrence of a greater-than-expected number of cancer cases within a group of people in a geographic area over a certain period.

The CDC (2013) defines a **cancer cluster** as "a greater-than-expected number of cancer cases that occurs within a group of people in a geographic area over a period of time." For a group of cancer cases to be considered a cancer cluster—rather than just a suspected cancer cluster—it must meet the following criteria, which correspond with the phrases in the definition:

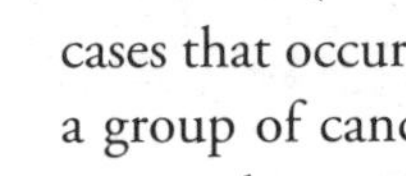

- *A greater-than-expected number*: "A greater-than-expected number is when the observed number of cases is higher than one would typically observe in a similar setting (in a group with similar population, age, race, or gender). This may involve comparison with rates for comparable groups of people over a much larger geographic area—e.g., an entire state" (CDC 2013).
- *Of cancer cases*: "All of the cases must involve the same type of cancer, or types of cancer scientifically proven to have the same cause" (CDC 2013).
- *That occurs within a group of people*: "The population in which the cancers are occurring is carefully defined by factors such as race/ethnicity, age, and gender, for purposes of calculating cancer rates" (CDC 2013).
- *In a geographic area*: "Both the number of cancer cases included in the cluster and calculation of the expected number of cases can depend on how we define the geographic area where the cluster occurred. The boundaries must be defined carefully. It is possible to 'create' or 'obscure' a cluster by selection of a specific area" (CDC 2013).
- *Over a period of time*: "The number of cases included in the cluster—and calculation of the expected number of cases—will depend on how we define the time period over which the cases occurred" (CDC 2013).

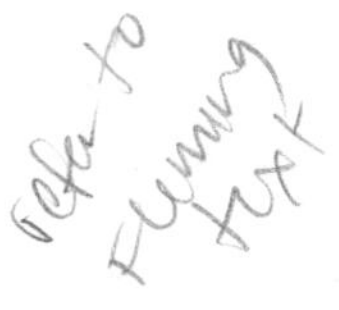

Two confirmed cancer clusters are briefly described in the paragraphs that follow. As you read the descriptions, note the similarities in the events.

The first cluster centered around Tom's River, in Dover Township, New Jersey, in the middle and late 1900s:

> In the mid-1990s, Tom's River physicians noticed an increase in cancers among children from the area. When childhood cancer rates were examined, it was discovered that between 1979 and 1995, leukemia and brain/central nervous system cancers among young children (under age 5) were up to 11 times higher than expected in some census tracts. A case-control study looked at possible environmental exposures to explain the higher cancers. There is evidence of historic contamination by volatile organic

compounds (VOCs) in some public drinking water wells. There is also a facility that emitted hazardous air pollutants; however, data on historic levels of air pollutants do not exist. The study found that for leukemia only, there was an association with prenatal exposure to some of the wells known to be contaminated with VOCs and with estimated prenatal exposure to contaminated air. (Connecticut Department of Public Health 2012, 3)

The second cluster was in Woburn, Massachusetts:

In 1979, Woburn residents noticed a cluster of childhood leukemia cases. This prompted investigations which discovered that two public drinking water wells were contaminated with trichloroethylene (TCE) and other organic compounds (presumably originating from nearby former industrial sites). Between 1969 and 1986, 21 cases of childhood leukemia were diagnosed in Woburn. Early studies concluded that the childhood leukemia rate in Woburn was elevated (2.3 times above expected) but could not establish any environmental causes. Later studies found potential associations between ingestion of contaminated drinking water and increased risk of childhood leukemia. However, not all of the leukemia cases could be explained by the contaminated wells because several cases occurred in children with no access to the wells. A case-control investigation conducted in 1997 found a higher risk of leukemia in children, but only in those exposed to TCE in utero. All of the studies were limited by the small numbers of cases and the incomplete exposure information. . . . While one of the companies was found liable for the Woburn pollution, the case was settled before a legal decision was reached regarding the cause for the leukemia cases. (Connecticut Department of Public Health 2012, 3)

Descriptive Epidemiology Indicators and Methods

incidence
The number of new cases or illnesses in a given period for a specified population.

prevalence
The total number of people who have a condition at a particular time, divided by the population at risk of having the condition.

Epidemiology uses a number of concepts to convey the significance of disease in populations. These concepts are summarized here and will be examined in greater detail throughout the book.

Two key indicators are incidence and prevalence. **Incidence** is "the number of instances or illnesses commencing, or of persons falling ill, during a given period in a specified population" (Porta 2014, 144). **Prevalence** is "the total number of individuals who have the condition (e.g., disease, exposure, attribute) at a particular time (or during a particular period) divided by the population at risk of having the condition" (Porta 2014, 223).

rate
A measure of the frequency with which an event occurs in a population over a specified period. Rates are useful for comparing disease frequency for different locations, at different times, or among different groups.

A **rate**, in epidemiology, is "an expression of the frequency with which an event occurs in a defined population, usually in a specified period of time" (Porta 2014, 239). The CDC (2012e) states: "Because rates put disease frequency in the perspective of the size of the population, rates are particularly useful for comparing disease frequency in different locations, at different times, or among different groups of persons with potentially different sized populations." In other words, a rate can be a "measure of risk" (CDC 2012e). For example, in the John Snow case study from earlier in the chapter, table 2 showed a rate of 4.2 cholera deaths per 1,000 people serviced by the Southwark and Vauxhall Company. That rate was calculated by dividing the number of cholera deaths in the Southwark and Vauxhall group (419) by the total population of the group (98,862) and then multiplying by 1,000. By comparing the resulting number (4.2) with the rate for the Lambeth Company (0.5), we can see that people who received their water from the Southwark and Vauxhall Company died from cholera at a significantly higher rate than those who received their water from the Lambeth Company.

case definition
A set of criteria that must be fulfilled to identify a person as a case of a particular disease.

The CDC (2012b) describes the basic epidemiologic approach in three parts: (1) counting cases or health events, (2) dividing by an appropriate denominator to establish rates, and (3) comparing rates over time and for different groups. The epidemiologist first must develop a **case definition**—a set of criteria used to establish what exactly a "case" is. Then, using the case definition, the epidemiologist finds and collects information about case patients; characterizes the cases collectively according to person, place, and time; and calculates the disease rate by dividing the number of cases by the size of the population. Finally, the epidemiologist compares the rate from this population to the rate for an appropriate comparison group, using analytic epidemiology techniques (CDC 2012b).

case report
A description of a patient or event that could lead to further investigation based on the case's uniqueness or magnitude; also called a *count*.

case series
A summary of characteristics for a consecutive listing of patients from one or more clinical settings.

Three important tools in the practice of descriptive epidemiology are case reports, case series, and cross-sectional studies. **Case reports**, also known as *counts*, are descriptions of patients or events that could lead to further investigation based on the cases' uniqueness or magnitude (Friis and Sellers 2014). A **case series** involves a summary of characteristics for a consecutive listing of patients from one or more clinical settings (Friis and Sellers 2014). A **cross-sectional study** aims to estimate the prevalence of a disease or exposure (Friis and Sellers 2014). Porta (2014, 64) further describes a cross-sectional study as one that "examines the relationship between diseases (or other health outcomes) and other variables of interest as they exist in a defined population at one particular time. The presence or absence of disease and the presence or absence of the other variables (or, if they are quantitative, their level) are determined in each member of the study population or in a representative sample at one particular time."

Work by Aucott and colleagues (2009, 79) dealing with Lyme disease diagnosis provides an example of a case series. The researchers conducted "a retrospective, consecutive case series of 165 patients presenting for possible early Lyme disease between August 1,

2002, and August 1, 2007, to a community-based Lyme referral practice in Maryland." All patients had acute symptoms of up to 12 weeks' duration. They were categorized according to CDC criteria, and data were collected on "presenting history, physical findings, laboratory serology, prior diagnoses and prior treatments." The case series showed a significant number of missed or delayed diagnoses, highlighting the challenges faced by physicians in areas with a high risk for Lyme disease (Aucott et al. 2009).

cross-sectional study
A study designed to estimate disease prevalence and examine the relationship between health outcomes and other variables in a defined population.

An example of a cross-sectional study is provided by Rehmet and colleagues (2002) in their research on influenza vaccination. The researchers conducted a telephone survey "to determine the influenza immunization rates in areas of the former East and West [Germany] during the 1999–2000 influenza season." The authors describe the methods—and some of the challenges—of their cross-sectional study as follows (Rehmet et al. 2002, 1442–1443):

> The target survey population included noninstitutionalized persons >18 years of age living in Germany. A standardized, pretested questionnaire was administered by telephone on November 8 and November 22, 1999. Sample households were chosen by random-digit dialing by using a computer-generated list of possible telephone numbers. Approximately half of the telephone numbers on the list had prefixes in the former East. However, the proportion of working phone numbers was lower in the former East, so the actual number of former East residents who answered the phone and agreed to participate was <50 percent of all participants. The person who initially answered the telephone was eligible to be interviewed; to be eligible, persons also had to be >18 years of age, live in a private household, and have sufficient knowledge of German to be able to understand and answer the questions. If persons <18 years of age answered the phone, they were asked if an adult was present in the household, and an attempt was made to interview that person. After verbal, informed consent was obtained from the participant, we administered a questionnaire that gathered information about demographics, individual risk factors for contracting influenza, history of vaccination, general attitude towards immunization, perceived efficacy and adverse effects of the influenza vaccine, as well as other factors that might influence whether a person was likely to have been vaccinated.

Based on this cross-sectional study, Rehmet and colleagues (2002, 1442) found that "previous influenza vaccination, positive attitudes towards immunization, and having a family physician increased the rate of vaccination; fear of adverse effects lowered the rate."

CASE STUDY

PERTUSSIS EPIDEMIC

The following case has been reproduced from the CDC (2014a). The report, prepared by Kathleen Winter, Carol Glaser, James Watt, and Kathleen Harriman, was posted on the CDC's Morbidity and Mortality Weekly Report *website (www.cdc.gov/mmwr) on December 5, 2014.*

PERTUSSIS EPIDEMIC—CALIFORNIA, 2014

On June 13, 2014, the California Department of Public Health (CDPH) declared that a pertussis epidemic was occurring in the state when reported incidence was more than five times greater than baseline levels. The incidence of pertussis in the United States is cyclical, with peaks every 3–5 years, as the number of susceptible persons in the population increases. The last pertussis epidemic in California occurred in 2010, when approximately 9,000 cases were reported, including 808 hospitalizations and 10 infant deaths, for a statewide incidence of 24.6 cases per 100,000 population (1). During January 1–November 26, 2014, a total of 9,935 cases of pertussis with onset in 2014 were reported to CDPH, for a statewide incidence of 26.0 cases per 100,000. CDPH is working closely with local health departments to prioritize public health activities, with the primary goal of preventing severe cases of pertussis, which typically occurs in infants. All prenatal care providers are being encouraged to provide tetanus, diphtheria, and acellular pertussis vaccine (Tdap) to pregnant women during each pregnancy, ideally at 27–36 weeks' gestation, as is recommended by the Advisory Committee on Immunization Practices (ACIP) (4), or refer patients to an alternative provider, such as a pharmacy or local public health department, to receive Tdap.

For this analysis, case report forms with preliminary data on demographics, symptoms, clinical course, and exposures were completed by local and state health department investigators through patient interviews and medical record reviews and were available for 8,562 (86%) cases. All cases met either the Council of State and Territorial Epidemiologists definition for confirmed pertussis, its definition for probable pertussis, or the CDPH definition for suspected pertussis (2).

Disease incidence in California among infants aged <12 months was 174.6 cases per 100,000 during January 1–November 26, 2014, and was significantly higher among Hispanic infants (rate ratio=1.7; 95% confidence interval [CI]=1.5–2.1) and lower among Asian/Pacific Islander infants (rate ratio=0.4; CI=0.3–0.6) than among white, non-Hispanic infants (Table 1). Of 6,790 cases with available data, 347 patients had been hospitalized, including 275 (79%) who were aged <12 months, of whom 214 (62% of those hospitalized) were aged <4 months. Among hospitalized infants aged <12 months with complete information, 33% required intensive care; few (24%) had received any doses of diphtheria, tetanus, and acellular pertussis vaccine (DTaP) (Table 2). One

(continued)

death was reported in an infant aged 5 weeks at the time of illness onset. Two additional fatal cases in infants who became ill in 2013 were also reported in early 2014; both were aged <5 weeks at the time of illness onset, and one was hospitalized for more than a year before succumbing to pertussis-related complications.

Of 211 (50%) infants aged <4 months whose mothers' Tdap immunization histories were available, only 35 (17%) had mothers who reported receiving Tdap at 27–36 weeks' gestation during their most recent pregnancy. Among mothers not vaccinated during pregnancy, 56 (36%) received Tdap within 7 days after delivery.

Disease incidence was also high among older children and adolescents, peaking at 137.8 cases per 100,000 among adolescents aged 15 years (Figure 1). Among the 2,006 cases in adolescents aged 14–16 years, five patients (0.2%) were hospitalized; four were admitted for ≤2 days, and one was admitted for 5 days. Among the 83% of adolescent cases aged 14–16 years with known vaccination histories, only 2.2% reported never receiving any doses of pertussis-containing vaccine. Of those vaccinated adolescents with complete data, 87% had previously received the Tdap booster vaccine, and the median length of time since prior Tdap dose was 3 years (range=0–7 years). Of the 1,321 (66%) adolescents aged 14–16 years with known race and ethnicity, rates were highest among non-Hispanic white (166.2 cases per 100,000) adolescents and lower among Hispanic (64.2 per 100,000), Asian/Pacific Islander (43.9 per 100,000) and non-Hispanic black (23.7 per 100,000) adolescents.

DISCUSSION

Because infants aged <12 months have the greatest risk for hospitalization and death from pertussis, public health strategies have been prioritized towards preventing disease in this age group. During the 2010 pertussis epidemic in California, the main strategy used to protect infants was "cocooning" (i.e., vaccinating contacts of infants so they do not transmit pertussis to the infant). However, this strategy is difficult to implement, and even if all anticipated contacts could be immunized, infants could still be exposed to infected persons in the community.

In 2011, data became available demonstrating efficient transplacental transfer of antipertussis antibodies to the fetus, which might protect vulnerable infants until they are old enough to receive the primary DTaP series beginning at aged 2 months. In that year, ACIP recommended that pregnant women who had never received Tdap receive a dose after 20 weeks' gestation (3). In 2012, ACIP reviewed data indicating that antipertussis antibody concentrations declined substantially 1 year after vaccination; therefore, ACIP recommended that Tdap be administered during the third trimester of every pregnancy. Since the immune response to Tdap peaks about 2 weeks after administration and the majority of maternal antibodies are acquired by the fetus at 36–40 weeks' gestation, Tdap is currently recommended at 27–36 weeks' gestation to optimize antibody transfer and protection at birth (4,5). Preliminary data indicate that infants born to vaccinated mothers have a lower risk for pertussis early in life (6).

(continued)

Very few mothers of infants with pertussis had received Tdap during pregnancy; many more were vaccinated after delivery, which does not confer any direct protection to the infant and is no longer a preferred strategy. Recently published data indicate that Tdap vaccination coverage among pregnant women was only 19.5% in 2012 across California Vaccine Safety Datalink sites (7). Similarly, in a survey conducted at 100 birthing hospitals in California during October 2013, only 25% of new mothers reported receiving Tdap during pregnancy, whereas an additional 44% received Tdap in the hospital after delivery (CDPH, unpublished data, 2013). However, efforts to increase vaccine coverage have been successful among Northern California Kaiser patients, and in the third quarter of 2014, an estimated 84% of pregnant women received Tdap vaccine in their third trimester (T. Flanagan; Northern California Kaiser; personal communications; November 26, 2014).

Prenatal care providers should vaccinate all pregnant patients with Tdap during the third trimester of each pregnancy, ideally at 27–36 weeks' gestation, as is recommended by ACIP (4). If Tdap cannot be administered on-site during routine prenatal care visits, CDPH encourages prenatal care providers to take the following steps: 1) provide the patient with a strong recommendation and patient-specific prescription for Tdap; 2) refer the patient to specific alternative sites for vaccine, such as pharmacies, primary care providers, or local health departments; and 3) assess Tdap status at follow-up visits to confirm and record receipt of vaccine. In addition, timely initiation of the primary DTaP infant series is essential for reducing severe disease in young infants. According to the American Academy of Pediatrics, DTaP can be administered to infants at an accelerated schedule, with the first dose administered as early as age 6 weeks, when pertussis is prevalent in the community. Even 1 dose of DTaP might offer some protection against serious pertussis disease in infants (8).

Hispanic infants age <12 months have the highest and Asian/Pacific Islanders of all ages have the lowest rates of disease compared with other racial and ethnic groups. However, the Hispanic overrepresentation among infants disappeared by age 1 year, and disease incidence among older children and adolescents was highest among non-Hispanic whites, similar to trends reported previously in California (1). Nationally, since the 1990s, Hispanic infants have been noted to have higher rates of reported disease and pertussis-related deaths compared with non-Hispanic infants (8). The causes of these disparities are unknown, and data are needed to assess the contributing factors. Current hypotheses attribute the disparities to larger household size and/or cultural practices that increase the number of persons in contact with young infants.

Notably, the peak age of disease incidence beyond infancy increased to age 14–16 years in 2014 compared with the peak among children aged 10 years during the 2010 pertussis epidemic (1). Children and teenagers born in the United State since 1997 have only received acellular pertussis vaccine, and the upper age of this cohort correlates with the peak age in incidence during both epidemic years. Data available since the 2010 epidemic indicate that immunity conferred by acellular vaccines, particularly when used for the primary series, wanes more rapidly than that conferred by

(continued)

older, whole-cell vaccines that were used in the United States from the 1940s to the 1990s. Because of vaccine safety concerns related to whole-cell pertussis vaccines, acellular pertussis vaccines were developed and recommended in 1992 for the 4th and 5th doses of the pertussis vaccine series and for all 5 doses in 1997. Acellular pertussis vaccines are less reactogenic than whole-cell vaccines, but the immunity conferred by them wanes more quickly. Most of the cases among adolescents aged 14–16 years were among those who had previously received Tdap ≥3 years earlier, suggesting that their illness was the result of waning immunity. It is likely that increased incidence will continue to be observed among this cohort in the absence of a new vaccine or more effective vaccination strategy. Although the highest burden of disease is currently being observed in adolescents aged 14–16 years, severe disease is uncommon at this age, and <0.5% of reported cases in this age group resulted in hospitalization. More data are needed to assess the potential benefit and timing of Tdap booster doses.

CDPH is working with local public health departments as well as prenatal and pediatric health care providers, with the primary goal of encouraging vaccination of pregnant women and infants. In addition, CDPH is providing free Tdap to local health departments and community health centers to support vaccination of uninsured and underinsured pregnant women and is working to identify and mitigate barriers to Tdap vaccination for pregnant women. CDPH has been working closely with California local health departments to modify guidance for managing the high burden of disease in older children and teenagers, including school outbreaks of pertussis, by prioritizing follow-up of patients and contacts who are at higher risk for developing severe disease (9).

As long as currently available acellular pertussis vaccines are in use, it is likely that the "new normal" will be higher disease incidence throughout pertussis cycles. The number of reported cases in 2014 has surpassed that of the 2010 epidemic and represents the most cases reported in California in nearly 70 years (1). However, it is important to put the current pertussis epidemic in historical perspective. In the immediate prevaccine era, there were approximately 157 reported cases of pertussis per 100,000 population in the United States, with 1.5 deaths per 1,000 infants (10). Therefore, despite the limitations of currently available pertussis vaccines, they continue to have an important impact on pertussis. Strategies to prevent the most severe cases of pertussis, which occur primarily in young infants, should be prioritized.

ACKNOWLEDGMENTS

Sixty-one California local health jurisdictions. James Cherry, MD, David Geffen School of Medicine, University of California, Los Angeles. Stacey Martin, MSc, Division of Bacterial Diseases, National Center for Immunization and Respiratory Diseases, CDC.

(continued)

REFERENCES

1. Winter K, Harriman K, Zipprich J, et al. California pertussis epidemic, 2010. J Pediatr 2012;161:1091–6.
2. California Department of Public Health. Pertussis: CDPH case definition. January 1, 2014. Available at http://www.cdph.ca.gov/healthinfo/discond/documents/cdph_pertussis%20case%20definition_1-2014.pdf.
3. CDC. Updated recommendations for use of tetanus toxoid, reduced diphtheria toxoid and acellular pertussis vaccine (Tdap) in pregnant women and persons who have or anticipate having close contact with an infant aged <12 months—Advisory Committee on Immunization Practices (ACIP), 2011. MMWR Morb Mortal Wkly Rep 2011;60:1424–6.
4. CDC. Updated recommendations for use of tetanus toxoid, reduced diphtheria toxoid, and acellular pertussis vaccine (Tdap) in pregnant women—Advisory Committee on Immunization Practices (ACIP), 2012. MMWR Morb Mortal Wkly Rep 2013;62:131–5.
5. Palmeira P, Quinello C, Silveira-Lessa AL, et al. IgG placental transfer in healthy and pathological pregnancies. Clin Dev Immunol 2011; October 1 [Epub ahead of print].
6. Dabrera G, Amirthalingam G, Andrews N, et al. A case-control study to estimate the effectiveness of maternal pertussis vaccination in protecting newborn infants in England and Wales, 2012–2013. Clin Infect Dis 2014; October 19 [Epub ahead of print].
7. Kharbanda EO, Vazquez-Benitez G, Lipkind H, et al. Receipt of pertussis vaccine during pregnancy across 7 Vaccine Safety Datalink Sites. Prev Med 2014; June 18 [Epub ahead of print].
8. Tanaka M, Vitek CR, Pascual FB, et al. Trends in pertussis among infants in the United States, 1980–1999. JAMA 2003;290:2968–75.
9. California Department of Public Health. CDPH pertussis quicksheet. Available at http://www.cdph.ca.gov/healthinfo/discond/documents/cdph_pertussis_quicksheet.pdf.
10. Cherry J, Brunnel P, Golden G. Report of the Task Force on Pertussis and Pertussis Immunization, 1988. Pediatrics 1988;81:933–84.

WHAT IS ALREADY KNOWN ON THIS TOPIC?

In the prevaccine and postvaccine eras, pertussis incidence has been cyclical and peaks every 3–5 years. Incidence of reported pertussis has been increasing in the United States since the 1980s despite widespread use of pertussis vaccines. Large outbreaks of pertussis occurred in California in 2010 and in other states during 2011–2012.

(continued)

WHAT IS ADDED BY THIS REPORT?

During January 1–November 26, a total of 9,935 cases of pertussis with onset in 2014 were reported in California, for an incidence of 26.0 cases per 100,000 population. The highest burden of disease is being observed in infants aged <12 months, especially Hispanic infants, and in non-Hispanic white teenagers aged 14–16 years, consistent with the upper age of the cohort of children who have only received acellular pertussis vaccines. Severe and fatal disease continues to occur almost exclusively in infants who are too young (age <2 months) to be vaccinated against pertussis. Few mothers of infants diagnosed with pertussis in California (17%) reported receiving tetanus, diphtheria, and acellular pertussis vaccine (Tdap) during the third trimester of pregnancy, as is recommended by the Advisory Committee on Immunization Practices.

WHAT ARE THE IMPLICATIONS FOR PUBLIC HEALTH PRACTICE?

Pertussis incidence is likely to continue to increase in the United States. Prevention efforts should be focused on preventing severe disease and death from pertussis in young infants. The preferred strategy is vaccination of pregnant women during the third trimester of each pregnancy to provide placental transfer of maternal antibodies to the infant. Prenatal care providers are encouraged to provide Tdap to pregnant women (considered best practice) or refer patients to obtain vaccine from an alternative provider, such as a pharmacy or local public health department. Efforts should be made to eliminate barriers to receiving vaccines from prenatal care providers.

Table 1 Number and rate of pertussis cases among infants aged <12 months, by race/ethnicity—California, 2014*

Race/Ethnicity	No.	Rate per 100,000	RR	(95% CI)
White, non-Hispanic	169	120.7	Referent	—
Hispanic, all races	551	207.0	1.7	(1.5–2.1)
Black, non-Hispanic	30	110.0	0.9	(0.6–1.4)
Asian/Pacific Islander, non-Hispanic	31	48.5	0.4	(0.3–0.6)
Other/Unknown	132			

Abbreviations: RR=rate ratio; CI=confidence interval.

* N=913. Rates based on population estimates obtained from the California Department of Finance.

(continued)

Figure 1: Incidence of pediatric pertussis, by age—California, 2014*

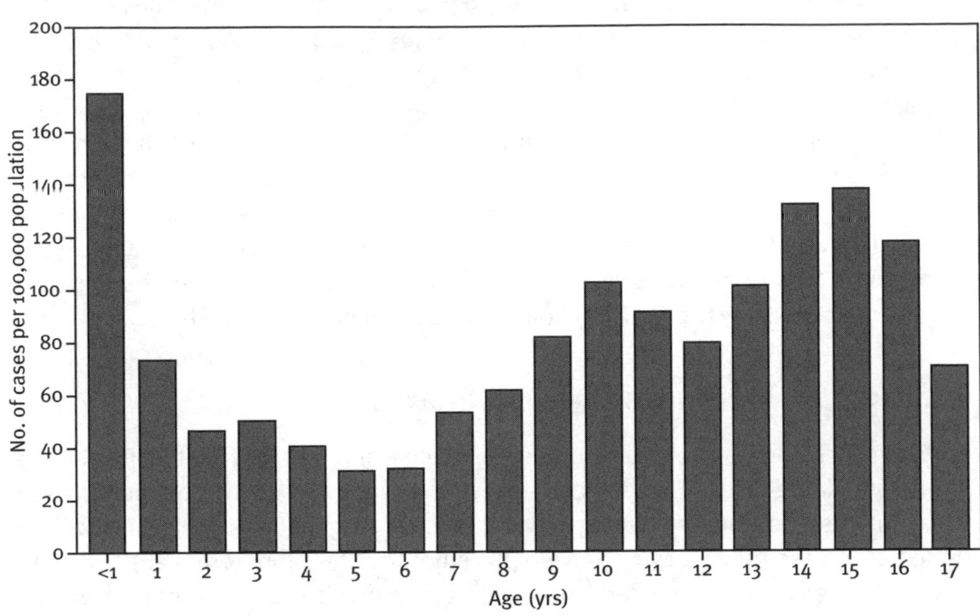

* Reported to the California Department of Public Health as of November 26, 2014.

The figure above is a bar chart showing incidence of pediatric pertussis, by age, in California during 2014. Disease incidence was also high among older children and adolescents, peaking at 137.8 cases per 100,000 among adolescents aged 15 years.

Table 2 Number and percentage of infants aged <12 months hospitalized with pertussis, by selected characteristics—California, 2014*

Characteristic	No.	(%)
Age group		
<2 mos	135	(49)
2 mos to <4 mos	79	(29)
4 mos to <6 mos	33	(12)
6 mos to <12 mos	28	(10)
Vaccination history†		
DTaP >7 days before onset	53	(24)
No DTaP or <7 days before onset	169	(76)

(continued)

Table 2
Number and percentage of infants aged <12 months hospitalized with pertussis, by selected characteristics—California, 2014*
(continued)

Characteristic	No.	(%)
Hospital course		
Median length of stay (days)§	3 (1–50)	
Admitted to intensive care unit¶	71	(33)
Intubated**	18	(8)
Died	1	(1)

Abbreviation: DTaP=diphtheria, tetanus, and acellular pertussis vaccine.

* N=275.

† Out of 222 with known vaccination status.

§ Out of 225 with complete data.

¶ Out of 216 with complete data.

** Out of 237 with complete data.

CASE STUDY DISCUSSION QUESTIONS

1. Describe the characteristics of person, place, and time in this case study.
2. Why might Hispanic infants have higher rates of pertussis and pertussis-related deaths compared to non-Hispanic infants?
3. Identify two reasons why a parent might choose not to have a child vaccinated.
4. Describe two ways to increase compliance with the pertussis vaccine in these two at-risk populations.

Epidemiologic and Demographic Transitions

Exhibits 3.7 and 3.8 list the ten leading causes of death in the United States both at the start of the twentieth century and at the end of the twentieth century. The differences in the two lists reflect what has been called an **epidemiologic transition**—"a shift in the pattern of morbidity and mortality from causes related primarily to infectious and communicable diseases to causes associated with chronic, degenerative diseases" (Friis and Sellers 2014, 743). The top three causes of death in 1900 were infectious in nature, whereas the top three causes in 1998, almost 100 years later, were chronic diseases.

epidemiologic transition
A shift in the pattern of morbidity and mortality away from causes related to infectious and communicable diseases and toward causes associated with chronic and degenerative diseases.

The CDC (2003) has noted that this epidemiologic transition took place first in the developed countries of North America and Europe and that other countries have

Exhibit 3.7
Leading Causes of Death in the United States, 1900

1. Pneumonia (all forms) and influenza
2. Tuberculosis (all forms)
3. Diarrhea, enteritis, and ulceration of the intestines
4. Diseases of the heart
5. Intracranial lesions of vascular origin
6. Nephritis
7. Accidents
8. Cancer and malignant tumors
9. Senility
10. Diphtheria

Source: Linder and Grove (1947).

progressed at different paces. Leading causes of death in developed countries, which tend to have low child mortality and delayed adult mortality, have included cardiovascular diseases, cancer, respiratory diseases, and injuries. Meanwhile, in less developed countries in Africa, for instance, child and adult mortality rates are higher, and leading causes of death have included infectious and parasitic diseases, respiratory infections, perinatal conditions, cardiovascular diseases, cancer, and injuries.

McKeown (2009), in his review of the epidemiologic transition, states: "Though it is true that the burden from infectious diseases has been surpassed in many countries by the burden from chronic disease and mental disorder, it is still the case in many countries and in many populations within countries that morbidity and mortality from infectious disease, poor nutrition, and perinatal complications dominate, with poverty being the most evident shared characteristic." McKeown (2009) continues: "We cannot assume that the evidence of the epidemiologic transition means we can redirect our attention and

Exhibit 3.8
Leading Causes of Death in the United States, 1998

1. Diseases of the heart
2. Malignant neoplasms
3. Cerebrovascular disease
4. Chronic obstructive pulmonary disease
5. Accidents and adverse effects
6. Pneumonia and influenza
7. Diabetes mellitus
8. Suicide
9. Nephritis
10. Chronic liver disease and cirrhosis

Source: Murphy (2000).

resources away from those determinants of death and disease that still threaten the lives and well-being of a large portion of the world's population. But we must also recognize that those same populations will be victims of the obesity, cardiovascular disease, hypertension, and diabetes epidemics that now characterize the US."

What factors determine whether a population would die in greater numbers from chronic diseases rather than infectious diseases? The developer of the epidemiologic transition theory, A. R. Omran (1971, 732), summarizes: "Conceptually, the theory of epidemiologic transition focuses on the complex change in patterns of health and disease *and* on the interactions between these patterns and their demographic, economic, and sociologic determinants and consequences."

demographic transition
The shift toward lower fertility rates and delayed mortality.

Accompanying the epidemiologic transition is **demographic transition**, a shift toward lower fertility rates and delayed mortality. Demographic transition was formerly attributed to technological change and industrialization but is probably more directly related to female literacy and changes in the status of women in society (Porta 2014).

Demographic transition is changing the shape of the global age distribution. Kinsella and Velkoff (2001) explain that the transition begins with declining infant and childhood mortality, in part because of effective public health measures. Lower childhood mortality contributes initially to a longer life expectancy and a younger population, in terms of average age. Declines in fertility rates generally follow, and improvements in adult health eventually lead to an older population. Developed countries had similar proportions of younger and older persons by 1990; for developing countries, age distribution is projected to have similar proportions by 2030 (Kinsella and Velkoff 2001).

population pyramid
A graphic presentation of the age and sex structure of a population.

Demographic transition is apparent in the population pyramids in exhibit 3.9. A **population pyramid** is a graphic presentation that aims to provide "a quick overall comprehension of age and sex structure in the population" (Porta 2014, 219). A high-fertility population will have a pyramid with a broad base (representing younger age groups) and a narrow apex (representing older age groups). Changes in the pyramid's shape over time reflect the shifting composition of the population, associated with changes in fertility and mortality at various ages (Porta 2014).

Friis (2012, 10) summarizes three stages of demographic transition that have affected age and sex distributions in developed societies:

> Stage 1 characterizes a population at the first stage of demographic transition when most of the population is young and fertility and mortality rates are high; overall, the population remains small. Stage 2 shows a drop in mortality rates that occurs during the demographic transition; at this stage, fertility rates remain high, and there is a rapid increase in population, particularly among the younger age groups. . . . Stage 3 reflects dropping fertility rates that cause a more even distribution of the population according to age and sex.

EXHIBIT 3.9 Population Pyramids for 1950, 1990, and 2030

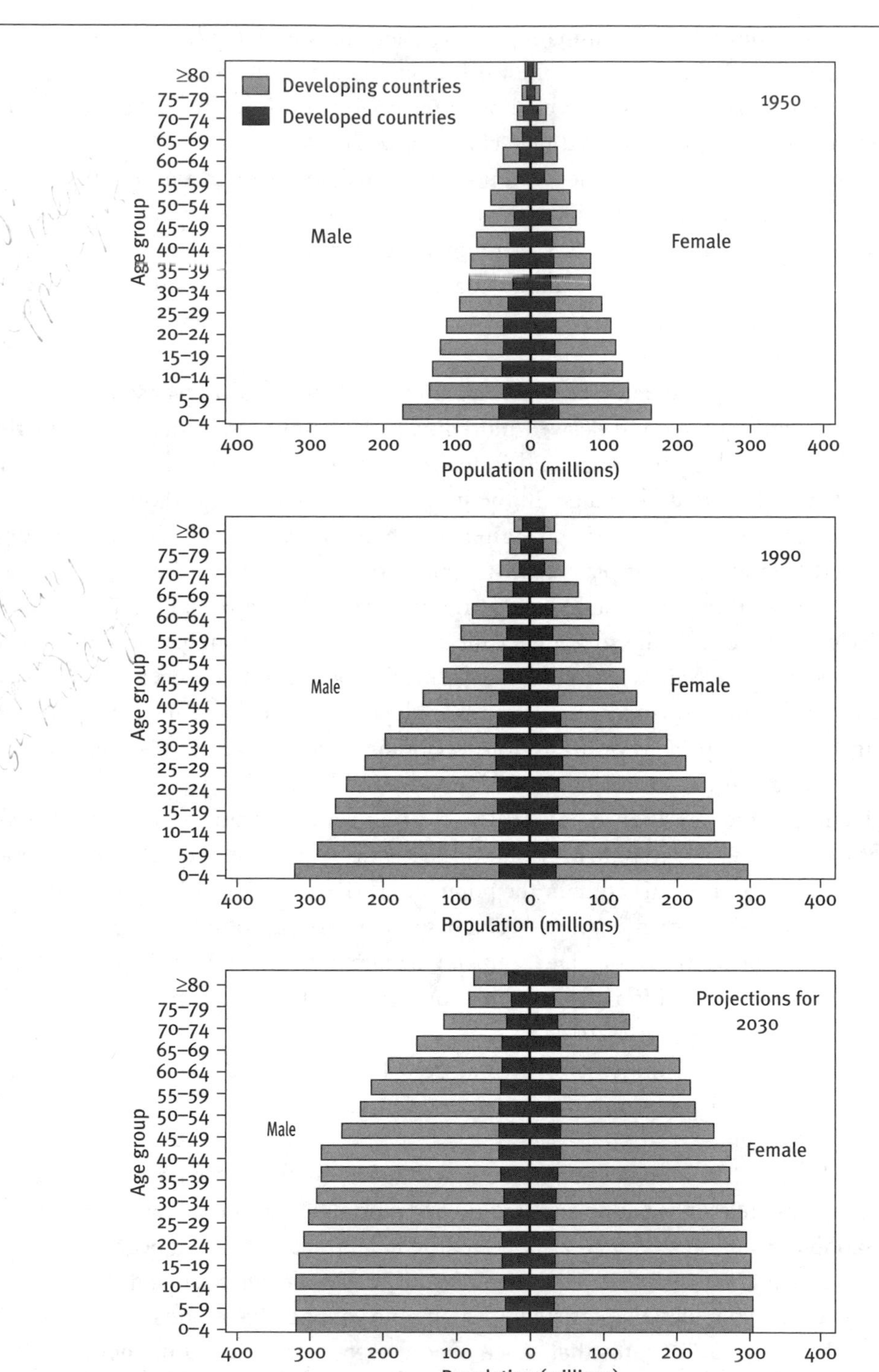

Source: Reprinted from CDC (2003).

EXERCISE: REVIEWING A COMMUNITY HEALTH ASSESSMENT FOR MANCHESTER, NEW HAMPSHIRE

Instructions

Locate *Believe in a Healthy Community*, a 2009 community health assessment for the city of Manchester, New Hampshire (available via www.manchesternh.gov/Departments/Health/Public-Health-Data). Read the selected sections, and answer the questions that follow.

Sections to Read

- *Introduction* (pages 1–5)
- *Healthy Aging: Age 65 and Older* (pages 55–66)
- *Healthy People in Healthy Neighborhoods* (pages 91–103)
- *People Prepared for Emerging Health Threats* (pages 105–14)
- *The Community Provides Input to This Needs Assessment* (pages 115–27)

Questions

Introduction

1. In this community health assessment, the greater Manchester community is called the Manchester Health Service Area (HSA). Describe the Manchester HSA, and explain how it is useful as a definition of "community."
2. What other communities within the greater Manchester area did the assessment also examine?
3. The greater Manchester area's health indicators are primarily compared against two different benchmark efforts. Name the two benchmarks, and explain why you think these benchmarks were used.
4. Describe at least two problems the assessment's authors faced in getting data for the assessment.
5. Explain what a "developmental indicator" means in the Manchester assessment.

Healthy Aging: Age 65 and Older

6. Data indicate that the city of Manchester's older adult (65 or older) population possesses a lower average level of educational attainment than the older adult

(continued)

population of the state as a whole. How might this fact affect the health of Manchester's older population?

Healthy People in Healthy Neighborhoods

7. Define the "built environment," and name two aspects of the built environment that were measured in this assessment.
8. What are some attributes of a positive social environment?

People Prepared for Emerging Health Threats

9. The report examined how Manchester residents with annual incomes less than $25,000 compared to community residents overall on several measures of health status and access to healthcare. How did that income bracket perform? What do you think are some reasons for the group's performance?

The Community Provides Input to This Needs Assessment

10. List five issues that focus group participants and key leaders identified as pressing community issues.

Source: A pilot project conducted by the New Hampshire Institute for Health Policy and Practice and the University of New Hampshire Department of Health Management and Policy, with funding from the University of New Hampshire Office of the Provost. Exercise developed by Rosemary M. Caron and Holly Tutko, 2011; used in HMP 501 Epidemiology and Community Medicine course.

Key Chapter Points

- British physician John Snow, considered the "father of epidemiology," conducted studies of cholera outbreaks both to discover the cause of disease and to prevent its recurrence.
- A natural experiment is one in which the experimenter does not control the manipulation of a study factor. Instead, the manipulation of the study factor occurs as a result of natural phenomena or policies.
- Descriptive epidemiology can identify patterns among cases and in populations by person, place, and time. It allows us to examine a health issue from varied perspectives, answering questions of what (health issue of concern), who

(person), where (place), when (time), and why/how (causes, risk factors, modes of transmission).

- "Person" attributes include age, sex, ethnicity/race, and socioeconomic status. "Because personal characteristics may affect illness, organization and analysis of data by 'person' may use inherent characteristics of people (for example, age, sex, race), biologic characteristics (immune status), acquired characteristics (marital status), activities (occupation, leisure activities, use of medications/tobacco/drugs), or the conditions under which they live (socioeconomic status, access to medical care)" (CDC 2012c).
- "Place" attributes may involve place of residence or any other geographic location relevant to disease occurrence. They may also refer not to a specific location at all but to a place category—for instance, urban versus rural settings.
- The study of "time" characteristics can reveal secular, or temporal, trends, which involve changes over long periods (usually years or decades) of time; cyclic or seasonal patterns; or the grouping of cases into clusters.
- *Incidence* refers to the number of cases or illnesses in a given period for a specified population.
- *Prevalence* refers to the total number of people who have a condition at a particular time, divided by the population at risk of having the condition.
- A rate, in epidemiology, is a measure of the frequency with which an event occurs in a population over a specified period. Rates are useful for comparing disease frequency for different locations, at different times, or among different groups.
- A case definition provides a set of criteria that must be fulfilled to identify a person as a case of a particular disease. It can be based on clinical or laboratory data (or both), or on a scoring system with points for each criterion matching the features of the disease.
- Case reports, case series, and cross-sectional studies are important tools in the practice of descriptive epidemiology.
- The epidemiologic transition is "a shift in the pattern of morbidity and mortality from causes related primarily to infectious and communicable diseases to causes associated with chronic, degenerative diseases" (Friis and Sellers 2014, 743).
- The demographic transition is a shift toward lower fertility rates and delayed mortality.
- A population pyramid is a graphic presentation of the age and sex structure of a population. Changes in the pyramid's shape over time reflect the shifting composition of the population.

Discussion Questions

1. Why is John Snow considered the "father of epidemiology"?
2. Describe how John Snow's work exemplifies a natural experiment.
3. What questions does descriptive epidemiology enable us to answer?
4. Provide examples of how descriptive epidemiology uses person, place, and time information.
5. Describe three factors that can account for place variation of disease.
6. Discuss case reports, case series, and cross-sectional studies.
7. Describe the epidemiologic transition and demographic transition.
8. Why did the leading causes of death change during the course of the 1900s?

References

Arias, E. 2010. "Vital and Health Statistics: United States Life Tables by Hispanic Origin." National Center for Health Statistics. Published October. www.cdc.gov/nchs/data/series/sr_02/sr02_152.pdf.

Aucott, J., C. Morrison, B. Munoz, P. C. Rowe, A. Schwarzwalder, and S. K. West. 2009. "Diagnostic Challenges of Early Lyme Disease: Lessons from a Community Case Series." *BMC Infectious Diseases* 9: 79.

Centers for Disease Control and Prevention (CDC). 2016a. "The Flu Season." Updated July 26. www.cdc.gov/flu/about/season/flu-season.htm.

———. 2016b. "Lyme Disease." Updated August 19. www.cdc.gov/lyme.

———. 2015a. "Epidemiology and Prevention of Vaccine-Preventable Diseases: Poliomyelitis." *Pink Book: Course Textbook*. Updated September 29. www.cdc.gov/vaccines/pubs/pinkbook/polio.html.

———. 2015b. "Epidemiology and Prevention of Vaccine-Preventable Diseases: Varicella." *Pink Book: Course Textbook*. Updated August 11. www.cdc.gov/vaccines/pubs/pinkbook/varicella.html.

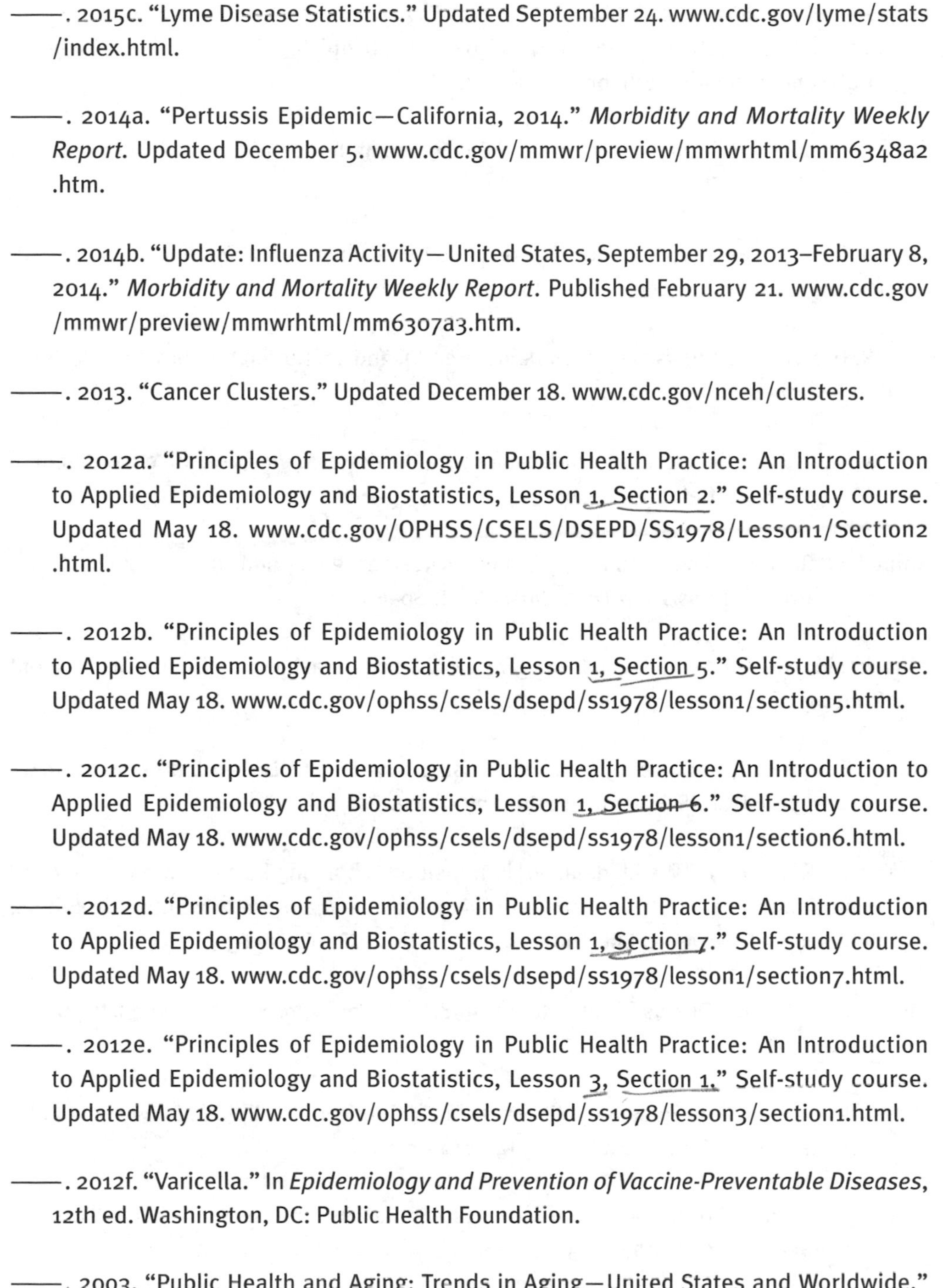

——. 2015c. "Lyme Disease Statistics." Updated September 24. www.cdc.gov/lyme/stats/index.html.

——. 2014a. "Pertussis Epidemic—California, 2014." *Morbidity and Mortality Weekly Report.* Updated December 5. www.cdc.gov/mmwr/preview/mmwrhtml/mm6348a2.htm.

——. 2014b. "Update: Influenza Activity—United States, September 29, 2013–February 8, 2014." *Morbidity and Mortality Weekly Report.* Published February 21. www.cdc.gov/mmwr/preview/mmwrhtml/mm6307a3.htm.

——. 2013. "Cancer Clusters." Updated December 18. www.cdc.gov/nceh/clusters.

——. 2012a. "Principles of Epidemiology in Public Health Practice: An Introduction to Applied Epidemiology and Biostatistics, Lesson 1, Section 2." Self-study course. Updated May 18. www.cdc.gov/OPHSS/CSELS/DSEPD/SS1978/Lesson1/Section2.html.

——. 2012b. "Principles of Epidemiology in Public Health Practice: An Introduction to Applied Epidemiology and Biostatistics, Lesson 1, Section 5." Self-study course. Updated May 18. www.cdc.gov/ophss/csels/dsepd/ss1978/lesson1/section5.html.

——. 2012c. "Principles of Epidemiology in Public Health Practice: An Introduction to Applied Epidemiology and Biostatistics, Lesson 1, Section 6." Self-study course. Updated May 18. www.cdc.gov/ophss/csels/dsepd/ss1978/lesson1/section6.html.

——. 2012d. "Principles of Epidemiology in Public Health Practice: An Introduction to Applied Epidemiology and Biostatistics, Lesson 1, Section 7." Self-study course. Updated May 18. www.cdc.gov/ophss/csels/dsepd/ss1978/lesson1/section7.html.

——. 2012e. "Principles of Epidemiology in Public Health Practice: An Introduction to Applied Epidemiology and Biostatistics, Lesson 3, Section 1." Self-study course. Updated May 18. www.cdc.gov/ophss/csels/dsepd/ss1978/lesson3/section1.html.

——. 2012f. "Varicella." In *Epidemiology and Prevention of Vaccine-Preventable Diseases*, 12th ed. Washington, DC: Public Health Foundation.

——. 2003. "Public Health and Aging: Trends in Aging—United States and Worldwide." *MMWR* 52 (06): 101–6.

Connecticut Department of Public Health. 2012. *Environmental Health Technical Brief: Cancer Clusters.* Published April. www.ct.gov/dph/lib/dph/environmental_health/eoha/pdf/cancer_cluster_tech_brief_final.pdf.

Doll, R., and A. B. Hill. 1950. "Smoking and Carcinoma of the Lung." *British Medical Journal* 2 (4682): 739–48.

Fenner, F., D. A. Henderson, I. Arita, Z. Jezek, and I. D. Ladnyi. 1988. *Smallpox and Its Eradication.* Geneva, Switzerland: World Health Organization.

Friis, R. H. 2012. *Essentials of Environmental Health*, 2nd ed. Burlington, MA: Jones & Bartlett Learning.

Friis, R. H., and T. A. Sellers. 2014. *Epidemiology for Public Health Practice*, 5th ed. Burlington, MA: Jones & Bartlett Learning.

Kannel, W. B. 2000. "The Framingham Study: Its 50-Year Legacy and Future Promise." *Journal of Atherosclerosis and Thrombosis* 6 (2): 60–66.

Kinsella, K., and V. A. Velkoff. 2001. *An Aging World: 2001.* Washington, DC: US Government Printing Office.

Linder, F. E., and R. D. Grove. 1947. *Vital Statistics Rates in the United States, 1900–1940.* Washington, DC: US Government Printing Office.

McKeown, R. E. 2009. "The Epidemiologic Transition: Changing Patterns of Mortality and Population Dynamics." *American Journal of Lifestyle Medicine* 3 (1 Suppl): 19S–26S. Published July. www.ncbi.nlm.nih.gov/pmc/articles/PMC2805833.

Murphy, S. L. 2000. "Deaths: Final Data for 1998." *National Vital Statistics Reports* 48 (11): 1–104.

Omran, A. R. 1971. "The Epidemiologic Transition: A Theory of the Epidemiology of Population Change." *Milbank Quarterly* 83 (4): 731–57.

Palloni, A., and E. Arias. 2004. "Paradox Lost: Explaining the Hispanic Adult Mortality Advantage." *Demography* 41 (3): 385–415.

Porta, M. (ed.). 2014. *A Dictionary of Epidemiology*, 6th ed. New York: Oxford University Press.

Rehmet, S., A. Ammon, G. Pfaff, N. Bocter, and L. R. Petersen. 2002. "Cross-Sectional Study on Influenza Vaccination: Germany, 1999–2000." *Emerging Infectious Diseases* 8 (12): 1442–47.

Sargent, R. P., R. M. Shepard, and S. A. Glantz. 2004. "Reduced Incidence of Admissions for Myocardial Infarction Associated with Public Smoking Ban: Before and After Study." *British Medical Journal* 328 (7446): 977–80.

Sorlie, P. D., E. Backlund, and J. B. Keller. 1995. "US Mortality by Economic, Demographic, and Social Characteristics: The National Longitudinal Mortality Study." *American Journal of Public Health* 85 (7): 949–56.

Twain, M. 1897. *Following the Equator.* Accessed January 11, 2017. www.gutenberg.org/files/2895/2895-h/2895-h.htm.

CHAPTER 4

PUBLIC HEALTH AND HEALTHCARE DATA

"Always remember, the data we use in epidemiology represent people. Our data have faces and are not the result of a laboratory controlled experiment."

—R. M. Caron

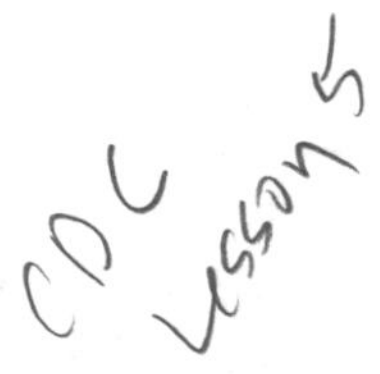

Learning Objectives

After completing this chapter, you should be able to

- ➤ describe the types of data used in epidemiology,
- ➤ describe the sources of the data,
- ➤ compare the strengths and limitations of public health and healthcare data,
- ➤ provide examples of the use of public health and healthcare data, and
- ➤ explain how confidentiality is maintained when dealing with such data.

Introduction

This chapter will discuss the types of public health and healthcare data used in assessing the health of populations; the sources of data; the strengths and limitations of the data; and the importance of confidentiality when dealing with personally identifiable information.

Why do people want to access data from public health and healthcare sources? The reasons are many, and they span a wide range of areas:

- Program development
- Program evaluation
- Intervention assessment
- Community planning
- Early event detection
- Grant applications
- Research for evidence-based practice
- General public interest

This chapter is not intended to be an all-inclusive compendium of the data sets used in public health and healthcare settings; instead, it aims to highlight the most representative data sets in use today.

Public Health Data

Evidence-based public health involves the use and application of the best available evidence—derived from epidemiologic, demographic, economic, and other relevant sources—for the development of public health policies and practices (Porta 2014).

The following sections describe key sources of public health data and a variety of resources for accessing and using such data.

evidence-based public health
The use of the best available evidence for the development of public health policies and practices.

Vital Statistics

Vital statistics provide "systematically tabulated information concerning births, marriages, divorces, separations and deaths based on registrations of these vital events" (Porta 2014, 292). The National Center for Health Statistics (NCHS), part of the Centers for Disease Control and Prevention (CDC), collects and disseminates the nation's official vital statistics via the National Vital Statistics System (NVSS), the "oldest and most successful example of intergovernmental data sharing in public health" (CDC 2016a). The CDC (2016a) further explains:

> These data are provided through contracts between NCHS and vital registration systems operated in the various jurisdictions legally responsible for the registration of vital events—births, deaths, marriages, divorces, and fetal deaths. Vital statistics data are also available online. In the United States, legal authority for the registration of these events resides individually with the 50 States, 2 cities (Washington, DC, and New York City), and 5 territories (Puerto Rico, the Virgin Islands, Guam, American Samoa, and the Commonwealth of the Northern Mariana Islands). These jurisdictions are responsible for maintaining registries of vital events and for issuing copies of birth, marriage, divorce, and death certificates.

Birth Data

The NCHS and the individual states' vital records bureaus cooperate to provide statistical information from birth certificates. Birth certificate data are necessary to calculate birth rates. Birth certificates also collect information about conditions present during pregnancy, **congenital malformations**, obstetric procedures, birth weight, length of gestation, and the demographic background of the mother (Friis and Sellers 2014). Exhibit 4.1 demonstrates the type of information that can be obtained through the collection and analysis of birth data. Such data are useful but may sometimes be unreliable, reflecting gaps in mothers' recall of events and the possible conditions and illnesses that were not detected at the time of birth (Friis and Sellers 2014).

congenital malformation
A physical anomaly present in a baby at birth.

The NVSS compiles and publishes birth and other vital statistics information that is mandated by federal law to be collected by each state (CDC 2015f). The NCHS and the states develop standard forms for the collection of data, outline procedures for the uniform registration of events, and provide materials to assist people in completing birth certificates. The NCHS shares the costs incurred by states in providing data for national use (CDC 2015f).

Exhibit 4.1
Birth Data for the United States, 2012

Number of births: 3,952,841
Birth rate: 12.6 births per 1,000 population
Fertility rate: 63.0 births per 1,000 women aged 15–44 years
Percent born with low birth weight: 8.0 percent
Percent of mothers unmarried: 40.7 percent

Source: Martin et al. (2013).

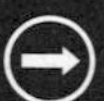

EXERCISE: ACCESSING US BIRTH DATA

Access the NVSS website (www.cdc.gov/nchs/nvss) and locate the most recent *National Vital Statistics Report* titled "Births: Final Data." Review the report and identify the following for the most recent year:

- Number of births
- Birth rate
- Fertility rate
- Percent born with low birth weight
- Percent of mothers unmarried

Mortality Data

Mortality data, also known as *death data*, are collected for each state and submitted to the NVSS. The collection of this data over multiple years allows for the identification of trends in cause of death by demographic and geographic area. Further, mortality data provide information about the population's leading causes of death, help determine a population's life expectancy, and allow for comparison of mortality trends with other populations (CDC 2016h).

Friis and Sellers (2014, 247, 251) write:

> Death certificate data in the United States include demographic information about the decedent and information about the cause of death, including the immediate cause and contributing factors. The death certificate is partially completed by the funeral director. The attending physician then completes the section on date and cause of death. If the death occurred as the result of accident, suicide, or homicide, or if the attending physician is unavailable, then the medical examiner or coroner completes and signs the death certificate. Once this is done, the local registrar checks the certificate for completeness and accuracy and sends a copy to the state registrar. The state registrar also checks for completeness and accuracy and sends a copy to the NCHS, which compiles and publishes national mortality rates (e.g., in Vital Statistics of the United States).

International Classification of Diseases (ICD)
A classification and coding system for diseases and other health problems, maintained by the World Health Organization and revised on a regular basis.

Data pertaining to causes of death are classified and coded according to the **International Classification of Diseases (ICD)**. The ICD is revised about once every ten years, and the latest edition, known as ICD-10, is the tenth. Regular revision helps the national mortality system to stay abreast of advances in medical science and changes in terminology (CDC 2016a). However, some revisions—such as changes in the classification of medical conditions or in the rules for selection of underlying causes of death—may complicate mortality trend data (CDC 2016a).

The use of mortality data has some inherent limitations. For example, errors may occur in the certification of cause of death. For many elder adults with chronic disease, a specific cause of death may be uncertain. Further inaccuracies may result from a lack of standardization of diagnostic criteria for physician reporting, ICD coding errors and changes in ICD codes, and the stigma associated with certain diseases (Friis and Sellers 2014).

Exhibit 4.2 shows the instructions from the NCHS for completing the cause-of-death section of a death certificate, as well as a completed example. Exhibit 4.3 demonstrates the type of information that can be obtained through the collection and analysis of death data.

EXERCISE: ACCESSING US MORTALITY DATA

Access the NVSS website (www.cdc.gov/nchs/nvss) and locate the most recent *National Vital Statistics Report* titled "Deaths: Final Data." Review the report and identify the following for the most recent year:

- Life expectancy for males and females
- The population groups that experienced a decrease in mortality
- Top three leading causes of death
- Top three leading causes of infant death

CDC *Vital Signs*

The CDC *Vital Signs* is a monthly report that presents recent public health data and calls to action concerning important issues. Available in English and Spanish, the report consists of a graphic fact sheet and website, social media tools, and the *Morbidity and Mortality Weekly Report (MMWR)* Early Release (CDC 2016k). *Vital Signs* provides information

Exhibit 4.2
Completing the Cause-of-Death Section of a Death Certificate

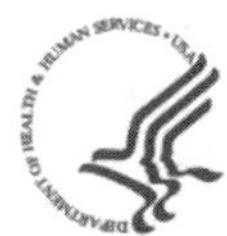

U.S. DEPARTMENT OF HEALTH AND HUMAN SERVICES
Centers for Disease Control and Prevention
National Center for Health Statistics

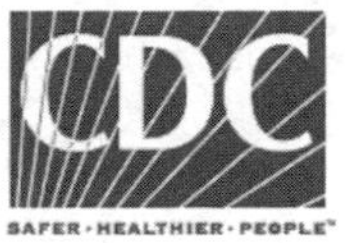

Instructions for Completing the Cause-of-Death Section of the Death Certificate

Accurate cause-of-death information is important:
- To the public health community in evaluating and improving the health of all citizens, and
- Often to the family, now and in the future, and to the person settling the decedent's estate.

The cause-of-death section consists of two parts. **Part I** is for reporting a chain of events leading directly to death, with the **immediate cause** of death (the final disease, injury, or complication directly causing death) on Line a and the **underlying cause** of death (the disease or injury that initiated the chain of morbid events that led directly and inevitably to death) on the lowest used line. **Part II** is for reporting all other significant diseases, conditions, or injuries that contributed to death but which did not result in the underlying cause of death given in Part I. **The cause-of-death information should be YOUR best medical OPINION.** A condition can be listed as "probable" even if it has not been definitively diagnosed.

Examples of properly completed medical certifications

CAUSE OF DEATH (See instructions and examples)

32. **PART I.** Enter the chain of events—diseases, injuries, or complications—that directly caused the death. DO NOT enter terminal events such as cardiac arrest, respiratory arrest, or ventricular fibrillation without showing the etiology. DO NOT ABBREVIATE. Enter only one cause on a line. Add additional lines if necessary.

		Approximate interval: Onset to death
IMMEDIATE CAUSE (Final disease or condition resulting in death) →	a. Rupture of myocardium	Minutes
	Due to (or as a consequence of):	
Sequentially list conditions, if any, leading to the cause listed on line a. Enter the UNDERLYING CAUSE (disease or injury that initiated the events resulting in death) LAST	b. Acute myocardial infarction	6 days
	Due to (or as a consequence of):	
	c. Coronary artery thrombosis	5 years
	Due to (or as a consequence of):	
	d. Atherosclerotic coronary artery disease	7 years

PART II. Enter other significant conditions contributing to death but not resulting in the underlying cause given in PART I.
Diabetes, Chronic obstructive pulmonary disease, smoking

33. WAS AN AUTOPSY PERFORMED? ■ Yes ☐ No

34. WERE AUTOPSY FINDINGS AVAILABLE TO COMPLETE THE CAUSE OF DEATH? ■ Yes ☐ No

35. DID TOBACCO USE CONTRIBUTE TO DEATH?
■ Yes ☐ Probably
☐ No ☐ Unknown

36. IF FEMALE:
■ Not pregnant within past year
☐ Pregnant at time of death
☐ Not pregnant, but pregnant within 42 days of death
☐ Not pregnant, but pregnant 43 days to 1 year before death
☐ Unknown if pregnant within the past year

37. MANNER OF DEATH
■ Natural ☐ Homicide
☐ Accident ☐ Pending Investigation
☐ Suicide ☐ Could not be determined

CAUSE OF DEATH (See instructions and examples)

32. **PART I.** Enter the chain of events—diseases, injuries, or complications—that directly caused the death. DO NOT enter terminal events such as cardiac arrest, respiratory arrest, or ventricular fibrillation without showing the etiology. DO NOT ABBREVIATE. Enter only one cause on a line. Add additional lines if necessary.

		Approximate interval: Onset to death
IMMEDIATE CAUSE (Final disease or condition resulting in death) →	a. Acute renal failure	5 days
	Due to (or as a consequence of):	
Sequentially list conditions, if any, leading to the cause listed on line a. Enter the UNDERLYING CAUSE (disease or injury that initiated the events resulting in death) LAST	b. Hyperosmolar nonketotic coma	8 weeks
	Due to (or as a consequence of):	
	c. Diabetes mellitus, noninsulin dependent	15 years
	Due to (or as a consequence of):	
	d.	

PART II. Enter other significant conditions contributing to death but not resulting in the underlying cause given in PART I.

33. WAS AN AUTOPSY PERFORMED? ☐ Yes ■ No

34. WERE AUTOPSY FINDINGS AVAILABLE TO COMPLETE THE CAUSE OF DEATH? ☐ Yes ■ No

35. DID TOBACCO USE CONTRIBUTE TO DEATH?
☐ Yes ☐ Probably
■ No ☐ Unknown

36. IF FEMALE:
■ Not pregnant within past year
☐ Pregnant at time of death
☐ Not pregnant, but pregnant within 42 days of death
☐ Not pregnant, but pregnant 43 days to 1 year before death
☐ Unknown if pregnant within the past year

37. MANNER OF DEATH
■ Natural ☐ Homicide
☐ Accident ☐ Pending Investigation
☐ Suicide ☐ Could not be determined

ITEM 32 - CAUSE OF DEATH

Take care to make the entry legible. Use a computer printer with high resolution, typewriter with good black ribbon and clean keys, or print legibly using permanent black ink in completing the cause-of-death section. **Do not abbreviate** conditions entered in section.

Part I (Chain of events leading directly to death)
- Only one cause should be entered on each line. Line a **MUST ALWAYS** have an entry. **DO NOT** leave blank. Additional lines may be added if necessary.
- If the condition on Line a resulted from an underlying condition, put the underlying condition on Line b, and so on, until the full sequence is reported. **ALWAYS** enter the **underlying cause of death** on the lowest used line in Part I.
- For each cause indicate the best estimate of the interval between the presumed onset and the date of death. The terms "unknown" or "approximately" may be used. General terms, such as minutes, hours, or days, are acceptable, if necessary. **DO NOT** leave blank.

(continued)

Exhibit 4.2
Completing the Cause-of-Death Section of a Death Certificate *(continued)*

• The terminal event (e.g., cardiac arrest or respiratory arrest) should not be used. If a mechanism of death seems most appropriate to you for Line a, then you must always list its cause(s) on the line(s) below it (e.g., cardiac arrest **due** to coronary artery atherosclerosis *or* cardiac arrest **due** to blunt impact to chest).
• If an organ system failure such as congestive heart failure, hepatic failure, renal failure, or respiratory failure is listed as a cause of death, always report its etiology on the line(s) beneath it (e.g., renal failure **due** to Type I diabetes mellitus).
• When indicating neoplasms as a cause of death, include the following: 1) primary site *or* that the primary site is unknown, 2) benign or malignant, 3) cell type *or* that the cell type is unknown, 4) grade of neoplasm, and 5) part or lobe of organ affected. Example: a primary well-differentiated squamous cell carcinoma, lung, left upper lobe.

Part II (Other significant conditions)
• Enter all diseases or conditions contributing to death that were not reported in the chain of events in Part I and that did not result in the **underlying cause of death**. See examples.
• If two or more possible sequences resulted in death, or if two conditions seem to have added together, report in Part I the one that, in your opinion, most directly caused death. Report in Part II the other conditions or diseases.

CHANGES TO CAUSE OF DEATH
If additional medical information or autopsy findings become available that would change the cause of death originally reported, the original death certificate should be amended by the certifying physician by **immediately** reporting the revised cause of death to the State Vital Records Office.

ITEMS 33 and 34 - AUTOPSY
• 33 - Enter "Yes" if either a partial or full autopsy was performed. Otherwise enter "No."
• 34 - Enter "Yes" if autopsy findings were available to complete the cause of death; otherwise enter "No." Leave item blank if no autopsy was performed.

ITEM 35 - DID TOBACCO USE CONTRIBUTE TO DEATH?
Check "Yes" if, in your opinion, the use of tobacco contributed to death. Tobacco use may contribute to deaths due to a wide variety of diseases; for example, tobacco use contributes to many deaths due to emphysema or lung cancer and some heart disease and cancers of the head and neck. Check "No" if, in your clinical judgment, tobacco use did not contribute to this particular death.

ITEM 36 - IF FEMALE, WAS DECEDENT PREGNANT AT TIME OF DEATH OR WITHIN PAST YEAR?
If the decedent is a female, check the appropriate box. If the female is either too old or too young to be fecund, check the "Not pregnant within past year" box. If the decedent is a male, leave the item blank. This information is important in determining pregnancy-related mortality.

ITEM 37 - MANNER OF DEATH
• Always check Manner of Death, which is important: 1) in determining accurate causes of death, 2) in processing insurance claims, and 3) in statistical studies of injuries and death.
• Indicate "Could not be determined" ONLY when it is impossible to determine the manner of death.

Common problems in death certification
The **elderly decedent** should have a clear and distinct etiological sequence for cause of death, if possible. Terms such as senescence, infirmity, old age, and advanced age have little value for public health or medical research. Age is recorded elsewhere on the certificate. When a number of conditions resulted in death, the physician should choose the single sequence that, in his or her opinion, best describes the process leading to death, and place any other pertinent conditions in Part II. If after careful consideration the physician cannot determine a sequence that ends in death, then the medical examiner or coroner should be consulted about conducting an investigation or providing assistance in completing the cause of death.

The **infant decedent** should have a clear and distinct etiological sequence for cause of death, if possible. "Prematurity" should not be entered without explaining the etiology of prematurity. Maternal conditions may have initiated or affected the sequence that resulted in infant death, and such maternal causes should be reported in addition to the infant causes on the infant's death certificate (e.g., Hyaline membrane disease **due to** prematurity, 28 weeks **due to** placental abruption **due to** blunt trauma to mother's abdomen).

When processes such as the following are reported, additional information about the etiology should be reported:

Abscess
Abdominal hemorrhage
Adhesions
Adult respiratory distress syndrome
Acute myocardial infarction
Altered mental status
Anemia
Anoxia
Anoxic encephalopathy
Arrhythmia
Ascites
Aspiration
Atrial fibrillation
Bacteremia
Bedridden
Biliary obstruction
Bowel obstruction
Brain injury
Brain stem herniation
Carcinogenesis
Carcinomatosis
Cardiac arrest
Cardiac dysrhythmia
Cardiomyopathy
Cardiopulmonary arrest
Cellulitis
Cerebral edema
Cerebrovascular accident
Cerebellar tonsillar herniation
Chronic bedridden state
Cirrhosis
Coagulopathy
Compression fracture
Congestive heart failure
Convulsions
Decubiti
Dehydration
Dementia (when not otherwise specified)
Diarrhea
Disseminated intravascular coagulopathy
Dysrhythmia
End-stage liver disease
End-stage renal disease
Epidural hematoma
Exsanguination
Failure to thrive
Fracture
Gangrene
Gastrointestinal hemorrhage
Heart failure
Hemothorax
Hepatic failure
Hepatitis
Hepatorenal syndrome
Hyperglycemia
Hyperkalemia
Hypovolemic shock
Hyponatremia
Hypotension
Immunosuppression
Increased intracranial pressure
Intracranial hemorrhage
Malnutrition
Metabolic encephalopathy
Multi-organ failure
Multi-system organ failure
Myocardial infarction
Necrotizing soft-tissue infection
Old age
Open (or closed) head injury
Pancytopenia
Paralysis
Perforated gallbladder
Peritonitis
Pleural effusions
Pneumonia
Pulmonary arrest
Pulmonary edema
Pulmonary embolism
Pulmonary insufficiency
Renal failure
Respiratory arrest
Seizures
Sepsis
Septic shock
Shock
Starvation
Subarachnoid hemorrhage
Subdural hematoma
Sudden death
Thrombocytopenia
Uncal herniation
Urinary tract infection
Ventricular fibrillation
Ventricular tachycardia
Volume depletion

If the certifier is unable to determine the etiology of a process such as those shown above, the process must be qualified as being of an unknown, undetermined, probable, presumed, or unspecified etiology so it is clear that a distinct etiology was not inadvertently or carelessly omitted.

The following conditions and types of death might seem to be specific or natural but when the medical history is examined further may be found to be complications of an injury or poisoning (possibly occurring long ago). Such cases should be reported to the medical examiner/coroner.

Asphyxia
Bolus
Choking
Drug or alcohol overdose/drug or alcohol abuse
Epidural hematoma
Exsanguination
Fall
Fracture
Hip fracture
Hyperthermia
Hypothermia
Open reduction of fracture
Pulmonary emboli
Seizure disorder
Sepsis
Subarachnoid hemorrhage
Subdural hematoma
Surgery
Thermal burns/chemical burns

REFERENCES
For more information on how to complete the medical certification section of the death certificate, refer to tutorial at **http://www.TheNAME.org** and resources including instructions and handbooks available by request from NCHS, Room 7318, 3311 Toledo Road, Hyattsville, Maryland 20782 or at **www.cdc.gov/nchs/about/major/dvs/handbk.htm.**

Issued: August 2004
04-0377 (8/04)

Source: Reprinted from CDC (2004).

Exhibit 4.3
Death Data for the United States, 2010

Number of deaths: 2,468,435
Death rate: 799.5 deaths per 100,000 population
Life expectancy: 78.7 years
Infant mortality rate: 6.15 deaths per 1,000 live births

Source: Murphy, Xu, and Kochanek (2013).

about such topics as screening for breast and colorectal cancer, tobacco and alcohol use, testing for HIV, heart disease, adolescent pregnancy, motor vehicle safety, foodborne disease, and hospital-associated infections (CDC 2016k). An example of a *Vital Signs* report is shown in exhibit 4.4.

Census Data

The mission of the US **Census Bureau** is "to serve as the leading source of quality data about the nation's people and economy." The organization's mission statement also emphasizes privacy and confidentiality, the sharing of the bureau's expertise globally, and transparency in conducting its work. The bureau is guided in pursuing this mission by its capable workforce, commitment to objective scientific methods, dedication to research-based innovation, and loyal commitment to its customers (US Census Bureau 2016a).

The following sections detail the types of information collected by the Census Bureau.

Census Bureau
A US government agency that provides data about the nation's people and economy. The bureau provides information through a decennial census of population and housing, an economic census, a census of governments, the American Community Survey, and economic indicators.

Decennial Census of Population and Housing

The decennial census of population and housing counts every resident in the United States. It occurs every ten years and is mandated by Article I, Section 2, of the US Constitution (US Census Bureau 2016a). The bureau explains, "The census tells us who we are and where we are going as a nation" (US Census Bureau 2016c). Communities use census data in deciding where to build roads, schools, hospitals, and other facilities. States use the data in redrawing congressional districts. Governments use the census to allot funds and support (US Census Bureau 2016c).

Economic Census

The Census Bureau also conducts an economic census every five years. The economic census gathers economic data and serves as the US government's official measure of American business and the economy (US Census Bureau 2016a).

Exhibit 4.4
Vital Signs Report on Pregnancy Among Younger Teens

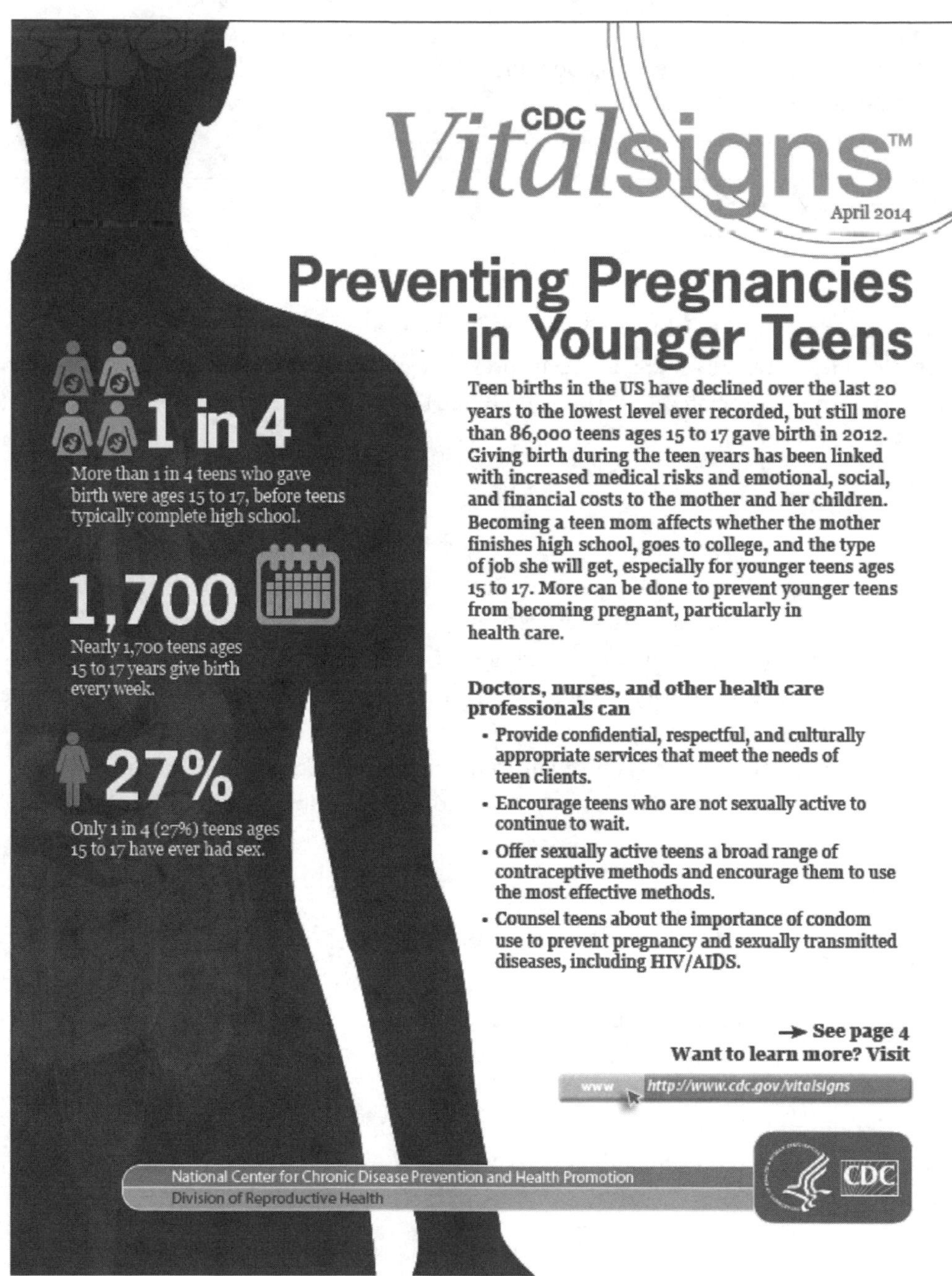
CDC Vitalsigns™
April 2014

Preventing Pregnancies in Younger Teens

Teen births in the US have declined over the last 20 years to the lowest level ever recorded, but still more than 86,000 teens ages 15 to 17 gave birth in 2012. Giving birth during the teen years has been linked with increased medical risks and emotional, social, and financial costs to the mother and her children. Becoming a teen mom affects whether the mother finishes high school, goes to college, and the type of job she will get, especially for younger teens ages 15 to 17. More can be done to prevent younger teens from becoming pregnant, particularly in health care.

1 in 4

More than 1 in 4 teens who gave birth were ages 15 to 17, before teens typically complete high school.

1,700

Nearly 1,700 teens ages 15 to 17 years give birth every week.

27%

Only 1 in 4 (27%) teens ages 15 to 17 have ever had sex.

Doctors, nurses, and other health care professionals can

- Provide confidential, respectful, and culturally appropriate services that meet the needs of teen clients.
- Encourage teens who are not sexually active to continue to wait.
- Offer sexually active teens a broad range of contraceptive methods and encourage them to use the most effective methods.
- Counsel teens about the importance of condom use to prevent pregnancy and sexually transmitted diseases, including HIV/AIDS.

→ See page 4

Want to learn more? Visit

www http://www.cdc.gov/vitalsigns

National Center for Chronic Disease Prevention and Health Promotion
Division of Reproductive Health

CDC

Source: Reprinted from CDC (2014b).

Census of Governments

Also every five years, the Census Bureau conducts a census of governments to examine state and local units of government. This census "identifies the scope and nature of the nation's state and local government sector; provides authoritative benchmark figures of public finance and public employment; classifies local government organizations, powers, and activities; and measures federal, state, and local fiscal relationships" (US Census Bureau 2016b).

American Community Survey

The American Community Survey (ACS) is an ongoing statistical survey that provides a variety of information—concerning jobs, education, veteran status, home ownership, and other areas—about the United States and its people. The survey samples a small percentage of the population every year, and its findings influence the distribution of billions of dollars of state and federal funds (US Census Bureau 2015). The ACS is the "premier source of information about America's changing population, housing, and workforce" (US Census Bureau 2016a).

Economic Indicator Reports

In addition to conducting its censuses and the ACS, the Census Bureau releases 14 reports on key economic indicators, each on a specific schedule (US Census Bureau 2016a).

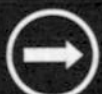

EXERCISE: USING THE AMERICAN COMMUNITY SURVEY

Use the American FactFinder website (http://factfinder.census.gov) to access the most recent ACS Five-Year Estimate for a state of your choosing. Investigate the following types of indicators:

- Predominant types of households
- Number of grandparents responsible for grandchildren under the age of 18
- Residence trends from one year ago
- Native population compared to foreign-born population entering the state
- School enrollment for high school, college, and graduate/professional programs

Repeat this exercise for two specific counties within the state you selected. How did the indicators differ between the county and state levels? What are the broader implications and questions raised for the county and the state?

Behavioral Risk Factor Surveillance System

The Behavioral Risk Factor Surveillance System (BRFSS) is a national system of health-related telephone surveys conducted under the oversight of the CDC. The surveys compile data at the state level about people's risk behaviors, health conditions, and use of preventive services (CDC 2016b). The BRFSS is especially important from a resource allocation standpoint, because individual states—each of which is unique and affected differently by the various social determinants of health—must understand the lifestyle practices and personal health behaviors contributing to premature morbidity and mortality. States have also used the BRFSS to address urgent and emerging health issues. In 2005, for instance, states on the US Gulf Coast used the BRFSS to assess the impact of Hurricane Katrina and Hurricane Rita (CDC 2014a).

The BRFSS was established in the early 1980s. Around that time, the relationships between personal health behaviors and chronic disease morbidity and mortality had become more widely recognized, and telephone surveys had emerged as a cheap and effective method for determining the prevalence of certain risk behaviors among populations. Telephone surveys were especially useful at the state and local levels, where the expertise and resources often were not available for in-person interviews (CDC 2014a).

The CDC (2014a) explains:

> Surveys were developed and conducted to monitor state-level prevalence of the major behavioral risks among adults associated with premature morbidity and mortality. The basic philosophy was to collect data on actual behaviors, rather than on attitudes or knowledge, that would be especially useful for planning, initiating, supporting, and evaluating health promotion and disease prevention programs.

When the BFSS was first established, 15 states participated in the monthly collection of data. The CDC developed a standard questionnaire that included such topics as alcohol use, diet, hypertension, physical inactivity, smoking, and use of seatbelts. Optional modules, which include additional sets of questions on specific topics, were made available in 1988. The BRFSS was expanded to a nationwide system in 1993, and the questionnaire was redesigned. The questionnaire now includes a mix of "fixed core" questions (asked every year) and "rotating core" questions (asked every other year), plus up to five "emerging core" questions on high-priority topics (CDC 2014a).

In 2008, the BRFSS piloted a cell phone survey, which enabled the system to reach population segments that had previously been inaccessible, thereby producing a more representative sample and higher-quality data (CDC 2014a). Aware that public health surveillance is likely to become more complex and multidimensional in the future, the BRFSS has launched a number of pilot studies and research initiatives to investigate additional approaches to interviewing and data collection.

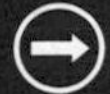

EXERCISE: USING BRFSS INTERACTIVE MAP DATA

Access the interactive map data at the BRFSS website (www.cdc.gov/brfss/gis/gis_maps.htm), and start by selecting the year 2002 and the category "Overweight and Obesity." Report the national status of this issue for 2002, and then repeat the process for the later years for which data are available. Note the trend over time, and discuss potential explanations.

Cancer Registries

A **cancer registry** is a central location, often in an academic setting or public health organization or hospital, that collects detailed information about the demographics of cancer patients and the treatments they receive. This information is extremely useful for research and healthcare management purposes.

cancer registry
A central location that collects information about cancer patients and the treatments they receive.

Cancer registry information can indicate, for instance, how the number of people with a specific cancer has increased or decreased since the previous year; whether people in a certain area of a state tend to find out they have breast cancer at a late stage, when the disease is harder to treat; and what groups of people are most likely to get a particular cancer. Groups such as state comprehensive cancer control coalitions can use this information to better understand cancer-related problems and figure out what steps should be taken. They may discover, for instance, that people lack sufficient cancer screening tests, that they are doing things that increase their cancer risk, or that conditions in their home or workplace are causing cancer. After the groups try to fix the problem, they can check new registry information to see if their solution is working (CDC 2015e).

HOW CANCER REGISTRIES WORK

Jennifer, a 55-year-old secretary, gets a routine mammogram, which shows she has a tumor about the size of a large pea in her left breast. Jennifer gets an operation at a hospital to remove the tumor, and afterward she gets chemotherapy treatments to make sure the cancer is all gone.

(continued)

Before the operation, Jennifer gave the hospital some information about herself, including her name, address, age, race and ethnicity, and health insurance company. Jennifer's doctors wrote down information about the tumor, like where it was located and how big it was, and what they did to treat it.

The hospital has its own cancer registry. A specially trained person called a *cancer registrar* looks at Jennifer's medical record and puts the information about her, her cancer, and her treatment into a computer using special codes. The cancer registrar also makes sure no important information is missing; if it is, he or she asks Jennifer's doctors or other hospital staff for the information. Once a year, the hospital registry sends this information to the central cancer registry in its state.

The state central cancer registry does its best to get information about every cancer case in the state. It reviews the information to make sure it's right and that no information is missing. Once a year, most state central cancer registries send information to CDC's National Program of Cancer Registries (NPCR), and some state and city cancer registries send information to the National Cancer Institute's Surveillance, Epidemiology, and End Results (SEER) program. The central cancer registries don't send any information that could identify a specific patient, like his or her name, street address, or Social Security number. The NPCR and SEER check the information again, and then the information is published every year in the *United States Cancer Statistics: Incidence and Mortality Web-Based Report* (USCS).

Source: Reprinted from CDC (2015f).

Cancer registry data have helped authorities discover, for instance, that women whose mothers took the drug *diethylstilbestrol* during pregnancy—mostly between 1947 and 1971—were increasingly likely to develop a rare type of reproductive cancer as they grew older (CDC 2013). Similarly, registry data showed that American Indians and Alaska natives, from 2001 to 2009, were more likely than non-Hispanic white people to develop certain types of cancers, including kidney, stomach, liver, and gallbladder (CDC 2016c).

The Surveillance, Epidemiology, and End Results (SEER) Program, a program of the National Cancer Institute, provides a wealth of information about cancer incidence and survival in the United States. Its registries collect data across such categories as patient demographics, tumor sites, courses of treatment, and follow-up for vital status, and they make that data available for researchers, clinicians, public health officials, policymakers, community groups, and the public (SEER 2016).

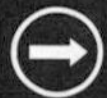

EXERCISE: ACCESSING CANCER REGISTRY STATISTICS

Access the US Cancer Statistics website (https://nccd.cdc.gov/uscs), go to the "Graphs" section of the page, and choose "Selected Cancers Ranked by State." Choose the earliest year of data presented (1999), select "All Cancer Sites Combined," and view the graph for males and females together. Report the ten top-ranked states, and then repeat this process for the most recent year of data available. Note the differences in the ranked states, and discuss possible reasons for the observations.

Geographic Information Systems

Geographic information systems (GIS) provide a powerful means for relating the incidence and prevalence of disease with place factors. The science and technology tools that make up GIS can help manage geographic relationships, integrate information, and identify trends over time, providing spatially referenced data to support informed decision making. The term *GIS* refers to both the hardware and software elements of the system of digital databases and layered maps (CDC 2016j; Mooney and Keesee 2014).

geographic information systems (GIS)
Science and technology tools that relate data to place factors, manage geographic relationships, and provide spatially referenced information to support decision making.

Exhibit 4.5 provides an example of a GIS map for heart disease death rates in the United States. The map displays heart disease death rates, for adults aged 35 or older, at the county level between the years 2011 and 2013. The shading indicates that counties with high heart disease death rates were largely concentrated in the southeastern part of the country, with lower rates to the west and north (CDC 2015b).

EXERCISE: ACCESSING GIS INFORMATION

Access the CDC's Interactive Atlas of Heart Disease and Stroke (http://nccd.cdc.gov/DHDSPAtlas), and complete the following steps:

Part A

1. Select a state or territory as your map area.
2. Use the data and filtering options to display all heart disease deaths for all races and genders, aged 35 or older, for the period of 2005–2007. Print the map.

(continued)

3. Repeat this process for each subsequent time period available (i.e., 2006–2008, 2007–2009, and so on).
4. Report on the trends in heart disease mortality over time.

Part B

1. For the same state or territory, use the interactive atlas to map three indicators of the social environment (e.g., poverty, unemployment rate, education less than high school). Print these maps and examine the indicators with respect to the maps you created for heart disease mortality. (Be sure to note the time period for the determinants of health.)
2. For your most recent heart disease mortality map from Part A, use the map overlay features to show the location of hospitals with cardiac intensive care; print the resultant map. Use the same process to locate short-term general hospitals with cardiac rehabilitation, and print that map as well.
3. Review your maps, let the data tell the story, and hypothesize what the indicators may be telling you about heart disease in your state or territory.

Exhibit 4.5
GIS Map of Heart Disease Death Rates

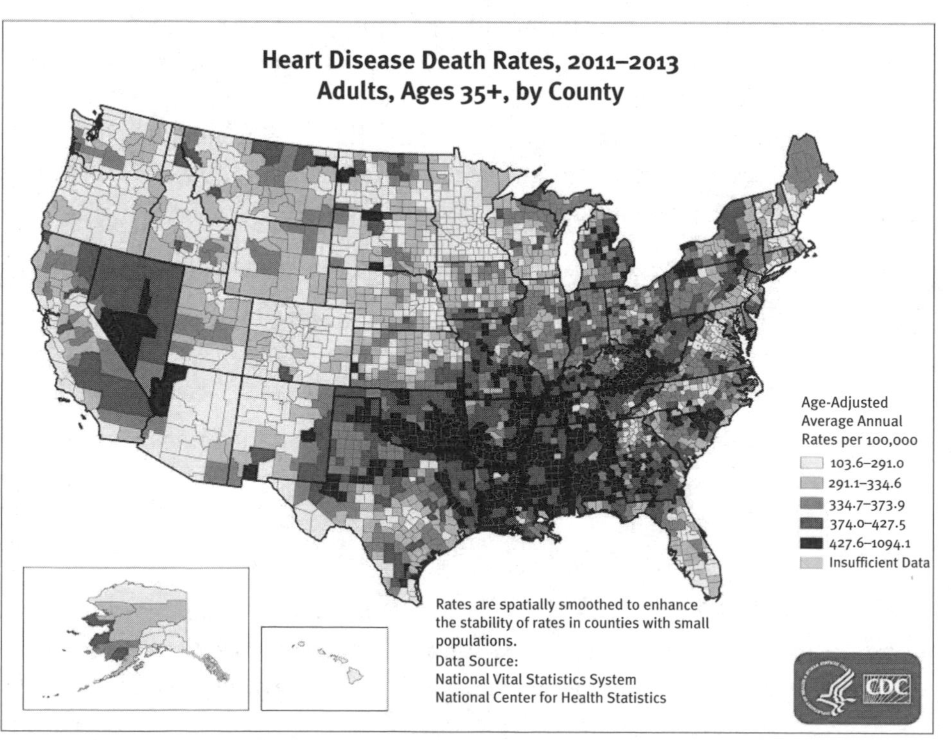

Source: Reprinted from CDC (2015b).

Syndromic Surveillance

Syndromic surveillance uses the signs and symptoms information collected by medical facilities upon the assessment of patients seeking care in an emergency room, ambulatory facility, or urgent care clinic. This information—which might include such measures as body temperature, presence of a rash, breathing rate, and pulse—is often reported to local health departments for trend analysis. Elevations in any of these measures might indicate exposure to an unusual agent. Syndromic surveillance was widely implemented following the anthrax attacks that occurred in the United States in 2001.

syndromic surveillance A form of surveillance that uses health and health-related data nearly in real time to provide information about the health of a community.

The Public Health Information Network (2015) summarizes syndromic surveillance efforts:

> Syndromic surveillance is a process that regularly and systematically uses health and health-related data in near "real-time" to make information available on the health of a community. This information includes statistics on disease trends and community health seeking behaviors that support essential public health surveillance functions in governmental public health authorities (PHAs). Syndromic surveillance is particularly useful to local, state, and federal PHAs for supporting public health situational awareness, emergency response management, and outbreak recognition and characterization. Patient encounter data from healthcare settings are a critical input for syndromic surveillance. Clinical data are provided by hospitals and urgent care centers to PHAs for all patient encounters (not a subset), and used by PHAs under authorities granted to them by applicable local and state laws.

Exercise: Considering Syndromic Surveillance

Describe a public health event that might warrant syndromic surveillance, and discuss how such surveillance would be conducted. Consider the following:

- Types of syndromes
- Sources of data
- Method by which the data would be received
- How the information should be analyzed
- Stakeholders to be informed
- Intervention
- Evaluation

Workplace Assessment and Surveillance

Much useful data can be obtained through the surveillance of workers and assessment of workplace health. Information about people's absences from work—both numbers and reasons—can be helpful in identifying emerging health issues (in effect, serving as an early warning system), developing appropriate interventions, and evaluating the effectiveness of those interventions (CDC 2015i). The CDC (2015i) states: "A successful intervention that improves employee health should also result in higher productivity and reduced number of work days missed, which will ultimately reduce organizational costs."

When examining employee time and attendance data, the number of sick days or sick hours and the reasons for absence should be carefully noted. How detailed is the reason for absence? Do the data distinguish between an employee who is sick and an employee who took sick time to care for an ill child? The tracking of absenteeism over time can reveal trends or changes in absenteeism rates—for instance, greater numbers of absences during cold and influenza season. Such information can be useful in planning policy changes or interventions such as flu shots (CDC 2015i).

Over-the-Counter Surveillance

over-the-counter (OTC) surveillance
A surveillance process driven by analysis of a community's over-the-counter medication purchases.

Another emerging source of data is **over-the-counter (OTC) surveillance**, which uses purchase analysis. Prior to seeking medical attention for an illness, people often will self-medicate by purchasing medications over the counter (McIsaac, Levine, and Goel 1998; Metzger et al. 2004; Vingilis, Brown, and Hennen 1999). Thus, OTC medication purchases can serve as an early indicator of community-wide illness.

For example, in Milwaukee in 1993, reports that local pharmacies had sold out of antidiarrheal medications offered one of the first signs of a large waterborne cryptosporidiosis outbreak in the area (MacKenzie et al. 1994; Morris, Naumova, and Griffiths 1998). Noting increases in sales of such medications as Immodium, Pepto Bismol, and Kaopectate, researchers suggested that prospective monitoring of OTC medication sales could have led to earlier detection of the outbreak (Morris, Naumova, and Griffiths 1998).

A study by Das and colleagues (2005) analyzed an OTC surveillance effort in New York City that tracked sales of medicines for influenza-like illness. Comparing the OTC sales trends with trends in emergency department (ED) visits for fever/influenza syndromes, the authors found that OTC surveillance can provide indications of community-wide illness but is likely to be less sensitive than the tracking of ED trends. These findings are illustrated in exhibit 4.6, which tracks OTC and ED measures through peak influenza seasons from 2002 to 2005.

Exhibit 4.6
Over-the-Counter Surveillance in New York City

Citywide trends and signals in over-the-counter (OTC) influenza-like illness category and emergency department (ED) fever/influenza category—New York City, August 1, 2002–March 31, 2005*

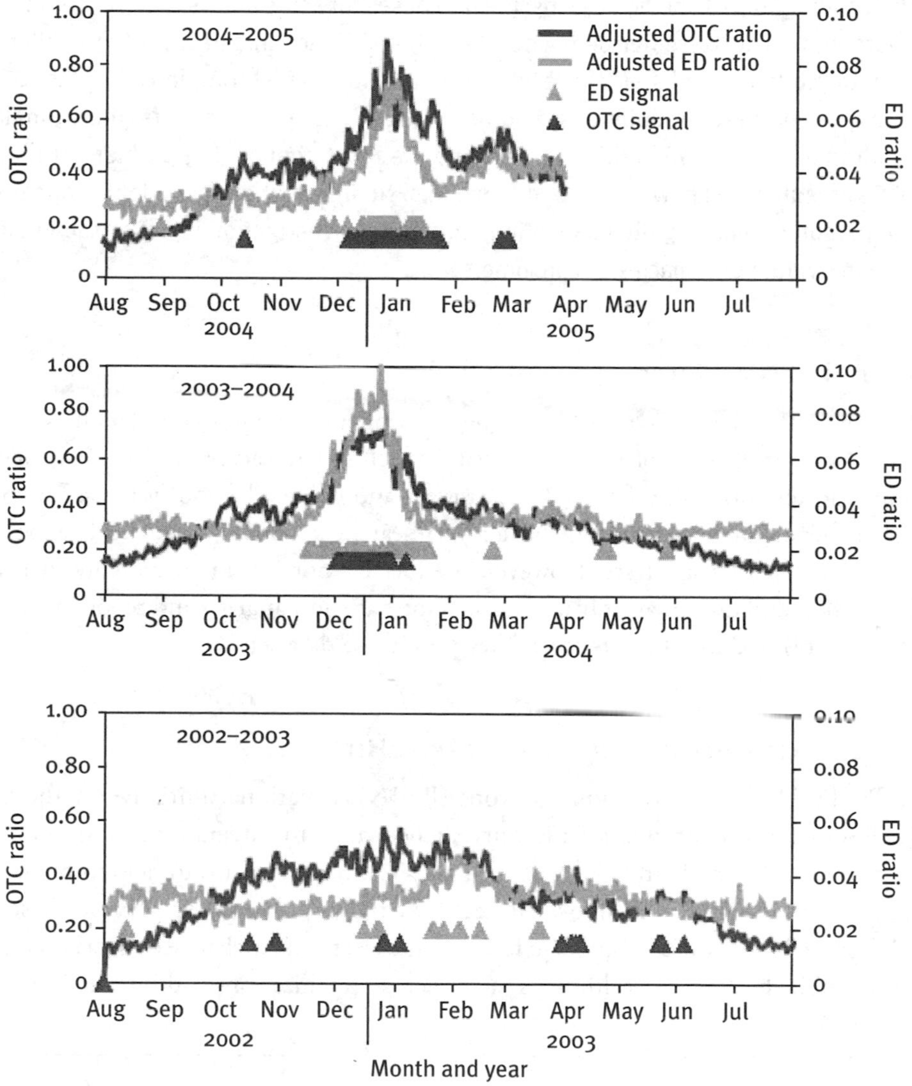

* The OTC ratio is adjusted for day of week and major national winter holidays and the day after these holidays (Thanksgiving, Christmas, New Years, and Martin Luther King observance day). The emergency department ratio is adjusted for day of week.

Source: Reprinted from Das et al. (2005).

Das and colleagues (2005) explain the limitations of OTC surveillance in this case:

> Multiple factors might contribute toward the challenges of OTC syndromic surveillance. The high rate of background sales unrelated to illness, which might include consumer "stockpiling" of OTC medicines, obscure purchases for acute illness. Differences in store hours and local consumer behavior add to the variance in sales, posing challenges to data modeling and spatial analysis to detect local clustering in OTC sales. Drugs comprise multiple formulations, and new drugs enter the market regularly, making syndrome categorization difficult. Perhaps the most challenging problem of routine OTC surveillance is how to respond to signals. No information is available concerning the person purchasing the medication, and direct investigation is not possible either with individual pharmacies or consumers.

Public-Use Data Files

Additional information is available through downloadable public-use data files from the CDC's National Center for Health Statistics, which provide access to data sets, documentation, and questionnaires from NCHS surveys and data collection systems. The public-use data files are prepared in a way that allows researchers to manipulate the data in formats appropriate for their analyses. However, the files do not include personally identifiable information, and users may only use the data for statistical analysis and reporting purposes (CDC 2016i). Exhibit 4.7 lists several key public-use data sets.

Public Health Information Network (PHIN)

The Public Health Information Network (PHIN), a national initiative of the CDC's Division of Health Informatics and Surveillance, aims to integrate the vast amounts of information collected by the public health and healthcare systems to help improve health management and advance the overall health of the population. To achieve these goals, PHIN provides tools and resources to facilitate the electronic exchange of data and information by public health and healthcare systems across organizations and jurisdictions. Secure

Exhibit 4.7
A Sampling of Public-Use Data Sets

National Health and Nutrition Examination Survey (www.cdc.gov/nchs/nhanes.htm)
National Health Care Surveys (www.cdc.gov/nchs/dhcs.htm)
National Health Interview Survey (www.cdc.gov/nchs/nhis.htm)
National Immunization Survey (www.cdc.gov/vaccines/imz-managers/coverage/nis/child)
National Survey of Family Growth (www.cdc.gov/nchs/nsfg.htm)
National Vital Statistics System (www.cdc.gov/nchs/nvss.htm)

data exchange practices must be established, for instance, so that data can be moved from clinical care organization to public health agency, from public health agency to public health agency, and from public health agency to other federal agencies. Thus, PHIN works to define functional and technical requirements for public health information exchange and to establish secure practices, standards, and policies for data exchange (CDC 2015g).

CDC WONDER

Another useful resource is CDC WONDER (Wide-Ranging Online Data for Epidemiologic Research), which provides convenient, menu-driven access for public health professionals and the general public to public health information generated by the CDC. The information provided in this database is intended to assist in decision making, research initiatives, program evaluation, and setting priorities related to health issues (CDC 2016f).

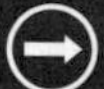

EXERCISE: USING CDC WONDER

Access the CDC WONDER website (http://wonder.cdc.gov), and complete the following steps:

1. Select the database titled "AIDS Public Use Data."
2. Follow the link to the National Center for HIV/AIDS, Viral Hepatitis, STD, and TB Prevention (NCHHSTP) Atlas, and view the map by state. You should see HIV diagnoses for adults and adolescents of all races/ethnicities and both sexes for the most recent year. What do you notice about this national map?
3. Next, adjust the query to show "Change over time" for HIV diagnoses for all races, ages, genders, and transmission types. Do the results change significantly? Describe the bar chart.
4. Select a specific state by double-clicking on the state on the map. Describe how HIV diagnoses for your selected state compare with those for the nation.
5. On the national map, adjust the settings so that counties are displayed. Now use the map to focus on Hillsborough County, New Hampshire. What is the population of Hillsborough County? What is the number of HIV cases? What is the rate of HIV diagnosis?
6. Now select Coos County, New Hampshire. What is the population of Coos County? What are the number of HIV cases and the rate of HIV diagnosis? Explain why the data are suppressed for Coos County.

CDC FastStats

CDC FastStats is a website that provides links to publications, statistics, and additional data sources for certain public health and health-related issues (CDC 2016e). Exhibit 4.8 provides an example of the FastStats data provided for asthma in the United States. In addition, the CDC provides lists of data and statistics by topic, tools and resources, and related organization information at www.cdc.gov/datastatistics.

Exhibit 4.8
CDC FastStats Data for Asthma

Morbidity: Adults (Aged 18 Years or Older)

- Number of adults who currently have asthma: 17.7 million
- Percent of adults who currently have asthma: 7.4%

[from "Summary Health Statistics for US Adults: National Health Interview Survey," 2014, table A-2]

Morbidity: Children (Under Age 18 Years)

- Number of children who currently have asthma: 6.3 million
- Percent of children who currently have asthma: 8.6%

[from "Summary Health Statistics for US Children: National Health Interview Survey, 2014," table C-1]

Physician Office Visits

- Number of visits to physician offices with asthma as primary diagnosis: 10.5 million

[from "National Ambulatory Medical Care Survey: 2012 Summary Tables," table 13]

Emergency Department Visits

- Number of visits to emergency departments with asthma as primary diagnosis: 1.8 million

[from "National Hospital Ambulatory Medical Care Survey: 2011 Emergency Department Summary Tables," table 12]

Mortality

- Number of deaths: 3,630
- Deaths per 100,000 population: 1.1

[from "Deaths: Final Data for 2013," tables 10, 11.]

Source: Adapted from CDC (2016d).

County Health Rankings & Roadmaps

The County Health Rankings & Roadmaps program, developed by the University of Wisconsin Population Health Institute and the Robert Wood Johnson Foundation, aims to build awareness of issues that affect health, provide reliable health data to communities, engage local leaders to implement change, and empower community leaders working to improve health (County Health Rankings & Roadmaps 2016a). The program describes its annual Rankings and Roadmaps components as follows:

> The annual County Health Rankings measure vital health factors, including high school graduation rates, obesity, smoking, unemployment, access to healthy foods, the quality of air and water, income, and teen births in nearly every county in America. The annual Rankings provide a revealing snapshot of how health is influenced by where we live, learn, work, and play. They provide a starting point for change in communities. That is why we also provide the Roadmaps that provide guidance and tools to understand the data and strategies that communities can use to move from education to action. The Roadmaps are helping communities bring people together from all walks of life to look at the many factors that influence health, focus on strategies that we know work, learn from each other, and make changes that will have a lasting impact on health. (County Health Rankings & Roadmaps 2016a)

The County Health Rankings are based on a population health model that emphasizes **health factors**—that is, factors that can potentially be improved to make communities healthier (County Health Rankings & Roadmaps 2016i). The factors are spread across four categories—clinical care, health behaviors, physical environment, and social and economic—and are outlined in exhibit 4.9 (County Health Rankings & Roadmaps 2016g).

health factors
Behaviors and conditions that influence health.

Exhibit 4.9
Health Factors Measured in County Health Rankings

Clinical Care	Health Behaviors	Physical Environment	Social and Economic
Access to care	Alcohol and drug use	Air and water quality	Community safety
Quality of care	Diet and exercise	Housing and transit	Education
	Sexual activity		Employment
	Tobacco use		Family and social support
			Income

Source: Adapted from County Health Rankings & Roadmaps (2016g).

health outcomes
Indicators of how healthy a community is.

The County Health Rankings (2016h) use two types of **health outcomes** to determine how healthy a county is. The first is length of life (mortality), which is measured by premature deaths (i.e., deaths before the age of 75). The second type of health outcome is quality of life (morbidity), which includes measures of people's physical and mental health, as well as birth outcomes (e.g., babies born with a low birth weight).

The County Health Rankings program advises that policies and programs can take different approaches to population health. Some might target health outcomes directly, whereas others might tackle the factors that contribute to those outcomes (County Health Rankings & Roadmaps 2016j). The program has identified a series steps—strongly emphasizing collaboration and communication—necessary to improve community health:

1. *Assess needs and resources.* "One of the first steps in local health improvement is to take stock of your community's needs, resources, strengths, and assets. You will want to understand what helps as well as what hinders progress toward improving your community's health" (County Health Rankings & Roadmaps 2016c). This step involves asking a number of questions: What data will help us understand the community? Where can we find such data? What do the data mean?
2. *Focus on what is important.* "Once you've accounted for your community's needs and resources, it's time to decide which problem(s) to tackle. . . . Taking time to set priorities will ensure that you direct your community's valuable and limited resources to the most important issues" (County Health Rankings & Roadmaps 2016f). This step involves asking, How many priorities are reasonable, and how can we narrow our focus?
3. *Choose effective policies and programs.* "Taking time to choose policies and programs that have been shown to work in real life and that are a good fit for your community will maximize your chances of success" (County Health Rankings & Roadmaps 2016d). Questions to consider at this step include how we can know if a strategy will work and how we should weigh innovative approaches relative to strategies backed by evidence.
4. *Act on what is important.* "Once you've decided what you want to do, the next step is to make it happen. Since there are no 'one size fits all' blueprints for success, communities build on inherent strengths, capitalize on available resources, and respond to unique needs" (County Health Rankings & Roadmaps 2016b). At this step, we have to consider how to move from planning to action and how to support our strategies.
5. *Evaluate actions.* "Evaluating your efforts is an important step in the process of improving your community's health. Evaluation helps you know if what

you're doing is working the way you intended and achieving the results you desire" (County Health Rankings & Roadmaps 2016e). This step involves asking where we might start with evaluation and how we can know if we are making a difference.

EXERCISE: COUNTY HEALTH RANKINGS & ROADMAPS IN PRACTICE

Access the County Health Rankings & Roadmaps website (www.countyhealthrankings.org), and complete the following steps:

Part A

1. Access the Rankings information for a state of your choosing.
2. View the state maps for health outcomes and health factors for the most recent year available, and compare the two. Which counties rank first and last?
3. Use the "Compare Counties" feature to examine the first- and last-ranked counties. Describe how the counties compare to the state as a whole for each health factor and health outcome.
4. View the state map for the clinical care health factor "Uninsured." Describe this indicator, identify the source of the data, and compare the rates in both counties.
5. Go the Action Center (www.countyhealthrankings.org/roadmaps/action-center), explore the sections dealing with public health and healthcare stakeholders, and review the key activities listed for these groups. Select three activities that you think could help improve the identified indicator (the uninsured) for the two counties. Explain your rationale, and describe how you think other stakeholders should be involved in addressing this issue.

Part B

1. Within the Roadmaps section of the website, access the Projects Showcase, and select one of the projects.
2. For your project, determine the health factors addressed, the desired health outcome, and the strategy implemented.
3. Discuss the challenges that needed to be overcome.
4. Describe the evaluation process and the resultant outcome.

Healthcare Data

For a complete assessment of the health of a population, public health data should be augmented by up-to-date information about the healthcare people receive. The US Department of Health and Human Services (HHS) makes much healthcare information available to the public via www.HealthData.gov. The site aims to make high-value data available to entrepreneurs, researchers, and policy makers in hopes of promoting better health outcomes for all (HealthData.gov 2016). The site includes data from such agencies as the Centers for Medicare & Medicaid Services (CMS), the Health Services and Resources Administration, the Agency for Healthcare Research and Quality, the National Cancer Institute, and the National Institutes of Health. For the data sets provided, the site indicates the agency responsible for the data, the type and date of the data, access level, and the geographic level for which the data are provided (e.g., county, state).

Healthcare data include both data from hospitals and data from other sources, such as government programs and insurance providers.

Hospital Data

Large amounts of hospital data are available through the American Hospital Association (AHA). The AHA provides a directory of hospitals in the United States, statistics regarding healthcare industry trends in community hospitals, hospital-specific data, and survey results for care systems and payments (AHA 2016). Other sources of hospital information include Medicare data, the *Dartmouth Atlas of Health Care*, discharge data, claims data, and the National Center for Veterans Analysis and Statistics.

Medicare Data

The CMS website www.Data.Medicare.gov provides data across a number of categories, and it incorporates information from a series of "Compare" data sets (Data.Medicare.gov 2016):

- Hospital Compare enables users to compare information about the quality of care received at Medicare-certified hospitals across the United States.
- Nursing Home Compare enables the comparison of quality-of-care information for every Medicare- and Medicaid-certified nursing home in the country.
- Home Health Compare provides information about the quality of care provided by Medicare-certified home health agencies.
- Dialysis Facility Compare presents information about the services and quality of care provided by Medicare-certified dialysis facilities.

The *Dartmouth Atlas* Project

Since 1996, the *Dartmouth Atlas of Health Care*, based at the Dartmouth Institute for Health Policy and Clinical Practice, has been a source of information about the US healthcare system and a useful tool for healthcare leaders, policymakers, the media, and others. The *Dartmouth Atlas* project "uses Medicare data to provide information and analysis about national, regional, and local markets, as well as hospitals and their affiliated physicians" (*Dartmouth Atlas* 2016). In doing so, the project has documented glaring variations in how medical resources are distributed and used, and it has contributed greatly to ongoing efforts to improve health and health systems across the United States.

EXERCISE: USING THE *DARTMOUTH ATLAS*

Access the *Dartmouth Atlas of Health Care* website (www.dartmouthatlas.org), and complete the following steps:

1. Navigate to the "Data by Hospital" section, and select a state.
2. Choose a representative hospital in an urban area of the state, and note the information provided.
3. Now choose a hospital in a rural area of the same state.
4. Compare the findings between the two hospitals, and discuss possible reasons for any differences.
5. In the "Key Issues" section of the site, read the "Reflections on Variations." Propose any additional explanations you might have for the variations in healthcare.

Hospital Discharge Data

Hospital discharge data, which describe the characteristics of inpatients who have been discharged from hospitals, can help with the study of important public health topics and assist with the development of policies and interventions. Much of this data had been made available through the National Hospital Discharge Survey (NHDS), which was conducted annually from 1965 to 2010. Today, the National Hospital Care Survey (NHCS) gathers inpatient information previously collected by the NHDS and integrates it with emergency department (ED), outpatient department (OPD), and ambulatory surgery center (ASC) data from the National Hospital Ambulatory Medical Care Survey. The CDC

(2015d) states: "The integration of these two surveys, along with the collection of personal identifiers (protected health information), will allow the linking of care provided to the same patient in the ED, OPD, ASC, and inpatient departments. It will also be possible to link the survey data to the National Death Index and Medicaid and Medicare data to obtain a more complete picture of patient care." The example in exhibit 4.10 demonstrates the utility of hospital discharge data.

Claims Data

Health claims data at the individual level, obtained through health plan providers, provide a valuable tool for assessing healthcare expenditures. Specifically, the CDC (2015h) recommends collecting the following information for each enrollee:

- Age
- Sex
- Employment status (employee, spouse, dependent, or retiree)
- Total healthcare costs
- Diagnosis codes (first or second code)
- Procedure codes (for preventive services use)
- Place of service

Exhibit 4.10 Hospitalization for Total Hip Replacement Among Inpatients Aged 45 and Over: United States, 2000–2010

Key findings from the National Hospital Discharge Survey:

- In 2010, 310,800 total hip replacements were performed among inpatients aged 45 or older.
- The number of total hip replacements among inpatients aged 45 or older increased from 138,700 to 310,800 between 2000 and 2010; during those same years, the rate, per 100,000 population, increased from 142.2 to 257.0.
- The age distribution of inpatients aged 45 or older who received total hip replacements changed significantly between 2000 and 2010; the percentage of total hip replacements increased for younger age groups and decreased for older age groups.
- The average length of stay after total hip replacement among inpatients aged 45 or older decreased from nearly 5 days in 2000 to just under 4 days in 2010.

Source: Adapted from Wolford, Palso, and Bercovitz (2015).

The CDC (2015a) further recommends calculating the following statistics (e.g., by employment status, by sex, by age) to help identify major contributors to healthcare expenditures:

1. Total healthcare costs (both percent of total costs and average cost per enrollee)
2. Percent of insured individuals receiving the following preventive services:
   - General exams
   - Physical exams
   - Diabetes screening
   - Influenza immunization
   - Pneumococcal immunization
   - General obstetrics/gynecology visit (females)
   - Breast cancer screening (females)
   - Cervical cancer screening (females)
   - Colon cancer screening

Claims data can be useful for the development of workplace wellness programs. The assessment of healthcare costs by individual demographic characteristics (e.g., age, sex) and by organizational demographic characteristics (e.g., division, work site) can help "identify target populations or worksites for which workplace health and safety programs should be developed to improve workplace conditions and the health and well-being of the workforce" (CDC 2015c).

National Center for Veterans Analysis and Statistics

The National Center for Veterans Analysis and Statistics (NCVAS) reports on the veteran population, the allocation of resources to help veterans, and the services veterans are using. The NCVAS (2016) develops statistical analyses and reports, develops estimates and projections related to the veteran population, operates a web portal to disseminate information, and leads data-sharing collaborations with other federal agencies.

Other Healthcare Data

Additional information related to healthcare comes from a variety of sources. The Social Security Administration (2016) collects large amounts of data about people's addresses, employers, wages, identifying information, and more. The Bureau of Labor Statistics (BLS), part of the US Department of Labor, is the main federal agency responsible for measuring labor market activity, working conditions, and price changes in the economy. Its mission is "to collect, analyze, and disseminate essential economic information to support public and private decision making" (BLS 2016). The Occupational Safety and Health Administration (OSHA), also part of the Department of Labor, makes data available as part of its mission "to assure safe and healthful working conditions for working men and women by setting and enforcing standards and by providing training, outreach, education, and assistance" (OSHA 2016). In addition, the US Census Bureau (2016d) keeps track of insurance coverage and purchases in the United States.

The Henry J. Kaiser Family Foundation (KFF) is a nonprofit organization that focuses on national health issues in the United States and on the US role in global health policy. The KFF operates policy analysis, journalism, and communications programs, including a news service called Kaiser Health News. Its information—which ranges from basic facts and figures to in-depth policy coverage—is available free of charge. The organization aims to "serve as a nonpartisan source of facts, analysis, and journalism for policymakers, the media, the health policy community, and the public" (KFF 2016).

The Trust for America's Health (TFAH) is a nonprofit and nonpartisan organization dedicated to "protecting the health of every community and working to make disease prevention a national priority" (TFAH 2016). The organization makes data available with the aim of helping to build a "public health defense that is strong enough to cover us from all points of attack—whether the threats are from a bioterrorist or Mother Nature" (TFAH 2016).

Health Insurance Portability and Accountability Act (HIPAA)
A US law that provides standards for the exchange, privacy, and security of health information. The HIPAA Privacy Rule protects "individually identifiable health information." The HIPAA Security Rule provides safeguards for electronic protected health information.

Health Information Privacy

In discussing the vast amounts of public health and healthcare data available, we must also note the ways that data sets containing personal identifying information are protected. In many cases, useful health-related information—for instance, information from physician medical records, community health centers, and local health departments—has been collected but is difficult to obtain for research purposes because of confidentiality concerns. This section highlights the aims of the Health Insurance Portability and Accountability Act and the role of institutional review boards.

The Health Insurance Portability and Accountability Act

Originally enacted in 1996, the **Health Insurance Portability and Accountability Act (HIPAA)** required the secretary of health and human services to publicize standards for the electronic exchange, privacy, and security of health information. The HIPAA Privacy

Rule, published in 2000, established a set of national standards for the protection of certain health information. Organizations that must comply with HIPAA's privacy standards are called "covered entities," and they include health plans, healthcare clearinghouses, and providers that conduct certain financial and administrative transactions electronically (HHS 2002).

The Privacy Rule protects "individually identifiable health information" that is transmitted in any manner, whether electronically, orally, or on paper. Such information is defined as follows:

> Information, including demographic data, that relates to:
>
> - the individual's past, present, or future physical or mental health or condition,
> - the provision of health care to the individual, or
> - the past, present, or future payment for the provision of health care to the individual,
>
> and that identifies the individual or for which there is a reasonable basis to believe it can be used to identify the individual. Individually identifiable health information includes many common identifiers (e.g., name, address, birth date, Social Security Number). (HHS 2016a)

The Privacy Rule provides federal protections for individually identifiable health information, and it recognizes patients' rights with respect to that information. However, the rule is also balanced so that it permits the disclosure of health information necessary for patient care, public health, and other important purposes (HHS 2016a). Another HIPAA rule, the Security Rule, provides a collection of administrative, physical, and technical safeguards for covered entities and their business associates to use to ensure the availability, confidentiality, and integrity of electronic protected health information (HHS 2016b).

Often, during public health emergencies, the authorities and personnel responsible for the public's safety will need access to protected health information in order to secure the safety and health of the population. The HIPAA Privacy Rule accommodates such situations by allowing involved entities to disclose the necessary protected information to legally authorized public health and safety professionals without authorization (HHS 2003). The HHS (2003) defines a *public health authority* as an agency or authority of the US government, a state, a territory, a political subdivision of a state or territory, or an Indian tribe that has responsibility for public health matters as part of its official mandate. The definition also applies to people or entities acting under a grant of authority from, or under a contract with, such an agency. Examples of public health authorities include state and local health departments, the CDC, the Food and Drug Administration (FDA), and OSHA. In such emergencies, covered entities are generally required to limit the disclosure of protected health information to the minimum amount necessary to accomplish the public health purpose. However, "covered entities are not required to make a minimum necessary determination for public health disclosures that are made pursuant to an individual's authorization, or for disclosures that are required by other law" (HHS 2003).

Additional public health areas for which the Privacy Rule permits disclosure of protected health information, without authorization, include the following (HHS 2003):

- Child abuse or neglect
- Quality, safety, or effectiveness of products or activities regulated by the FDA
- People at risk of contracting or spreading a disease
- Workplace medical surveillance

Institutional Review Boards

Any research (e.g., clinical investigations) involving human subjects that is conducted or sponsored by the CDC must be approved by an institutional review board (IRB) prior to its beginning. The research must comply with the US Department of Health and Human Services' Policy for Protection of Human Research Subjects (CDC 2016g). The IRBs help ensure that subjects' personal health information is handled responsibly.

Key Chapter Points

- Public health and healthcare data can assist with program development and evaluation, community planning, early event detection, research for evidence-based practice, and a variety of other purposes.
- Epidemiologists use public health data to conduct the core functions of public health—assessment, policy development, and assurance—and to assist with the development of interventions to fulfill the public health mission.
- Vital statistics provide systematically tabulated information about such events as births, marriages, separations, divorces, and deaths.
- Federal law in the United States mandates the national collection and publication of births and other vital statistics data. The federal National Vital Statistics System is the result of cooperation between the National Center for Health Statistics and the individual states to provide access to statistical information from birth certificates.

- Data pertaining to cause of death are classified and coded according to the International Classification of Diseases system, which is revised about every ten years. Regular revision helps the national mortality system stay abreast of advances in medical science and changes in terminology.
- The Census Bureau's mission is "to serve as the leading source of quality data about the nation's people and economy" (US Census Bureau 2016a). The bureau provides information through a decennial census of population and housing, an economic census, a census of governments, the American Community Survey, and economic indicators.
- The Behavioral Risk Factor Surveillance System is a national system of health-related telephone surveys conducted under the oversight of the Centers for Disease Control and Prevention. The surveys compile data at the state level about people's risk behaviors, health conditions, and use of preventive services.
- Cancer registries collect and store detailed information about cancer patients and the treatments they receive. The registries are useful, for instance, in determining how rates for certain cancers have changed over time or vary by location.
- Geographic information systems, or GIS, relate the incidence and prevalence of disease with place factors. GIS can help manage geographic relationships, integrate information, and identify trends over time, providing spatially referenced data to support informed decision making. The term *GIS* comprises both hardware and software elements.
- Syndromic surveillance uses the signs and symptoms information collected by medical facilities upon the assessment of patients seeking care in an emergency room, ambulatory facility, or urgent care clinic. This information can be reported to local health departments for trend analysis.
- Surveillance of workers and assessment of workplace health can help with identifying emerging diseases and developing effective interventions.
- Because people often use over-the-counter medications before or instead of seeking medical care, OTC medication sales may serve as an early indicator of community-wide illness.
- The National Center for Health Statistics offers downloadable public-use data files, which provide access to data sets, documentation, and survey questionnaires.
- The CDC's Public Health Information Network aims to integrate the vast amounts of information collected by the public health and healthcare systems to help improve health management and advance the overall health of the population.
- Additional CDC resources include CDC WONDER (Wide-Ranging Online Data for Epidemiologic Research), which provides menu-driven access to public health

information, and the FastStats website, which provides quick access to statistics of importance to public health.

- The County Health Rankings & Roadmaps program aims to build awareness of issues that affect health, provide reliable health data to communities, and help community leaders make improvements in health. The annual County Health Rankings measure such factors as education, obesity, smoking, unemployment, air and water quality, income, and teen births in nearly every county in the United States. The Roadmaps provide guidance, tools, and strategies for action.
- Health factors, as identified in the County Health Rankings, represent the behaviors and conditions that influence health. Health outcomes represent how long people live and how healthy they feel while alive.
- The US Department of Health and Human Services makes much healthcare information available to the public via www.HealthData.gov. The site includes data from such agencies as the Centers for Medicare & Medicaid Services, the Agency for Healthcare Research and Quality, and the National Institutes of Health.
- The American Hospital Association provides a directory of hospitals in the United States, statistics regarding healthcare industry trends in community hospitals, hospital-specific data, and survey results for care systems and payments.
- The CMS website www.Data.Medicare.gov provides data across a number of categories. The "Compare" data sets enable comparisons between hospitals, nursing homes, home health agencies, and dialysis facilities.
- The *Dartmouth Atlas of Health Care* uses Medicare data to provide information and analysis for healthcare leaders, policymakers, the media, and others.
- Hospital discharge data describe the characteristics of inpatients who have been discharged from hospitals. Information of this type has been made available through the National Hospital Discharge Survey and, more recently, the National Hospital Care Survey.
- Health claims data at the individual level, obtained through health plan providers, provide a valuable tool for assessing healthcare expenditures.
- The National Center for Veterans Analysis and Statistics reports on the veteran population, the allocation of resources to help veterans, and the services veterans are using.
- Health data that would be useful for a given issue may be difficult to obtain for research purposes because of confidentiality concerns.
- The Health Insurance Portability and Accountability Act aims to protect patients' medical records and other health information provided to health plans, doctors, hospitals, and other providers. The HIPAA Privacy Rule provides federal protections for "individually identifiable health information." The HIPAA Security Rule provides administrative, physical, and technical safeguards to

ensure the availability, confidentiality, and integrity of electronic protected health information.

- The HIPAA Privacy Rule aims to protect information but also permits the disclosure of health information necessary for patient care, public health, and other important purposes.

Discussion Questions

1. Describe the significance of evidence-based public health.
2. What are the strengths and limitations of using birth and death data for public health purposes?
3. Identify a strength and a limitation of the Behavioral Risk Factor Surveillance System.
4. Describe two examples of useful data collected via surveillance methods.
5. Name three examples of healthcare data sets. What are the strengths and limitations of those data sets?
6. What is the purpose of public-use data?
7. Discuss the significance of HIPAA, the HIPAA Privacy Rule, and the HIPAA Security Rule.
8. Give an example of exceptions to the HIPAA protections.
9. Access the Behavioral Risk Factor Surveillance System data for your state, and discuss how healthcare access varies by age, gender, and race.
10. Access the County Health Rankings data for your state, and select two neighboring counties. Compare the health outcomes, and hypothesize as to what might account for any differences.

References

American Hospital Association (AHA). 2016. "AHA Data and Directories." Accessed September 19. www.aha.org/research/rc/stat-studies/data-and-directories.shtml.

Bureau of Labor Statistics (BLS). 2016. "About BLS." Updated April 18. www.bls.gov/bls/infohome.htm.

Centers for Disease Control and Prevention (CDC). 2016a. "About the National Vital Statistics System." Updated January 4. www.cdc.gov/nchs/nvss/about_nvss.htm.

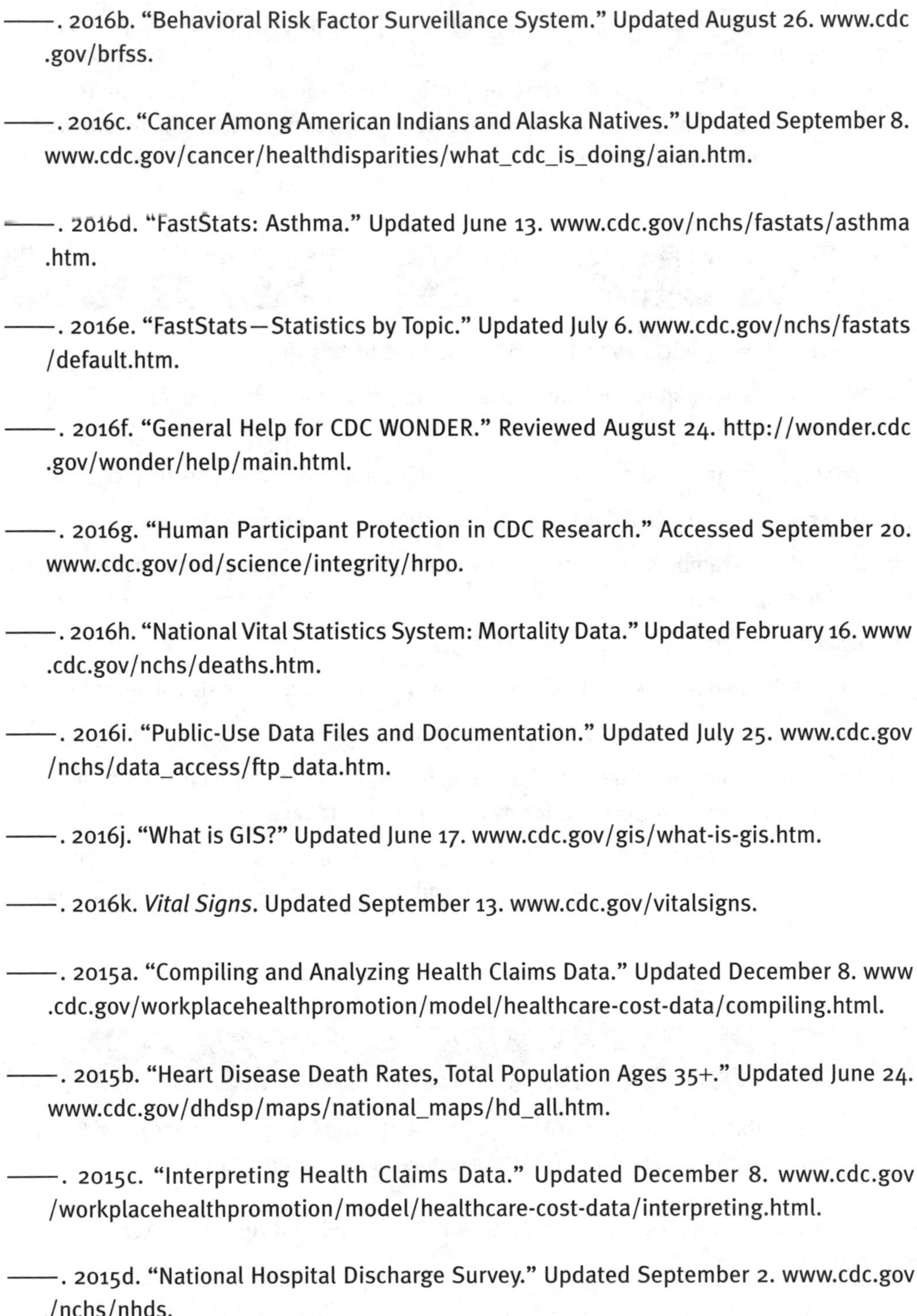

———. 2016b. "Behavioral Risk Factor Surveillance System." Updated August 26. www.cdc.gov/brfss.

———. 2016c. "Cancer Among American Indians and Alaska Natives." Updated September 8. www.cdc.gov/cancer/healthdisparities/what_cdc_is_doing/aian.htm.

———. 2016d. "FastStats: Asthma." Updated June 13. www.cdc.gov/nchs/fastats/asthma.htm.

———. 2016e. "FastStats—Statistics by Topic." Updated July 6. www.cdc.gov/nchs/fastats/default.htm.

———. 2016f. "General Help for CDC WONDER." Reviewed August 24. http://wonder.cdc.gov/wonder/help/main.html.

———. 2016g. "Human Participant Protection in CDC Research." Accessed September 20. www.cdc.gov/od/science/integrity/hrpo.

———. 2016h. "National Vital Statistics System: Mortality Data." Updated February 16. www.cdc.gov/nchs/deaths.htm.

———. 2016i. "Public-Use Data Files and Documentation." Updated July 25. www.cdc.gov/nchs/data_access/ftp_data.htm.

———. 2016j. "What is GIS?" Updated June 17. www.cdc.gov/gis/what-is-gis.htm.

———. 2016k. *Vital Signs*. Updated September 13. www.cdc.gov/vitalsigns.

———. 2015a. "Compiling and Analyzing Health Claims Data." Updated December 8. www.cdc.gov/workplacehealthpromotion/model/healthcare-cost-data/compiling.html.

———. 2015b. "Heart Disease Death Rates, Total Population Ages 35+." Updated June 24. www.cdc.gov/dhdsp/maps/national_maps/hd_all.htm.

———. 2015c. "Interpreting Health Claims Data." Updated December 8. www.cdc.gov/workplacehealthpromotion/model/healthcare-cost-data/interpreting.html.

———. 2015d. "National Hospital Discharge Survey." Updated September 2. www.cdc.gov/nchs/nhds.

———. 2015e. "National Program of Cancer Registries." Updated October 19. www.cdc.gov/cancer/npcr/value/registries.htm.

———. 2015f. "National Vital Statistics System: Birth Data." Updated September 29. www.cdc.gov/nchs/births.htm.

———. 2015g. "PHIN Tools and Resources." Updated September 10. www.cdc.gov/phin/index.html.

———. 2015h. "Potential Health Claims Data." Updated December 8. www.cdc.gov/workplacehealthpromotion/model/healthcare-cost-data/claims-data.html.

———. 2015i. "Workplace Health Promotion: Employee Time and Attendance." Updated December 7. www.cdc.gov/workplacehealthpromotion/model/employee-level-assessment/attendance.html.

———. 2014a. "About the Behavioral Risk Factor Surveillance System." Updated July 31. www.cdc.gov/brfss/about/about_brfss.htm.

———. 2014b. "Preventing Pregnancies in Younger Teens." *Vital Signs*. Published April. www.cdc.gov/vitalsigns/pdf/2014-04-vitalsigns.pdf.

———. 2013. "Increased Risk of Rare Cancer as DES Daughters Age." Updated September 3. www.cdc.gov/cancer/dcpc/research/articles/des_risk.htm.

———. 2004. *Instructions for Completing the Cause-of-Death Section of the Death Certificate*. Published August. www.cdc.gov/nchs/data/dvs/blue_form.pdf.

County Health Rankings & Roadmaps. 2016a. "About." Accessed September 16. www.countyhealthrankings.org/about-project.

———. 2016b. "Act on What's Important." Accessed September 16. www.countyhealthrankings.org/roadmaps/action-center/act-whats-important.

———. 2016c. "Assess Needs & Resources." Accessed September 16. www.countyhealthrankings.org/roadmaps/action-center/assess-needs-resources.

———. 2016d. "Choose Effective Policies & Programs." Accessed September 16. www.countyhealthrankings.org/roadmaps/action-center/choose-effective-policies-programs.

——. 2016e. "Evaluate Actions." Accessed September 16. www.countyhealthrankings.org/roadmaps/action-center/evaluate-actions.

——. 2016f. "Focus on What's Important." Accessed September 16. www.countyhealthrankings.org/roadmaps/action-center/focus-whats-important.

——. 2016g. "Health Factors." Accessed September 16. www.countyhealthrankings.org/our-approach/health-factors.

——. 2016h. "Health Outcomes." Accessed September 16. www.countyhealthrankings.org/our-approach/health-outcomes.

——. 2016i. "Our Approach." Accessed September 16. www.countyhealthrankings.org/our-approach.

——. 2016j. "Policies and Programs." Accessed September 16. www.countyhealthrankings.org/our-approach/policies-and-programs.

Dartmouth Atlas of Health Care. 2016. "Understanding the Efficiency and Effectiveness of the Health Care System." Accessed September 19. www.dartmouthatlas.org.

Das, D., K. Metzger, R. Heffernan, S. Balter, D. Weiss, and F. Mostashari. 2005. "Monitoring Over-the-Counter Medication Sales for Early Detection of Disease Outbreaks—New York City." *MMWR Supplement*. Published August 26. www.cdc.gov/mmWR/preview/mmwrhtml/su5401a9.htm.

Data.Medicare.gov. 2016. "About This Site." Accessed September 19. https://data.medicare.gov/about.

Friis, R. H., and T. A. Sellers. 2014. *Epidemiology for Public Health Practice*, 5th ed. Burlington, MA: Jones & Bartlett Learning.

HealthData.gov. 2016. "About." Accessed September 16. www.healthdata.gov.

Kaiser Family Foundation (KFF). 2016. "About Us." Accessed September 19. http://kff.org/about-us.

MacKenzie, W. R., N. J. Hoxie, M. E. Proctor, M. S. Gradus, K. A. Blair, D. E. Peterson, J. J. Kazmierczak, D. G. Addiss, K. R. Fox, and J. B. Rose. 1994. "A Massive Outbreak in Milwaukee of *Cryptosporidium* Infection Transmitted Through the Public Water Supply." *New England Journal of Medicine* 331 (3): 161–67.

Martin, J. A., B. E. Hamilton, M. J. K. Osterman, S. C. Curtin, and T. J. Mathews. 2013. "Births: Final Data for 2012." *National Vital Statistics Reports* 62 (9): 1–68.

McIsaac, W. J., N. Levine, and V. Goel. 1998. "Visits by Adults to Family Physicians for the Common Cold." *Journal of Family Practice* 47 (5): 366–69.

Metzger, K. B., A. Hajat, M. Crawford, and F. Mostashari. 2004. "How Many Illnesses Does One Emergency Department Visit Represent? Using a Population-Based Telephone Survey to Estimate the Syndromic Multiplier." *MMWR* 53 (Suppl.): 106–11.

Mooney, T., and K. Keesee. 2014. "Spatial Analysis of Obesity: Geographic Information Systems and Descriptive Epidemiology." Centers for Disease Control and Prevention. Accessed September 15, 2016. www.cdc.gov/careerpaths/scienceambassador/documents/ms-spatial-analysis-of-obesity-2014.pdf.

Morris, R. D., E. N. Naumova, and J. K. Griffiths. 1998. "Did Milwaukee Experience Waterborne Cryptosporidiosis Before the Large Documented Outbreak in 1993?" *Epidemiology* 9 (3): 264–70.

Murphy, S. L., J. Xu, and K. D. Kochanek. 2013. "Deaths: Final Data for 2010." *National Vital Statistics Reports* 61 (4): 1–118.

National Center for Veterans Analysis and Statistics (NCVAS). 2016. "About Us." Updated April 8. www.va.gov/vetdata/about_us.asp.

Occupational Safety and Health Administration (OSHA). 2016. "About OSHA." Accessed September 19. www.osha.gov/about.html.

Porta, M. (ed.). 2014. *A Dictionary of Epidemiology*, 6th ed. New York: Oxford University Press.

Public Health Information Network. 2015. *PHIN Messaging Guide for Syndromic Surveillance: Emergency Department, Urgent Care, Inpatient and Ambulatory Care Settings.* Published April 21. www.cdc.gov/nssp/documents/guides/syndrsurvmessagguide2_messagingguide_phn.pdf.

Social Security Administration. 2016. "Office of Open Government Select Datasets." Accessed September 19. www.ssa.gov/open/data.

Surveillance, Epidemiology, and End Results (SEER) Program. 2016. "Overview of the SEER Program." Accessed September 20. http://seer.cancer.gov/about/overview.html.

Trust for America's Health (TFAH). 2016. "About the Trust for America's Health." Accessed September 19. http://healthyamericans.org/about.

US Census Bureau. 2016a. "About the Bureau." Updated September 9. www.census.gov/about/what.html.

——. 2016b. "Census of Governments." Updated March 2. www.census.gov/govs/cog.

——. 2016c. "Decennial Census of Population and Housing." Accessed September 14. www.census.gov/programs-surveys/decennial-census.html.

——. 2016d. "Health Insurance." Accessed September 19. www.census.gov/topics/health/health-insurance.html.

——. 2015. "American Community Survey (ACS)." Updated June 22. www.census.gov/programs-surveys/acs/about.html.

US Department of Health and Human Services (HHS). 2016a. "Summary of the HIPAA Privacy Rule." Accessed September 19. www.hhs.gov/hipaa/for-professionals/privacy/laws-regulations.

——. 2016b. "Summary of the HIPAA Security Rule." Accessed September 20. www.hhs.gov/hipaa/for-professionals/security/laws-regulations.

——. 2003. "Disclosures for Public Health Activities." Updated April 3. www.hhs.gov/hipaa/for-professionals/privacy/guidance/disclosures-public-health-activities/index.html.

——. 2002. "Who Must Comply with HIPAA Privacy Standards?" Published December 19. www.hhs.gov/hipaa/for-professionals/faq/190/who-must-comply-with-hipaa-privacy-standards/index.html.

Vingilis, E., U. Brown, and B. Hennen. 1999. "Common Colds: Reported Patterns of Self-Care and Health Care Use." *Canadian Family Physician* 45: 2644–46, 2649–52.

Wolford, M. L., K. Palso, and A. Bercovitz. 2015. "Hospitalization for Total Hip Replacement Among Inpatients Aged 45 and Over: United States, 2000–2010." National Center for Health Statistics Data Brief No. 186. Published February. www.cdc.gov/nchs/products/databriefs/db186.htm.

CHAPTER 5

EPIDEMIOLOGIC MEASURES

"When you can measure what you are speaking about, and express it in numbers, you know something about it; but when you cannot measure it, when you cannot express it in numbers, your knowledge is of a meager and unsatisfactory kind."

—Lord Kelvin (1883)

Learning Objectives

After completing this chapter, you should be able to

- explain the purpose of analytic epidemiology,
- describe various types of rates and the information they provide, and
- calculate rates and interpret their indication.

Introduction

analytic epidemiology The branch of epidemiology that uses studies to examine associations—often, putative or hypothesized causal relationships—concerning the health effects of various risk factors, characteristics, and exposures.

Analytic epidemiology is the branch of epidemiology that uses studies to examine associations—often, putative or hypothesized causal relationships—concerning the health effects of various risk factors, characteristics, and exposures (Last 2001). Whereas descriptive studies help us to develop hypotheses and answer questions of *who, what, where,* and *when,* analytic studies enable us to test hypotheses and answer questions of *why* and *how* (CDC 2012a, 2012b). Analytic studies complement descriptive studies, with the aim of determining causes or risk factors for illness and evaluating the effectiveness of interventions (CDC 2013). An important component of analytic studies is the use of quantitative measures (e.g., rates) to determine the significance of a finding.

Measures and numbers help us improve our descriptions of important health issues and enable us to make meaningful comparisons between populations. Without sufficient numbers, we will likely have difficulty reaching useful conclusions. Imagine, as an example, that both Florida and New York experience 10,000 deaths in the 80–85 age group in a given year. Based on just that information, how do we know which state might have a problem? We are unable to say, because we need more quantitative data (e.g., the total population of the age group in each state) to assess the situation.

Rates—measures of the frequency with which events occur in a certain population over a specified period—are critical to the study of epidemiology. The Centers for Disease Control and Prevention (CDC) explains: "Because rates put disease frequency in the perspective of the size of the population, rates are particularly useful for comparing disease frequency in different locations, at different times, or among different groups of persons with potentially different-sized populations." In other words, "A rate is a measure of risk" (CDC 2012c).

This chapter looks closely at the concept of rates and examines three classes: crude rates, specific rates, and adjusted rates. It also demonstrates how rates can be used to approach issues like the Florida and New York question posed earlier.

crude rate A summary measure based on the actual number of events in a population over a certain period.

Crude Rates

A **crude rate** is a summary rate based on the actual number of events that occur in a population during a given period (Friis and Sellers 2014). Examples of crude rates include the crude birth rate, fertility rate, crude death rate, infant mortality rate, and maternal mortality rate.

crude birth rate The number of live births during a certain time period divided by the resident population at the midpoint of that period.

Types of Crude Rates

The **crude birth rate** is a population-based measure of live births during a certain time period (CDC 2012f). Friis and Sellers (2014, 127) define the crude birth rate as "the number of live births during a specified period of time (e.g., one calendar year) per the resident population during the midpoint of the time period (expressed as rate per 1,000)." The crude birth rate serves as a useful measure of population growth and as an index for comparison between developed and developing countries; it is typically higher in less developed regions (Friis and Sellers 2014). The formula for crude birth rate can be written as follows (Porta 2014, 26):

$$\text{Crude birth rate} = \frac{\begin{array}{c}\text{Number of live births to residents}\\ \text{in an area in a calendar year}\end{array}}{\text{Average or midyear population in the area in that year}} \times 1{,}000$$

The **general fertility rate**, shown in exhibit 5.1, is similar to the crude birth rate but more refined. Its denominator is limited to the number of women of childbearing age—defined as ages 15 to 44 years in most jurisdictions, though it may sometimes extend to the age of 49. The general fertility formula can be written as follows (Porta 2014, 118):

general fertility rate The number of live births during a certain time period divided by the number of women of childbearing age.

$$\text{General fertility rate} = \frac{\text{Number of live births in an area during a year}}{\begin{array}{c}\text{Midyear female population age 15} - 44\\ \text{in the same area in same year}\end{array}} \times 1{,}000$$

Exhibit 5.1 General Fertility Rate in the United States, 1925–2009

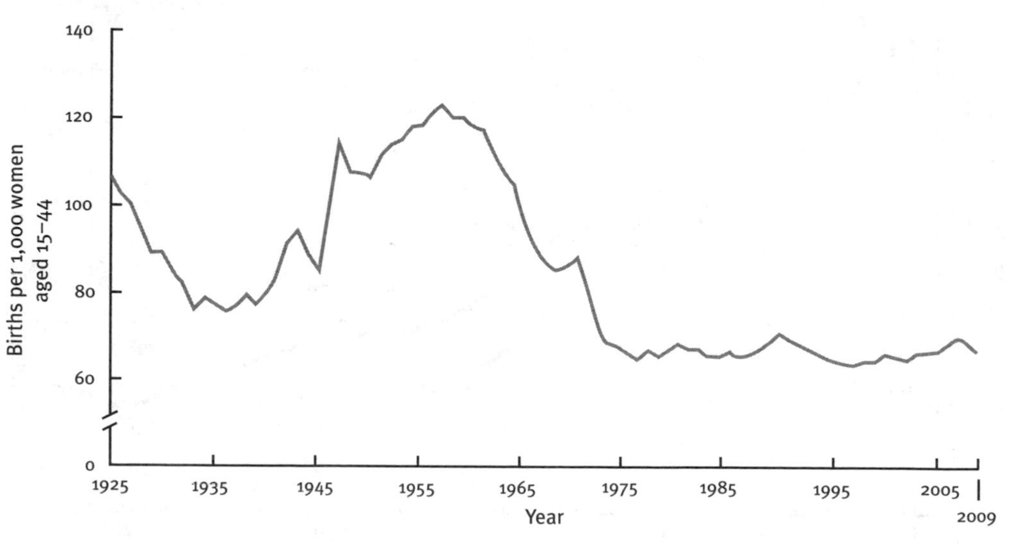

Source: Reprinted from Sutton, Hamilton, and Mathews (2011).

crude death rate
The proportion of a population that dies during a certain period.

The **crude death rate**, shown in exhibit 5.2, approximates the proportion of a population that dies during a certain period (Friis and Sellers 2014). It provides an estimate of the **person-time** death rate—that is, the death rate per 10^n person-years—and can be expressed mathematically as follows (Porta 2014, 69):

$$\text{Crude death rate} = \frac{\text{Number of deaths during a specified period}}{\text{Number of persons at risk of dying during the period}} \times 10^n$$

person-time
A concept that allows for the combination of people and time in the denominator for incidence or mortality rates when individuals, for varying periods, are at risk of developing disease or dying.

The concept of person-time (e.g., person-years) allows for the combination of people and time in the denominator for incidence or mortality rates when individuals, for varying periods, are at risk of developing disease or dying. Porta (2014, 213–214) explains: "With this approach, each subject contributes only as many years of observation to the population at risk as the period over which that subject has been observed to be at risk of the disease; a subject observed over 1 year contributes 1 person-year, a subject observed over a 10-year period contributes 10 person-years."

The use of person-time enables the measurement of incidence rates over extended and variable time periods (Porta 2014). The **person-time incidence rate** for an event, such as a disease or death, can be calculated as follows (Porta 2014, 214):

EXHIBIT 5.2
Crude Death Rate, Number of Deaths, and Age-Adjusted Death Rate in the United States, 1935–2010

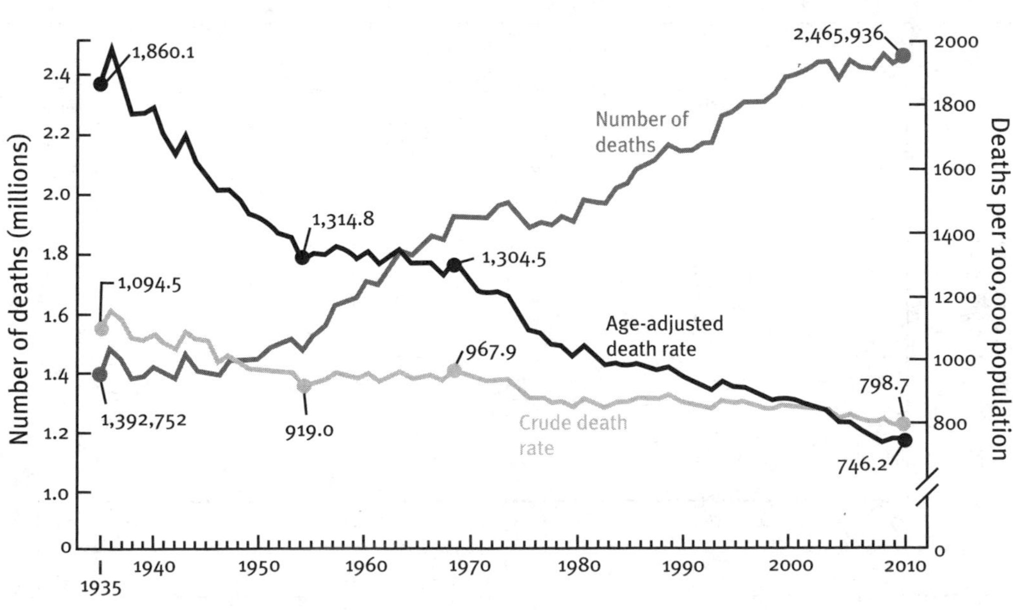

Source: Reprinted from Hoyert (2012).

$$\text{Person-time incidence rate} = \frac{\text{Number of events during the interval}}{\text{Number of person-time units at risk observed during the interval}}$$

person-time incidence rate
The number of events during a time period divided by the number of person-time units at risk observed during that period.

Though useful to epidemiologists, the use of person-time incidence rates can be confusing to general audiences. To make the rates more easily understandable, the CDC (2012d) recommends simply replacing "person-years" with "persons per year." For instance, "2.5 new cases of heart disease per 1,000 persons per year" will be more widely understood than "2.5 per 1,000 person-years."

The **infant mortality rate** indicates the yearly rate of deaths in children less than one year old, and it is calculated as follows (Porta 2014, 147):

infant mortality rate
The yearly rate of deaths in children less than one year old.

$$\text{Infant mortality rate} = \frac{\text{Number of deaths in a year of children less than 1 year of age}}{\text{Number of live births in the same year}} \times 1{,}000$$

It measures the risk of dying during the first year of life for infants who were born alive (Friis and Sellers 2014).

The **maternal mortality rate**, shown in exhibit 5.3, represents the risk of women dying from causes related to pregnancy and childbirth. The World Health Organization's definition of *maternal mortality* includes deaths during pregnancy or within 42 days of delivery, whereas other definitions may extend as far as a year after delivery (Porta 2014). Factors known to affect maternal mortality include age, socioeconomic status, nutritional status, and access to healthcare (Friis and Sellers 2014). The maternal mortality rate can be expressed using the following formula (Porta 2014, 178):

maternal mortality rate
A rate that represents the risk of women dying from causes related to pregnancy and childbirth.

$$\text{Maternal mortality rate} = \frac{\text{Number of deaths from puerperal causes in a given geographic area during a given year}}{\text{Number of live births that occurred among the population of the given geographic area during the same year}} \times \begin{matrix}1{,}000 \\ \text{(or 100,000)}\end{matrix}$$

Puerperal causes are those causes that are related to complications of pregnancy, childbirth, and the period following the delivery of a baby. The population of women exposed to the risk of dying from puerperal causes includes anyone who was pregnant during the period being observed. However, because that number is unknown, the conventional denominator for computing maternal mortality rates is the number of live births.

Exhibit 5.3
Maternal Mortality Rate in the United States Through the 1900s

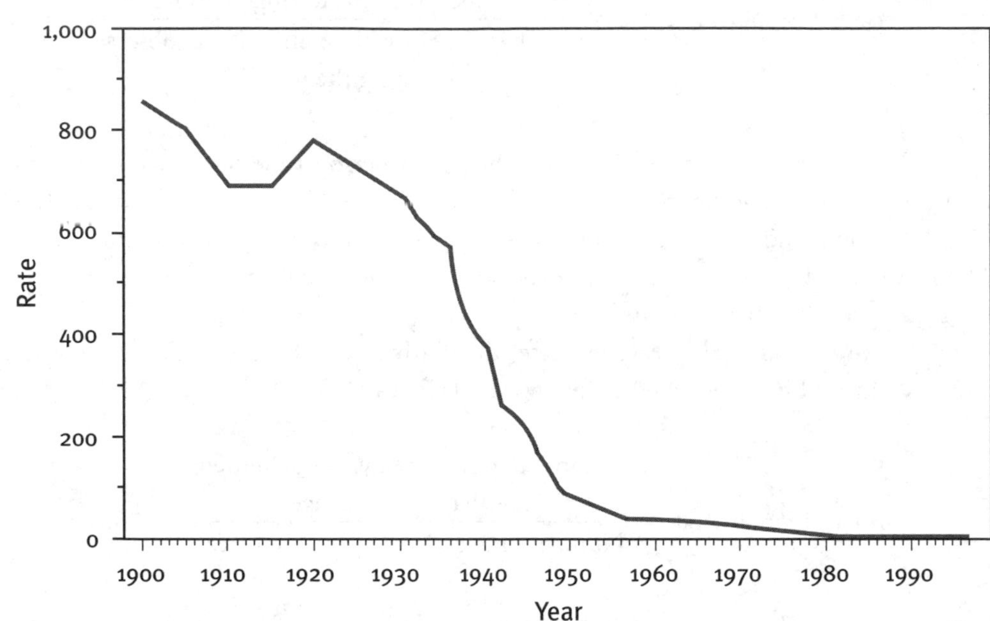

* Per 100,000 live births.

Source: Adapted from CDC (1999).

Limitations of Crude Rates

Crude rates are useful but should be cautiously interpreted. For the example introduced at the start of the chapter, the use of crude rates to compare mortality data in Florida and New York might cause us to overlook differences in the populations that are the result of systematic factors, such as differences in age or gender distribution. To correct for these influencing factors, two other types of rates—specific and adjusted—should be calculated (Friis and Sellers 2014).

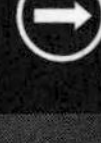

EXERCISE: WORKING WITH CRUDE RATES

Review the crude rate formulas presented in this chapter, and complete the following calculations.

1. In 2003, the estimated US population was 290,809,777, and a total of 2,419,921 deaths occurred. Calculate the crude mortality rate per 100,000 population.

(continued)

2. In 2003, 28,025 infants died, and 4,089,950 children were born. Calculate the infant mortality rate per 1,000 births.
3. As of July 1, 2006, the estimated US population was 299,398,484. The age distribution of the US female population is shown in the accompanying table. Given that 4,265,555 registered births occurred during 2006, calculate the general fertility rate per 1,000 women.

Age Group	Female Population
15–19	10,389,322
20–24	10,201,150
25–29	10,125,210
30–34	9,726,116
35–39	10,535,872
40–44	11,280,796
45–49	11,568,552
50–54	12,758,665
55–59	13,542,147
60–64	14,635,889
65–69	13,521,564
70–74	12,398,215
75–79	11,521,478

Source: CDC (2012e).

Note: Answers for this exercise are provided at the end of the chapter.

Specific Rates

Specific rates differ from crude rates in that they are based on particular subgroups of the population. The subgroups may be defined, for instance, in terms of age, race, or sex, or they may refer to the entire population but focus specifically on a single illness or cause of death. Examples of specific rates include cause-specific rates and age-specific rates (Friis and Sellers 2014).

specific rate
A summary measure based on a particular subgroup of the population. The subgroups may be defined, for instance, in terms of age, race, or sex, or they may refer to the entire population but focus specifically on a single illness or cause of death.

Types of Specific Rates

Cause-specific rates describe events, such as deaths, according to their causes (Porta 2014). A cause-specific mortality rate, for instance, might provide information about the

cause-specific rate
A kind of rate that describes events, such as deaths, according to their cause.

frequency of death due to HIV infection (Friis and Sellers 2014). A cause-specific rate can be expressed mathematically as follows (Friis and Sellers 2014, 138):

$$\text{Cause-specific rate} = \frac{\text{Mortality (or frequency of a given disease)}}{\text{Population size at midpoint of time period}} \times 100{,}000$$

age-specific rate
A rate for a particular age group.

An **age-specific rate** is a rate for a particular age group. When expressed in a formula, the numerator and denominator refer to the same age group, as in this example (Porta 2014, 5):

$$\begin{array}{l}\text{Age-specific death rate} \\ \text{(age 25–34)}\end{array} = \frac{\begin{array}{c}\text{Number of deaths among residents} \\ \text{age 25–34 in an area in a year}\end{array}}{\begin{array}{c}\text{Average (for midyear) population} \\ \text{age 25–34 in the area in that year}\end{array}} \times 100{,}000$$

proportional mortality ratio (PMR)
The number of deaths within a population resulting from a specific cause or disease, divided by the total number of deaths in that population.

The **proportional mortality ratio (PMR)** is the number of deaths within a population resulting from a specific cause or disease, divided by the total number of deaths in that population (Friis and Sellers 2014). The PMR is expressed as a percentage and can be calculated as follows (Friis and Sellers 2014, 142):

$$\text{Proportional mortality ratio} = \frac{\begin{array}{c}\text{Mortality due to a specific cause during} \\ \text{a time period}\end{array}}{\begin{array}{c}\text{Mortality due to all causes during} \\ \text{the same time period}\end{array}} \times 100$$

case fatality rate
The proportion of cases of a particular condition that are fatal within a specified period.

The **case fatality rate** is the proportion of cases of a particular condition that are fatal within a specified period (Porta 2014). The case fatality rate is normally expressed as a percentage and calculated in the following manner (Porta 2014, 36):

$$\text{Case fatality rate} = \frac{\begin{array}{c}\text{Number of deaths from a disease} \\ \text{(in a given period)}\end{array}}{\begin{array}{c}\text{Number of diagnosed cases of that disease} \\ \text{(in the same time period)}\end{array}} \times 100$$

Limitations of Specific Rates

Specific rates provide a better indicator of risk than crude rates do, especially for rates specific to certain subsets of the population. However, Friis and Sellers (2014, 139) state, "A disadvantage of specific rates is the difficulty in visualizing the 'big picture' in those situations where specific rates for several factors are presented in complex tables."

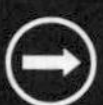

EXERCISE: WORKING WITH SPECIFIC RATES

Review the specific rate formulas presented in this chapter, and complete the following calculations.

1. Using the table provided below, calculate the unintentional-injury-specific mortality rate for the entire US population in 2002. Identify what type of rate it is.

All-Cause and Unintentional Injury Mortality and Estimated Population by Age Group, for Both Sexes and for Males Alone—United States, 2002

	All Races, Both Sexes			All Races, Males		
Age Group (Years)	**All Causes**	**Unintentional Injuries**	**Estimated Pop. (x1,000)**	**All Causes**	**Unintentional Injuries**	**Estimated Pop. (x1,000)**
Total	2,443,387	106,742	288,357	1,199,264	69,257	141,656
0–4	32,892	2,587	19,597	18,523	1,577	10,020
5–14	7,150	2,718	41,037	4,198	1,713	21,013
15–24	33,046	15,412	40,590	24,416	11,438	20,821
25–34	41,355	12,569	39,928	28,736	9,635	20,203
35–44	91,140	16,710	44,917	57,593	12,012	22,367
45–54	172,385	14,675	40,084	107,722	10,492	19,676
55–64	253,342	8,345	26,602	151,363	5,781	12,784
65+	1,811,720	33,641	35,602	806,431	16,535	14,772
Not stated	357	85	0	282	74	0

Source: CDC (2012e).

2. Using the same table, calculate the all-cause mortality rate for people in the 25–34 age group. Identify what type of rate it is.
3. Using the same table, calculate the all-cause mortality rate among males, and identify what type of rate it is.
4. Using the same table, calculate the unintentional-injury-specific mortality among males in the 25–34 age group, and identify what type of rate it is.
5. In 2001, a total of 15,555 homicide deaths occurred among males, and 4,753 homicide deaths occurred among females. The estimated 2001 midyear

(continued)

populations for males and females were 139,813,000 and 144,984,000, respectively. Calculate the homicide-related death rates for males and for females. Identify what type of rate they are.

6. Using the data from the previous question, calculate the ratio of the homicide-specific mortality rate for males to the rate for females. Describe your findings as if you were presenting information to a policy maker.
7. An epidemic of hepatitis A has been traced to green onions from a specific restaurant. A total of 555 cases were identified, and 3 of the case patients died as a result of their infections. Calculate the case fatality rate.
8. In the following table, calculate the missing PMRs for the 25–44 age group for diseases of the heart and assaults (homicide).

Numbers, Proportions (Percentages), and Rankings for Leading Causes of Death—United States, 2003

	All Ages			Ages 25–44 Years		
	Number	Percentage	Rank	Number	Percentage	Rank
All causes	2,443,930	100		128,924	100	
Diseases of heart	684,462	28	1	16,283	—	3
Malignant neoplasms	554,643	22.7	2	19,041	14.8	2
Cerebrovascular disease	157,803	6.5	3	3,004	2.3	8
Chronic lower respiratory diseases	126,128	5.2	4	401	0.3	*
Accidents (unintentional injuries)	105,695	4.3	5	27,844	21.6	1
Diabetes mellitus	73,965	3	6	2,662	2.1	9
Influenza and pneumonia	64,847	2.6	7	1,337	1	10
Alzheimer's disease	63,343	2.6	8	0	0	*
Nephritis, nephrotic syndrome, nephrosis	33,615	1.4	9	305	0.2	*
Septicemia	34,243	1.4	10	328	0.2	*
Intentional self-harm (suicide)	30,642	1.3	11	11,251	8.7	4

(continued)

	All Ages			Ages 25–44 Years		
	Number	**Percentage**	**Rank**	**Number**	**Percentage**	**Rank**
Chronic liver disease and cirrhosis	27,201	1.1	12	3,288	2.6	7
Assault (homicide)	17,096	0.7	13	7,367	—	5
HIV disease	13,544	0.5	*	6,879	5.3	6
All other	456,703	18.7		29,480	22.9	

* Not among top-ranked causes

Source: CDC (2012e).

Note: Answers for this exercise are provided at the end of the chapter.

Adjusted Rates

Another type of summary measure is an **adjusted rate**, which involves the use of statistical procedures to account for differences in the composition of populations. Rates are commonly adjusted for age, because older populations tend to be associated with greater risks of morbidity and mortality. An older population will likely have a higher crude mortality rate than a younger population, and differences associated with age will likely mask other differences between the populations being compared (Friis and Sellers 2014). Rates that have been adjusted, or standardized, can allow for more useful comparisons. Porta (2014, 268) defines *standardization* as "a set of techniques, based on weighted averaging, used to remove as much as possible the effects of differences in age or other confounding variables when comparing two or more populations."

adjusted rate
A summary measure that has been adjusted or standardized through the use of statistical procedures to account for differences in the composition of populations.

The adjustment of rates can be either direct or indirect. Porta (2014, 269) describes the direct method as follows:

> The specific rates in a study population are averaged, using as weights the distribution of a specified standard population. The directly standardized rate represents what the crude rate would have been in the study population if that population had the same distribution as the standard population with respect to the variable(s) for which the adjustment or standardization was carried out.

By contrast, the indirect method is used to compare study populations for which the specific rates are unknown or statistically unstable. Porta (2014, 269) writes:

The specific rates in the standard population are averaged, using as weights the distribution of the study population. The ratio of the crude rate for the study population to the weighted average so obtained is the standardized mortality (or morbidity) ratio, or SMR.

standardized mortality ratio (SMR)
The ratio of the number of deaths observed in a study population to the number that would be expected if that population had the same specific rates as the standard population.

The **standardized mortality ratio (SMR)** is the ratio of the number of deaths observed in a study population to the number that would be expected if that population had the same specific rates as the standard population (Porta 2014). A similar ratio, the standardized morbidity ratio, serves the same purpose for morbidity. The SMR can be expressed as a percentage and is calculated as follows (Friis and Sellers 2014, 150):

$$\text{Standardized mortality ratio (SMR)} = \frac{\text{Observed deaths}}{\text{Expected deaths}} \times 100$$

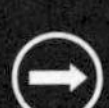

An answer greater than 1.0, or 100 percent, would warrant further investigation, because it would indicate that the observed number of deaths was greater than what was expected.

EXERCISE: WORKING WITH ADJUSTED RATES

Answer the following questions concerning adjusted rates.

1. Examine the mortality data for Alaska and Florida, provided below. Based on the data, would you recommend that people from Florida move to Alaska to reduce their risk of death?

All-Cause Mortality by Age Group—Alaska and Florida, 2002

	ALASKA			FLORIDA		
Age Group (Years)	**Population**	**Deaths**	**Death Rate (per 100,000)**	**Population**	**Deaths**	**Death Rate (per 100,000)**
<1	9,938	55	553.4	205,579	1,548	753
1–4	38,503	12	31.2	816,570	296	36.2
5–9	50,400	6	11.9	1,046,504	141	13.5
10–14	57,216	24	41.9	1,131,068	219	19.4
15–19	56,634	43	75.9	1,073,470	734	68.4
20–24	42,929	63	146.8	1,020,856	1,146	112.3

(continued)

	ALASKA			FLORIDA		
Age Group (Years)	Population	Deaths	Death Rate (per 100,000)	Population	Deaths	Death Rate (per 100,000)
25–34	84,112	120	142.7	2,090,312	2,627	125.7
35–44	107,305	280	260.9	2,516,004	5,993	238.2
45–54	103,039	427	414.4	2,225,957	10,730	482
55–64	52,543	480	913.5	1,694,574	16,137	952.3
65–74	24,096	502	2,083.30	1,450,843	28,959	1,996
75–84	11,784	645	5,473.50	1,056,275	50,755	4,805.10
85+	3,117	373	11,966.60	359,056	48,486	13,503.70
Unknown	NA	0	NA	NA	43	NA
Total	3,030	3,030	472.2	16,687,068	167,814	1,005.70
Age-adjusted rate:			794.1			787.8

Source: CDC (2012e).

2. Interpret the age-adjusted death rate for Alaska and Florida using the data provided.
3. The number of observed deaths due to lung cancer in New Hampshire during 2005 was 583. The expected number of deaths was 375. Calculate the standardized mortality ratio. Does the answer warrant further investigation?

Note: Answers for this exercise are provided at the end of the chapter.

Key Chapter Points

- Analytic epidemiology is the branch of epidemiology that uses studies to examine associations—often, putative or hypothesized causal relationships—concerned with the health effects of various risk factors, characteristics, and exposures.
- In epidemiology, a rate is a measure of the frequency with which an event occurs in a population over a specified period. "Because rates put disease frequency

in the perspective of the size of the population, rates are particularly useful for comparing disease frequency in different locations, at different times, or among different groups of persons with potentially different-sized populations" (CDC 2012c).

- A crude rate is a summary rate based on the actual number of events that occur in a population during a given period.
- The crude birth rate is a population-based measure of live births during a certain time period.
- The general fertility rate, like the crude birth rate, uses the number of live births as its numerator, but its denominator is limited to the number of women of childbearing age.
- The crude death rate approximates the proportion of a population that dies during a certain period.
- The concept of person-time (e.g., person-years) allows for the combination of people and time in the denominator for incidence or mortality rates when individuals, for varying periods, are at risk of developing disease or dying.
- The infant mortality rate indicates the yearly rate of deaths in children less than one year old.
- The maternal mortality rate represents the risk of women dying from causes related to pregnancy and childbirth.
- Crude rates are useful but should be cautiously interpreted. Two other types of rates—specific and adjusted—can help account for differences in populations that are the result of systematic factors, such as variations in age or gender distribution.
- Specific rates are based on particular subgroups of the population. The subgroups may be defined, for instance, in terms of race, age, or sex, or they may refer to the entire population but focus specifically on a single illness or cause of death.
- Cause-specific rates describe events, such as deaths, according to their causes.
- An age-specific rate is a rate for a particular age group.
- The proportional mortality ratio (PMR) is the number of deaths within a population resulting from a specific cause or disease divided by the total number of deaths in that population.
- The case fatality rate is the proportion of cases of a particular condition that are fatal within a specified period.
- Adjusted rates are summary measures calculated with the use of statistical procedures to account for differences in the composition of populations. Rates are commonly adjusted for age, because older populations tend to be associated with greater risks of morbidity and mortality. Rates can be adjusted through direct or indirect methods.
- The standardized mortality ratio is the ratio of the number of deaths observed in a study population to the number that would be expected if that population had the same specific rates as the standard population.

Discussion Questions

1. How do analytic epidemiology and descriptive epidemiology complement each other?
2. What are the differences between crude, specific, and adjusted rates?
3. Describe the importance of each type of rate described in this chapter. Consider, for example, why we might want to know the crude birth rate for a community.

Answers to Chapter Exercises

Working with Crude Rates

1. (2,419,921 / 290,809,777) × 100,000 = 832.1 deaths per 100,000 population.
2. (28,025 / 4,089,950) × 1,000 = 6.85 deaths per 1,000 population.
3. (4,265,555 / 62,258,466) × 1,000 = 68.5 per 1,000 population.

Working with Specific Rates

1. (106,742 / 288,357,000) × 100,000 = 37.0 unintentional-injury-related deaths per 100,000 population. This is a cause-specific mortality rate.
2. (41,355 / 39,928,000) × 100,000 = 103.6 deaths per 100,000 population (aged 25–34). This is an age-specific mortality rate.
3. (1,199,264 / 141,656,000) × 100,000 = 846.6 deaths per 100,000 males. This is a sex-specific mortality rate.
4. (9,635 / 20,203,000) × 100,000 = 47.7 unintentional-injury-related deaths per 100,000 population (males, aged 25–34). This is a cause-, age-, and sex-specific mortality rate.
5. Homicide-related death rate for males: (15,555 / 139,813,000) × 100,000 = 11.1 homicide deaths per 100,000 males. Homicide-related death rate for females: (4,753 / 144,984,000) × 100,000 = 3.3 homicide deaths per 100,000 females. These are cause- and sex-specific mortality rates.
6. 11.1 / 3.3 = 3.4 to 1. Because the homicide rate among males is more than three times higher than the homicide rate among females, specific intervention programs should target males and females differently.
7. (3 / 555) × 100 = 0.5%.
8. PMR for diseases of the heart: (16,283 / 128,924) × 100 = 12.6%. PMR for assault: (7,367 / 128,924) × 100 = 5.7%.

Working with Adjusted Rates

1. No, the reason that Alaska's total mortality rate is so much lower than Florida's is that Alaska's population is considerably younger. Indeed, for seven age groups, the age-specific mortality rates in Alaska are actually higher than in Florida.
2. To eliminate the distortion caused by different underlying age distributions in the two states, statistical techniques have been used to adjust or standardize the rates in the populations being compared. Alaska's age-adjusted mortality rate (794.1 per 100,000) was higher than Florida's (787.8 per 100,000), which is not surprising given that 7 of 13 age-specific mortality rates were higher in Alaska than Florida.
3. 583/375=1.5. Yes, this answer warrants further investigation.

References

Centers for Disease Control and Prevention (CDC). 2013. "Descriptive and Analytic Studies." Accessed September 21. www.cdc.gov/globalhealth/healthprotection/fetp/training_modules/19/desc-and-analytic-studies_ppt_final_09252013.pdf.

——. 2012a. "Principles of Epidemiology in Public Health Practice: An Introduction to Applied Epidemiology and Biostatistics, Lesson 1, Section 6." Self-study course. Updated May 18. www.cdc.gov/ophss/csels/dsepd/ss1978/lesson1/section6.html.

——. 2012b. "Principles of Epidemiology in Public Health Practice: An Introduction to Applied Epidemiology and Biostatistics, Lesson 1, Section 7." Self-study course. Updated May 18. www.cdc.gov/ophss/csels/dsepd/ss1978/lesson1/section7.html.

——. 2012c. "Principles of Epidemiology in Public Health Practice: An Introduction to Applied Epidemiology and Biostatistics, Lesson 3, Section 1." Self-study course. Updated May 18. www.cdc.gov/ophss/csels/dsepd/ss1978/lesson3/section1.html.

——. 2012d. "Principles of Epidemiology in Public Health Practice: An Introduction to Applied Epidemiology and Biostatistics, Lesson 3, Section 2." Self-study course. Updated May 18. www.cdc.gov/ophss/csels/dsepd/SS1978/Lesson3/Section2.html.

——. 2012e. "Principles of Epidemiology in Public Health Practice: An Introduction to Applied Epidemiology and Biostatistics, Lesson 3, Section 3." Self-study course. Updated May 18. www.cdc.gov/ophss/csels/dsepd/SS1978/Lesson3/Section3.html.

——. 2012f. "Principles of Epidemiology in Public Health Practice: An Introduction to Applied Epidemiology and Biostatistics, Lesson 3, Section 4." Self-study course. Updated May 18. www.cdc.gov/ophss/csels/dsepd/ss1978/lesson3/section4.html.

——. 1999. "Achievements in Public Health, 1990–1999: Healthier Mothers and Babies." Published October 1. www.cdc.gov/mmwr/preview/mmwrhtml/mm4838a2.htm.

Friis, R. H., and T. A. Sellers. 2014. *Epidemiology for Public Health Practice*, 5th ed. Burlington, MA: Jones & Bartlett Learning.

Hoyert, D. L. 2012. "75 Years of Mortality in the United States, 1935–2010." National Center for Health Statistics data brief. Published March. www.cdc.gov/nchs/data/databriefs/db88.pdf.

Kelvin, L. 1883. "Electrical Units of Measurement." Lecture, London, May 3. Accessed via http://zapatopi.net/kelvin/quotes.

Last, J. M. (ed.). 2001. *A Dictionary of Epidemiology*, 4th ed. New York: Oxford University Press.

Porta, M. (ed.). 2014. *A Dictionary of Epidemiology*, 6th ed. New York: Oxford University Press.

Sutton, P. D., B. E. Hamilton, and T. J. Mathews. 2011. "Recent Decline in Births in the United States, 2007–2009." National Center for Health Statistics data brief. Published March. www.cdc.gov/nchs/products/databriefs/db60.htm.

CHAPTER 6

ANALYTIC EPIDEMIOLOGY STUDY DESIGN

"Epidemiology is in large part a collection of methods for finding things out on the basis of scant evidence, and this by its nature is difficult."

—Alex Broadbent (2011)

CDC lesson 3

Learning Objectives

After completing this chapter, you should be able to

- identify the characteristics of analytic epidemiology studies,
- describe the strengths and limitations of analytic epidemiology studies, and
- interpret the measure of association for analytic epidemiology studies.

Introduction

Analytic epidemiology involves the use of observational and experimental studies to answer that most difficult of questions: *What is responsible for the health outcome of interest?* Whereas descriptive epidemiology helps us form hypotheses about the factors that could be contributing to disease, analytic epidemiology allows for those hypotheses to be tested and for associations between causes and outcomes to be measured. In a sense, analytic epidemiology represents the culmination of the disease detective work begun by its partner, descriptive epidemiology.

Exhibit 6.1 shows the various types of study designs for the two branches of epidemiology. We discussed the descriptive epidemiology designs—case reports, case series, and cross-sectional studies—in chapter 3. This chapter will focus on the analytic epidemiologic study designs and their respective measures of association. We will begin with the study designs within the observational branch, in which the epidemiologist observes

Exhibit 6.1
Epidemiology Study Designs

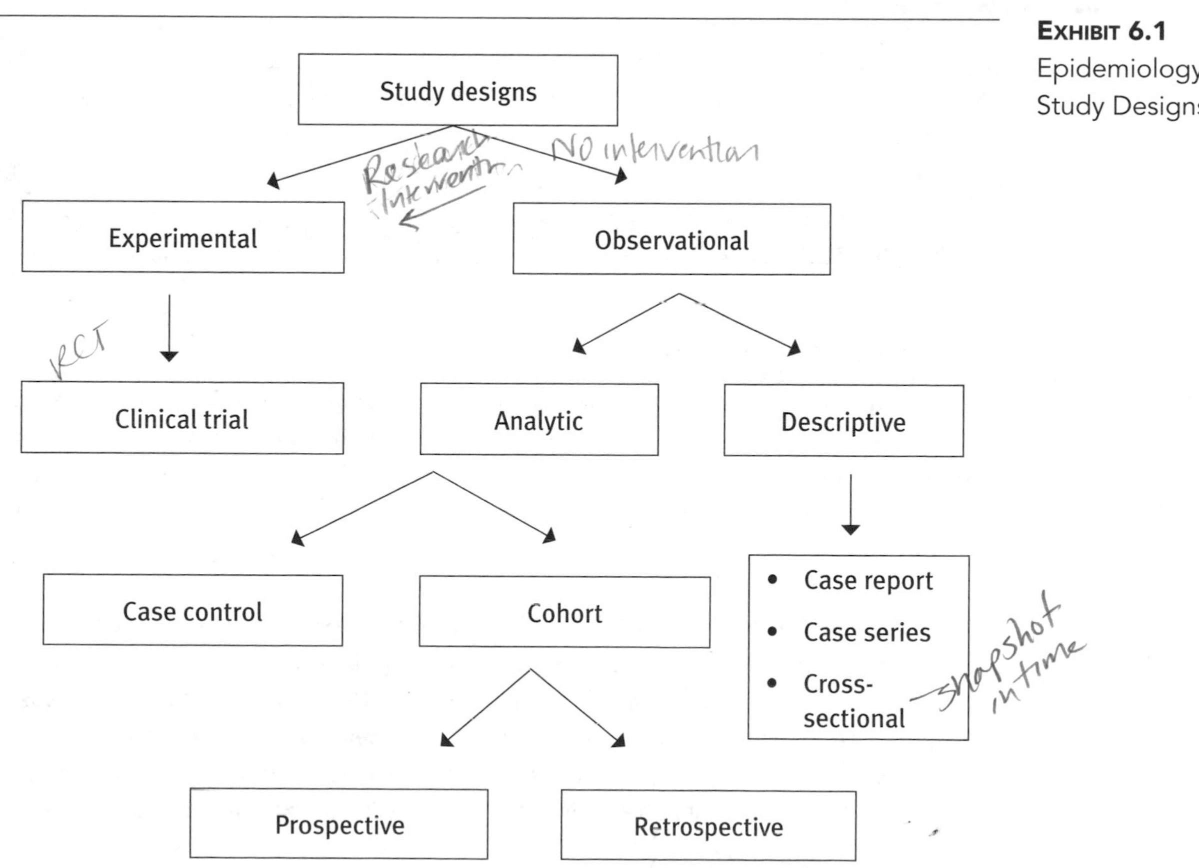

the relationship between exposure and disease but does not intervene in the process. We will discuss experimental studies, in which the epidemiologist does intervene, later in the chapter.

ETHICAL CONDUCT IN RESEARCH

Because of the nature of an epidemiologist's work with human subjects, ethical concerns are of the highest priority in epidemiology. The Presidential Commission for the Study of Bioethical Issues, commonly known as the Bioethics Commission, is an advisory panel comprising the nation's leaders in medicine, science, ethics, religion, law, and engineering. The commission promotes policy and practice to ensure that scientific research, the delivery of healthcare, and innovations are conducted in a manner that is socially and ethically responsible. This body serves in an advisory role to the president of the United States (Presidential Commission for the Study of Bioethical Issues 2016). In addition, the research conducted by the Centers for Disease Control and Prevention (CDC) is guided by ethical principles that emphasize respect for persons, beneficence, and justice (CDC 2010).

Case-Control Studies

case-control study
An observational study in which investigators select a case group (with a particular disease or outcome) and a control group and then compare previous exposures between the two groups.

A **case-control study** is an observational study of a group of people with a disease or other outcome of interest—called the case group—and a suitable control group of people without the disease (Porta 2014). Once both the case group and control group have been selected, investigators compare previous exposures between the two groups. The CDC (2012a) explains:

> The control group provides an estimate of the baseline or expected amount of exposure in that population. If the amount of exposure among the case group is substantially higher than the amount you would expect based on the control group, then illness is said to be associated with that exposure. . . . The key in a case-control study is to identify an appropriate control group, comparable to the case group in most respects, in order to provide a reasonable estimate of the baseline or expected exposure.

The case-control study design is useful for studying diseases that are not common and for examining a single outcome that could be related to multiple causes. It is also feasible when resources (e.g., time, money) are limited (CDC 2013). The basic structure of the case-control study design is illustrated in exhibit 6.2.

Friis and Sellers (2014, 303) elaborate:

> The case-control study seeks to identify possible causes of the disease by finding out how the two groups differ with respect to an exposure (or suspected risk factor). That is, because disease does not occur randomly, the case group must have been exposed to some risk factor, either voluntarily (e.g., through diet, exercise, or smoking) or involuntarily (e.g., through such factors as cosmic radiation, air pollution, occupational hazards, or genetic constitution). Therefore, a comparison of the frequency of exposure among cases and controls may permit inferences regarding their difference in disease status.

Case groups can be assembled with the help of such resources as a tumor or disease registry or listings from a vital statistics bureau (Friis and Sellers 2014). Control groups can be assembled from patients from the same hospital as the cases, relatives of the cases, or people from the same population as the cases (Friis and Sellers 2014). An important feature of the case-control study design is **matching**—that is, the process of making sure that the case group and control group have the same characteristics except for the exposure of interest (Porta 2014).

matching
The process of making sure that the case group and control group have the same characteristics except for the exposure of interest.

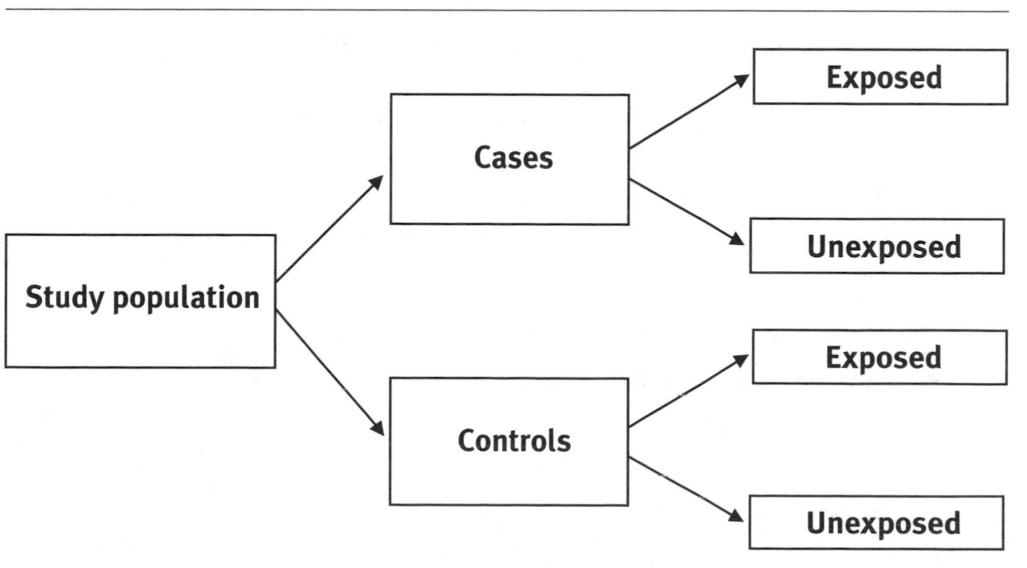

Exhibit 6.2
The Case-Control Study Design

Measure of Association for a Case-Control Study

2×2 table
A tool for evaluating the association between exposure and disease.

odds ratio (OR)
The measure of association for a case-control study, representing the odds of exposure to a particular disease for the case group relative to the control group.

A key tool for evaluating the association between exposure and disease in a case-control study is the **2×2 table**, shown in exhibit 6.3. The table is useful for calculating the **odds ratio (OR)**, which is the measure of association for a case-control study.

The OR helps investigators evaluate whether the odds of exposure to the disease for the case group are different from the odds of exposure for the control group (Friis and Sellers 2014). It is calculated using the following formula from the 2×2 table:

$$OR = \frac{(A \times D)}{(B \times C)}$$

An OR of 1.0 indicates that the cases and controls have equal odds of exposure to the disease; it therefore suggests that a particular exposure is not a risk factor for the disease being studied. An OR of 2.0, however, indicates that the cases were twice as likely to be exposed to the disease; it therefore suggests that the factor is associated with twice the risk of disease. An OR less than 1.0 would indicate a "protective" factor that lowers the risk of disease (Friis and Sellers 2014).

Friis and Sellers (2014) summarize the advantages of case-control studies as follows:

- They typically use smaller sample sizes than surveys.
- They are relatively easy and quick to complete.
- They are cost effective.
- They are useful for the study of rare disease and multiple exposures.

Friis and Sellers (2014) also observe the following limitations:

- The timing of an exposure–disease relationship is difficult to determine because information is collected about events that occurred in the past.
- The studies provide an indirect estimate of risk.
- The representativeness of cases and controls is often unknown.

Exhibit 6.3
2×2 Table

		Disease Status		
Exposure Status		**Yes**	**No**	**Total**
	Yes	A	B	A+B
	No	C	D	C+D
	Total	A+C	B+D	

A = Exposure and disease present
B = Exposure present, but disease not present
C = No exposure, but disease present
D = No exposure, no disease
A+C = Total number with disease
B+D = Total number without disease
A+B = Total number exposed
C+D = Total number with no exposure

EXERCISE: CREATING A 2×2 TABLE AND CALCULATING AN ODDS RATIO

An outbreak of tuberculosis occurred among prison inmates in China. Of the 162 inmates who developed the disease, 35 resided in the west wing of the building. Among 126 controls, 5 resided in that wing. Develop a 2×2 table, calculate the odds ratio, and interpret your findings.

Source: Adapted from CDC (2012b).

Note: Answers to this exercise appear at the end of the chapter.

SAMPLE EXCERPTS FROM CASE-CONTROL STUDIES

The following abstract has been reproduced from a study by Payne and colleagues (2003) that was published in the CDC's *Emerging Infectious Diseases* journal. The

(continued)

study, titled "Vero Cytotoxin–Producing Escherichia coli O157 Gastroenteritis in Farm Visitors, North Wales," provides an example of the case-control study design and the use of odds ratios to inform policy recommendations:

> An outbreak of Vero cytotoxin–producing *Escherichia coli* O157 (VTEC O157) gastroenteritis in visitors to an open farm in North Wales resulted in 17 primary and 7 secondary cases of illness. *E. coli* O157 Vero cytotoxin type 2, phage type 2 was isolated from 23 human cases and environmental animal fecal samples. A case-control study of 16 primary case-patients and 36 controls (all children) showed a significant association with attendance on the 2nd day of a festival, eating ice cream or cotton candy (candy floss), and contact with cows or goats. On multivariable analysis, only the association between illness and ice cream (odds ratio [OR] = 11.99, 95% confidence interval [CI] 1.04 to 137.76) and cotton candy (OR = 51.90, 95% CI 2.77 to 970.67) remained significant. In addition to supervised handwashing, we recommend that foods on open farms only be eaten in dedicated clean areas and that sticky foods be discouraged.

An excerpt from a case-control study by Zhong and colleagues (1999, 607), examining the role of environmental tobacco smoke (ETS) in the development of lung cancer in Chinese women, further illustrates the methodology:

> A population-based, case-control study was conducted to evaluate the relationship between lung cancer and exposure to ETS among nonsmoking women living in Shanghai, China. Five-hundred and four women diagnosed with incident, primary lung cancer between February 1992 and January 1994 were identified through the population-based Shanghai Cancer Registry. A control group of 601 nonsmoking women was selected randomly from the Shanghai Residential Registry, and was approximately frequency-matched to the age distribution of the lung cancer cases. Information on lifetime domestic and occupational exposure to ETS was obtained through face-to-face interviews. Adjusted odds ratios (OR) and 95% confidence intervals (CI) were estimated by unconditional logistic regression . . . The OR for ever exposed to ETS from spouses was 1.1 (95% CI: 0.8–1.5), and the OR for ever exposed to ETS at work was 1.7 (95% CI: 1.3–2.3). Furthermore, the OR increased with increasing number of hours of daily exposure to ETS in the workplace and with increasing number of smoking co-workers. No associations were found for exposure to ETS during childhood. . . . The main findings of the present study are that long-term occupational exposure to ETS, both alone or in combination with exposures at home, conferred an increased risk of lung cancer among women who never smoked.

Cohort Studies

A **cohort** is a well-defined group of people who have a common characteristic or experience—for instance, a group of people who were born in the same year (CDC 2015). Porta (2014, 49) defines a *cohort* in a broad sense as "any designated group of persons who are followed or traced over a period of time."

cohort
A well-defined group of people who have a common characteristic or experience.

In a **cohort study**, also called a *longitudinal study* or *follow-up study*, participants are classified according to their exposure status and then followed over time to ascertain the outcome. The CDC (2012a) explains:

cohort study
An observational study in which participants are classified according to their exposure status and then followed over time to ascertain the outcome.

> In a cohort study, the epidemiologist records whether each study participant is exposed or not, and then tracks the participants to see if they develop the disease of interest. . . . After a period of time, the investigator compares the disease rate in the exposed group with the disease rate in the unexposed group. The unexposed group serves as the comparison group, providing an estimate of the baseline or expected amount of disease occurrence in the community. If the disease rate is substantively different in the exposed group compared to the unexposed group, the exposure is said to be associated with illness.

Porta (2014, 50) defines a *cohort study* more specifically as "the analytic epidemiological study in which subsets of a defined population can be identified who are, have been, or in the future may be exposed or not exposed—or exposed in different degrees—to a factor or factors hypothesized to influence the occurrence of a given outcome." A key feature of a cohort study is the observation of large numbers of people over a long period (often years), with comparison of incidence rates in groups of different exposure levels.

Cohort studies contribute greatly to our understanding of cause and effect. Unlike case-control studies, they can be used to determine multiple outcomes based on a single exposure; hence, they are useful when rare exposures are of interest. In addition, cohort studies ensure temporality—in other words, they ensure that the exposure occurs before the observed outcome (CDC 2013).

Cohort studies can be prospective or retrospective. A **prospective cohort study** groups participants according to their past or current exposure and then follows them going forward, into the future, to determine if an outcome occurs (CDC 2013). It allows for a direct test of one's hypothesis (Friis and Sellers 2014). Exhibit 6.4 illustrates the study design for a prospective cohort study.

prospective cohort study
A cohort study that groups participants according to their past or current exposure and then follows them going forward to determine if an outcome occurs.

A **retrospective cohort study** is similar to a prospective cohort study in that an investigator calculates and compares rates of disease in the exposed and unexposed groups; however, a retrospective study is conducted when both the exposure and the outcomes have already occurred in the past (CDC 2012a). Porta (2014, 249) defines a retrospective study as "a research design used to test etiologic hypotheses in which inferences about

retrospective cohort study
A cohort study that is conducted when both the exposure and the outcomes have already occurred in the past.

EXHIBIT 6.4
Prospective Cohort Study Design

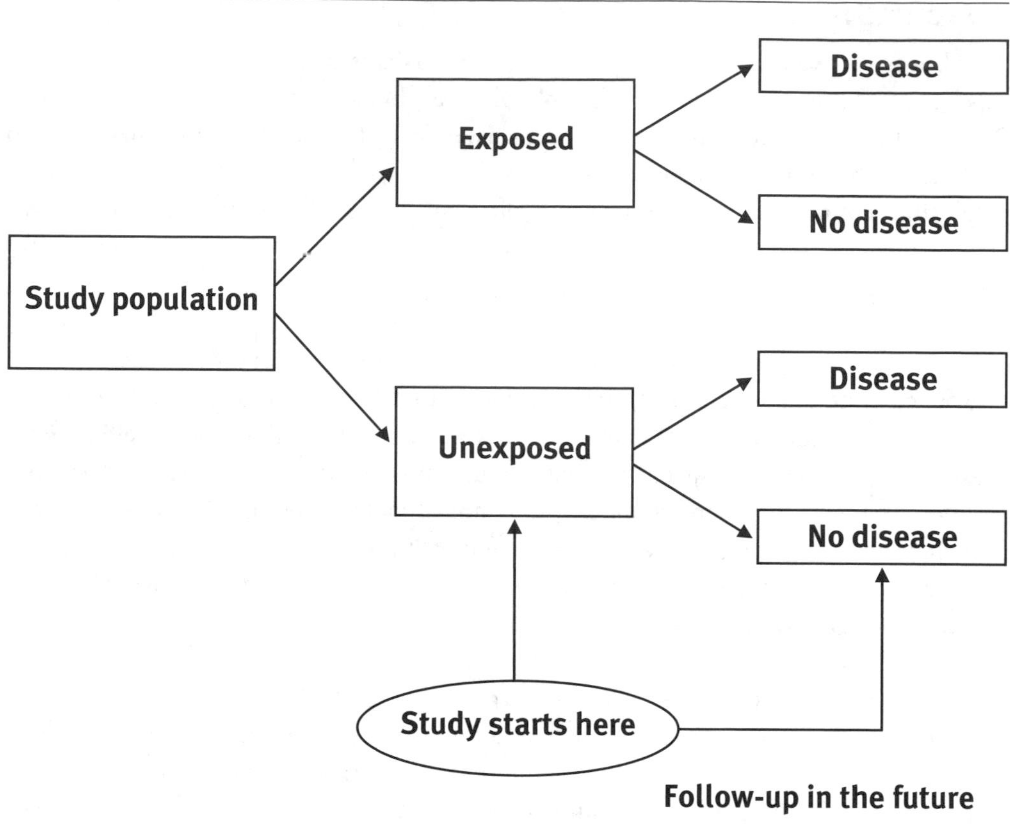

exposure to the putative causal factor(s) are derived from data relating to characteristics of the person under study or to events or experiences in their past." In a retrospective cohort study, some of the people under study have the disease or other outcome of interest, and their characteristics and past experiences are compared with those of unaffected persons. Exhibit 6.5 illustrates the study design for a retrospective cohort study.

relative risk (RR)
The measure of association for a cohort study, expressed as the incidence of disease in the exposed group divided by the incidence of disease in the nonexposed group.

MEASURE OF ASSOCIATION FOR A COHORT STUDY

The measure of association for a cohort study is the **relative risk (RR)**, which can be expressed as the incidence of disease in the exposed group divided by the incidence of disease in the nonexposed group (CDC 2013). The CDC (2012b) states:

> A risk ratio, also called relative risk, compares the risk of a health event (disease, injury, risk factor, or death) among one group with the risk among another group. It does so by dividing the risk (incidence proportion, attack rate) in group 1 by the risk (incidence proportion, attack rate) in group 2. The two groups are typically differentiated by such

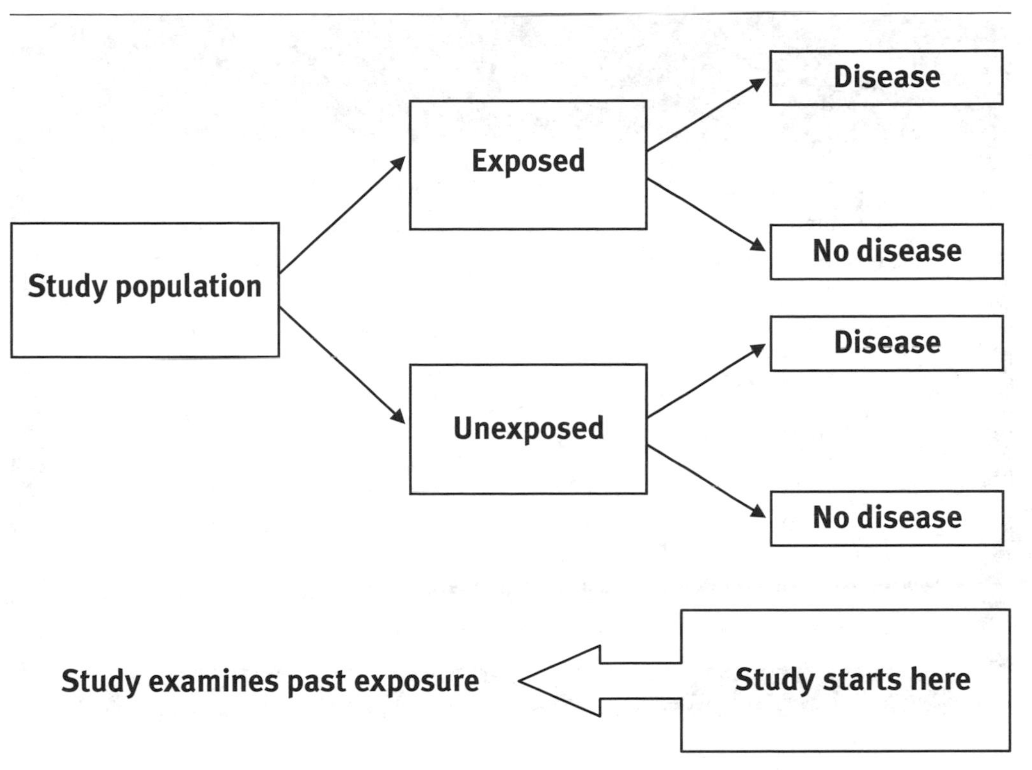

Exhibit 6.5 Retrospective Cohort Study Design

demographic factors as sex (e.g., males versus females) or by exposure to a suspected risk factor (e.g., did or did not eat potato salad). Often, the group of primary interest is labeled the exposed group, and the comparison group is labeled the unexposed group.

Porta (2014, 252) defines the RR as "the ratio of two risks, usually of exposed and not exposed."

An RR of 1.0 indicates that the risk of disease among the exposed group is no different from the risk among the nonexposed group. An RR of 2.0 suggests that the risk among the exposed group is twice as high, whereas an RR of 0.5 indicates that the risk among the exposed group is half that of the nonexposed group (Friis and Sellers 2014).

Like the odds ratio, the RR can be calculated using a 2×2 table (shown previously in exhibit 6.3). The formula is as follows (Friis and Sellers 2014):

$$OR = \frac{\frac{A}{A+B}}{\frac{C}{C+D}}$$

EXERCISE: CALCULATING RELATIVE RISK

During an outbreak in Oregon in 2002, varicella (chickenpox) was diagnosed in 18 of 152 vaccinated children and 3 of 7 unvaccinated children (CDC 2012b). Use the 2×2 table that follows to calculate the relative risk, and then interpret your findings.

	Varicella	No Varicella	Total
Vaccinated	18	134	152
Unvaccinated	3	4	7
Total	21	138	159

Source: Adapted from CDC (2012b); data from Tugwell et al. (2004).

Note: Answers to this exercise appear at the end of the chapter.

SAMPLE EXCERPTS FROM A COHORT STUDY

The Framingham Heart Study (FHS) followed a group of people from the town of Framingham, Massachusetts, with the aim of identifying factors that contribute to the development of cardiovascular disease. Descriptions of the various stages of the study provide a detailed example of the cohort study design (FHS 2016a):

- The Original Cohort of the study "consisted of 5,209 respondents of a random sample of 2/3 of the adult population of Framingham, Massachusetts, 30 to 62 years of age by household, in 1948" (FHS 2016a).
- The Offspring Cohort was initiated in 1971 when researchers recognized the need for a prospective epidemiologic study of young adults. This cohort comprised "5,124 men and women, consisting of the offspring of the Original Cohort and their spouses" (FHS 2016a).

(continued)

- The Third Generation Cohort developed after researchers asked offspring participants to update information about their children. "To assess interest in participation prior to the start of clinic exams, 5,500 letters and response cards were sent in November 2001 to prospective third generation participants who had at least one parent in the Offspring Study and would be at least 20 years old by the close of the first exam cycle" (FHS 2016a).
- Omni Cohorts were initiated in 1994 to provide a better representation of the increasingly diverse Framingham community. "The original Omni Cohort consisted of 507 men and women of African-American, Hispanic, Asian, Indian, Pacific Islander, and Native American origins, who at the time of enrollment were residents of Framingham and the surrounding towns. Omni Cohort 1 continues to be examined and followed" (FHS 2016a).

The Framingham Heart Study has produced a number of research findings that have shaped public health practice and healthcare delivery. In 1960, for example, cigarette smoking was found to increase the risk of heart disease, and in 1970, high blood pressure was linked to the risk of stroke. Obesity was identified as a risk factor for heart failure in 2002, and sleep apnea was tied in 2010 to increased risk of stroke (FHS 2016b).

Friis and Sellers (2014) summarize the advantages of cohort studies as follows:

- They can help directly estimate risk for disease.
- They ensure temporality of exposure and outcome.
- They are suitable for studying multiple outcomes and rare exposures.

Friis and Sellers (2014) also point out the following limitations:

- They take a long time to complete (potentially decades).
- They are more costly than case-control studies.
- Some subjects may be unavailable for follow-up.

Experimental Studies

experimental study
A study in which the researcher determines the exposure for the subjects and then tracks the subjects to observe the effects of the exposure.

The **experimental study** design differs from the observational study design in one significant aspect: In the experimental study design, the researcher intervenes in the assignment of who receives the exposure. Whereas researchers conducting observational studies simply observe and do not directly intervene, those conducting experimental studies exercise greater control over the research process. Porta (2014, 103) defines an experimental study as "a study in which the investigator intentionally alters one or more factors and controls the other study conditions in order to analyze the effects of so doing"—or, more simply, as "a study in which conditions are under the direct control of the investigator."

The CDC (2012a) states:

> In an experimental study, the investigator determines through a controlled process the exposure for each individual (clinical trial) or community (community trial) and then tracks the individuals or communities over time to detect the effects of the exposure. For example, in a clinical trial of a new vaccine, the investigator may randomly assign some of the participants to receive the new vaccine, while others receive a placebo shot. The investigator then tracks all participants, observes who gets the disease that the new vaccine is intended to prevent, and compares the two groups (new vaccine vs. placebo) to see whether the vaccine group has a lower rate of disease.

clinical trial
An experimental research activity that involves administering a test regimen to people to evaluate its effectiveness and safety.

prophylactic trial
A type of clinical trial seeking to evaluate the effectiveness of a treatment intended to prevent disease.

therapeutic trial
A type of clinical trial seeking to evaluate the effectiveness of a treatment in improving a patient's health.

A **clinical trial** is an experimental research activity that involves administering a test regimen to people to evaluate its effectiveness and safety (Porta 2014). Clinical trials can be prophylactic or therapeutic. A **prophylactic trial** seeks to evaluate the effectiveness of a treatment intended to prevent disease (Friis and Sellers 2014). For instance, a prophylactic trial might test a vaccine, vitamin supplement, or prevention program. In contrast, a **therapeutic trial** seeks to evaluate the effectiveness of a treatment in bringing about improvement in a patient's health (Friis and Sellers 2014). A therapeutic trial might evaluate, for instance, a new curative drug or surgical procedure.

A **randomized controlled trial (RCT)** is generally considered the most scientifically rigorous method of hypothesis testing in epidemiology. In an RCT, subjects are randomly assigned to groups—usually called *test* (or *study*) and *control* groups—and they either receive or do not receive an experimental procedure or intervention. Results are assessed through the comparison of rates of disease, death, recovery, or other outcomes for the two groups (Porta 2014).

Among the key features of a clinical trial are the random assignment of subjects into groups and the blinding of subjects to study conditions (Friis and Sellers 2014). Assignment to test and control groups through **randomization**—that is, by chance—helps ensure that the two groups will be comparable except in the regimen that is given to them (Porta 2014). **Blinding**, or *masking*, involves making participants unaware of the group to which subjects have been assigned. In a single-blind trial, either the subjects or the observers are kept ignorant of the subjects' group assignment. In a double-blind trial, both the subjects and the observers are kept ignorant (Porta 2014).

Experimental studies have a number of important ethical considerations. Researchers should protect the interests of subjects, and the benefits of participation should outweigh the risks (Friis and Sellers 2014). The concept of **informed consent**—the subject's knowing, voluntary agreement to participate—is central to the conduct of ethical research. Porta (2014, 149) defines *informed consent* as the "voluntary consent given by a subject or a responsible proxy (e.g., a parent) for participation in a study, immunization program, treatment regimen, etc., after being informed of the purpose, methods, procedures, potential benefits and potential harms, and, when relevant, the degree of uncertainty about such outcomes." Porta (2014, 149) continues: "The essential criteria of informed consent are that the subject has both knowledge and comprehension, that consent is freely given without duress or undue influence, and that the right of withdrawal at any time is clearly communicated to the subject."

Friis and Sellers (2014) describe the advantages of experimental studies as follows:

- They give the investigator significant control over the amount, timing, and frequency of exposure and the period of patient observation.
- The randomization of patients reduces the possibility that the test and control groups will have significantly different characteristics.

Friis and Sellers also describe the following limitations:

- Experimental studies are often conducted in artificial settings.
- Researchers may have difficulty enforcing adherence to protocol.
- Researchers may be confronted with ethical dilemmas.

SAMPLE ABSTRACT FROM AN EXPERIMENTAL STUDY

The following is an abstract from an experimental study titled "Randomized Controlled Trial Targeting Obesity-Related Behaviors: Better Together Healthy Caswell County" by Zoellner and colleagues (2013), published in the CDC's *Preventing Chronic Disease* journal:

Introduction

Collaborative and multilevel interventions to effectively address obesity-related behaviors among rural communities with health disparities can be challenging,

(continued)

randomized controlled trial (RCT)
An epidemiologic experiment in which subjects are randomly assigned to test and control groups, which either receive or do not receive an intervention, and outcomes from the two groups are compared.

randomization
The assignment of individuals to test and control groups by chance, with the aim of ensuring that the two groups will be comparable except in the regimen that is given to them.

blinding
The act of making participants in a study unaware of the group to which subjects have been assigned; also called *masking*.

informed consent
A subject's knowing, voluntary agreement to participate in a study.

and traditional research approaches may be unsuitable. The primary objective of our 15-week randomized controlled pilot study, which was guided by community-based participatory research (CBPR) principles, was to determine the effectiveness of providing twice-weekly access to group fitness classes, with and without weekly nutrition and physical activity education sessions, in Caswell County, North Carolina, a rural region devoid of medical and physical activity resources.

Methods

Participants were randomly divided into 2 groups: Group 1 was offered fitness sessions and education in healthful eating and physical activity; group 2 was offered fitness sessions only. Outcome measures were assessed at baseline and immediately after the intervention. Standardized assessment procedures, validated measures, and tests for analysis of variance were used.

Results

Of 91 enrolled participants, most were African American (62%) or female (91%). Groups were not significantly different at baseline. Group 1 experienced significantly greater improvements in body mass index ($F=15.0$, $P < .001$) and waist circumference ($F=7.0$, $P=.01$), compared with group 2. Both groups significantly increased weekly minutes of moderate physical activity ($F=9.4$, $P<.003$). Participants in group 1 also had significantly greater weight loss with higher attendance at the education ($F=14.7$, $P<.001$) and fitness sessions ($F=18.5$, $P<.001$).

Conclusion

This study offers effective programmatic strategies that can reduce weight and increase physical activity and demonstrates feasibility for a larger scale CBPR obesity trial targeting underserved residents affected by health disparities. This study also signifies successful collaboration among community and academic partners engaged in a CBPR coalition.

Source: Reprinted from Zoellner et al. (2013).

bias
Systematic deviation from the truth, or any processes that contribute to such deviation.

Bias and Confounding

When conducting and interpreting epidemiologic studies, researchers must remain aware of the possibilities of bias and confounding. **Bias** is the systematic deviation of results or inferences from the truth; the term also refers to any processes that contribute to such deviation (Porta 2014). Bias can result from errors in the study's design or conception, or in the collection, analysis, interpretation, publication, or review of data (Porta 2014). **Confounding** is distortion that occurs when the outcomes being observed are influenced by associations with factors other than the one being studied.

confounding
Distortion that occurs when the outcomes being observed are influenced by associations with factors other than the one being studied.

Information Bias

Two main types of bias are information bias and selection bias. **Information bias** is a flaw in the measurement of exposure or outcome data that results in differences in the quality of information between the comparison groups (Porta 2014).

information bias
A flaw in the measurement of exposure or outcome data that results in differences in the quality of information between comparison groups.

One form of information bias is **recall bias**, systematic error that results from differences in the accuracy or completeness of people's memories of past events (Porta 2014). For example, a mother whose child had a serious illness is more likely than the mother of a healthy child to remember details of past experiences with X-ray services when the child was in utero (Porta 2014). Information bias may also take the form of **interviewer bias** or **abstractor bias**. Interviewer bias might occur if an interviewer has a tendency to probe more thoroughly for a certain finding in a case than in a control. In a similar manner, an abstractor might pore over records more thoroughly in a case than in a control (Friis and Sellers 2014). A final example of information bias is **prevarication bias**, or lying, which may occur if participants have ulterior motives when answering questions (Friis and Sellers 2014).

recall bias
Systematic error resulting from differences in the accuracy or completeness of people's memories of past events.

Friis and Sellers (2014) suggest the following techniques to reduce information bias:

- Use memory aids.
- Keep interviewers blind to the participant's study status.
- Provide standardized training and protocols for researchers.
- Keep participants blind to the study's goals.

interviewer bias
A form of information bias related to an interviewer's gathering of data or influencing of responses.

abstractor bias
A form of information bias related to the way a data abstractor reviews and interprets records.

Selection Bias

Selection bias is distortion resulting from systematic differences in characteristics between people who take part in a study and people who do not (Last 2001). For instance, selection bias might exist if the subjects in a survey are limited to volunteers or to people who are present at a particular place and time. It might also exist if a study of disease looks only at hospital cases under the care of a physician, excluding people not sick enough to require hospital care, people who die before hospital admission, or people excluded by cost, geography, or other factors (Last 2001).

prevarication bias
A form of information bias that occurs when participants answer questions dishonestly.

selection bias
Distortion resulting from systematic differences in characteristics between people who take part in a study and people who do not.

Friis and Sellers (2014) suggest the following techniques to reduce selection bias:

- Establish an explicit definition for eligibility for selection.
- Enroll all cases at a specified time and in a specified geographic region.
- Aim for high participation rates.
- Ensure that the sample is representative of the larger population.

Confounding

Confounding involves the presence of an extraneous factor that is associated both with the exposure and the outcome (Last 2001). Porta (2014, 55) explains: "Confounding occurs when all or part of the apparent association between the exposure and the outcome is in fact accounted for by other variables that affect the outcome and are not themselves affected by the exposure." For example, a study of the effect of aspirin on the risk of stroke might be confounded if aspirin is more likely to be prescribed to people with heart disease (Porta 2014). Matching and randomization help prevent confounding in epidemiologic studies (Friis and Sellers 2014).

Hill's Criteria

Hill's criteria
A series of epidemiologic criteria for causal association introduced by Sir Austin Bradford Hill in 1965. The criteria are strength, consistency, specificity, temporality, dose–response relationship, biological plausibility, coherence, experiment, and analogy.

Epidemiology is a science that strives to elucidate the causal relationship between exposures and outcomes. This chapter has highlighted many of the useful tools available via analytic epidemiology to further define that relationship, and we will conclude with the set of criteria introduced by the British medical statistician Sir Austin Bradford Hill. Introduced in 1965, **Hill's criteria**, also called Hill's considerations for causation, represent the first complete statement of epidemiologic criteria for causal association (Last 2001). The criteria for a causal association between a factor and a disease are as follows (Porta 2014):

1. *Strength.* The size of the risk, as measured by appropriate statistical estimates, provides the basis for the strength criterion.
2. *Consistency.* An association meeting the consistency criterion should remain apparent when tested in different settings using different methods.
3. *Specificity.* This criterion is present when a single putative cause produces a specific effect.
4. *Temporality.* Exposure must always precede the outcome.
5. *Dose–response relationship.* This criterion is present when an increasing level of exposure is associated with increasing risk.

6. *Biological plausibility.* The association is consistent with current understanding of pathobiological processes.
7. *Coherence.* The association is consistent with existing theory and knowledge.
8. *Experiment.* The condition can be altered by an appropriate experimental regimen.
9. *Analogy.* Similar relations have been established previously.

EXERCISE: IDENTIFYING STUDY TYPES

Identify each of the following studies as either (A) an experimental study, (B) a cohort study, (C) a case control study, (D) a cross-sectional study, or (E) not an analytical or epidemiologic study.

1. A representative sample of residents was telephoned and asked how much they exercise each week and whether they currently have or have ever been diagnosed with heart disease.
2. Occurrence of cancer was identified between April 1991 and July 2002 for 50,000 troops who served in the first Gulf War (1990–1991) and 50,000 troops who served elsewhere during the same period.
3. People diagnosed with new-onset Lyme disease were asked how often they walk through woods, use insect repellant, wear short sleeves and pants, and engage in other behaviors. Twice as many patients without Lyme disease from the same physician's practice were asked the same questions, and the responses in the two groups were compared.
4. A study's subjects were children enrolled in a health maintenance organization. At the age of two months, each child was randomly given one of two types of a new vaccine against rotavirus infection. Parents were called by a nurse two weeks later and asked whether the children had experienced any of a list of side effects.

Source: Adapted from CDC (2012a).

Note: Answers to this exercise appear at the end of the chapter.

Key Chapter Points

- Analytic epidemiology uses observational and experimental studies to answer the question, *What is responsible for the health outcome of interest?*
- Because of the nature of an epidemiologist's work with human subjects, ethical concerns are of the highest priority.
- In observational studies, the epidemiologist observes the relationship between exposure and disease but does not intervene in the process.
- In a case-control study, a group of people with a disease or other outcome of interest—called the case group—is compared with a suitable control group of people without the disease.
- Matching involves making sure that the case group and control group have the same characteristics except for the exposure of interest.
- A 2 × 2 table helps epidemiologists evaluate the association between exposure and disease.
- The measure of association for a case-control study is the odds ratio. The OR helps investigators evaluate whether the odds of exposure to the disease for the case group are different from the odds of exposure for the control group. It can be calculated using a 2 × 2 table.
- In a cohort study, participants are classified according to their exposure status and then followed over time to ascertain the outcome.
- A prospective cohort study groups participants according to their past or current exposure and then follows them going forward to determine if an outcome occurs. A retrospective cohort study is conducted when both the exposure and the outcomes have already occurred in the past.
- The measure of association for a cohort study is the relative risk. It can be expressed as the incidence of disease in the exposed group divided by the incidence of disease in the nonexposed group. It can be calculated using a 2 × 2 table.
- In contrast to researchers conducting observational studies, researchers conducting experimental studies intervene in the assignment of who receives the exposure. They exercise greater control over the research process.
- A clinical trial is an experimental research activity that involves administering a test regimen to people to evaluate its efficacy and safety.
- A prophylactic trial seeks to evaluate the effectiveness of a treatment intended to prevent disease. A therapeutic trial seeks to evaluate the effectiveness of a treatment in bringing about improvement in a patient's health.
- In a randomized controlled trial, subjects are randomly assigned to groups—usually called *test* and *control* groups—and either receive or do not receive an experimental procedure or intervention. Results are assessed through the comparison of rates of disease, death, recovery, or other outcomes.

- Assignment of subjects to test and control groups through randomization—that is, by chance—helps ensure that the groups will be comparable except in the regimen that is given to them for the study.
- Blinding involves making participants unaware of the group to which subjects have been assigned. In a single-blind trial, either the subjects or the observers are kept ignorant of the subjects' group assignment. In a double-blind trial, both the subjects and the observers are kept ignorant.
- The concept of informed consent—the subject's knowing, voluntary agreement to participate—is central to the conduct of ethical research. "The essential criteria of informed consent are that the subject has both knowledge and comprehension, that consent is freely given without duress or undue influence, and that the right of withdrawal at any time is clearly communicated to the subject" (Porta 2014, 149).
- When conducting and interpreting epidemiologic studies, researchers should be aware of the possibilities of bias and confounding.
- Information bias is a flaw in the measurement of exposure or outcome data that leads to differences in the quality of information between the comparison groups. Forms of information bias include recall bias, interviewer bias, and prevarication bias.
- Selection bias creates distortion through systematic differences in characteristics between people who take part in a study and people who do not.
- Confounding is a distortion that occurs "when all or part of the apparent association between the exposure and the outcome is in fact accounted for by other variables that affect the outcome and are not themselves affected by the exposure" (Porta 2014, 55).
- In 1965, the British medical statistician Sir Austin Bradford Hill introduced a set of epidemiologic criteria for causal association. Hill's criteria are strength, consistency, specificity, temporality, dose–response relationship, biological plausibility, coherence, experiment, and analogy.

Discussion Questions

1. What are the advantages and limitations of each study design described in this chapter?
2. Explain why case-control studies are useful in studying rare diseases.
3. Describe how the measure of association is calculated and interpreted for a case-control study and for a cohort study.
4. How does an experimental study differ from an observational study?

5. Describe the different types of bias.
6. What are some ways to minimize the problems of bias and confounding?

Answers to Chapter Exercises

Creating a 2 x 2 Table and Calculating an Odds Ratio

		Disease Status—Tuberculosis		
Exposure Status—West Wing Residence		Yes	No	Total
	Yes	35	5	40
	No	127	121	248
	Total	162	126	288

$$\mathrm{OR} = \frac{(35 \times 121)}{(5 \times 127)} = 6.7$$

Exposure to residing in the west wing of the prison is associated with 6.7 times the risk of developing tuberculosis.

Calculating Relative Risk

Risk of varicella among vaccinated children = 18 / 152 = 0.118 = 11.8%
Risk of varicella among unvaccinated children = 3 / 7 = 0.429 = 42.9%
RR = 0.118 / 0.429 = 0.28
The RR of less than 1.0 indicates a decreased risk for the vaccinated children.

Identifying Study Types

1. D; 2. B; 3. C; 4. A

References

Broadbent, A. 2011. "Philosopher Offers a Different Perspective in Thinking About Epidemiologic Topics." *Epimonitor*. Accessed September 27, 2016. http://epimonitor.net/Philosopher_Offers_Different_Perspective.htm.

Centers for Disease Control and Prevention (CDC). 2015. "Epidemiology Glossary." Updated January 21. www.cdc.gov/reproductivehealth/data_stats/glossary.html.

——. 2013. "Descriptive and Analytic Studies." Accessed September 21. www.cdc.gov/globalhealth/healthprotection/fetp/training_modules/19/desc-and-analytic-studies_ppt_final_09252013.pdf.

——. 2012a. "Principles of Epidemiology in Public Health Practice: An Introduction to Applied Epidemiology and Biostatistics, Lesson 1, Section 7." Self-study course. Updated May 18. www.cdc.gov/ophss/csels/dsepd/ss1978/lesson1/section7.html.

——. 2012b. "Principles of Epidemiology in Public Health Practice: An Introduction to Applied Epidemiology and Biostatistics, Lesson 3, Section 5." Self-study course. Updated May 18. www.cdc.gov/ophss/csels/dsepd/SS1978/Lesson3/Section5.html.

——. 2010. "Human Research Protections Policy." Published July 29. www.cdc.gov/od/science/integrity/docs/cdc-policy-human-research-protections.pdf.

Framingham Heart Study (FHS). 2016a. "Participants." Accessed September 29. www.framinghamheartstudy.org/participants/index.php.

——. 2016b. "Research Milestones." Accessed September 29. www.framinghamheartstudy.org/about-fhs/research-milestones.php.

Friis, R. H., and T. A. Sellers. 2014. *Epidemiology for Public Health Practice*, 5th ed. Burlington, MA: Jones & Bartlett Learning.

Last, J. M. (ed.). 2001. *A Dictionary of Epidemiology*, 4th ed. New York: Oxford University Press.

Payne, C. J. I., M. Petrovic, R. J. Roberts, A. Paul, E. Linnane, M. Walker, D. Kirby, A. Burgess, R. M. M. Smith, T. Cheasty, G. Willshaw, and R. L. Salmon. 2003. "Vero Cytotoxin–Producing Escherichia coli O157 Gastroenteritis in Farm Visitors, North Wales." *Emerging Infectious Diseases*. Published May. wwwnc.cdc.gov/eid/article/9/5/02-0237.

Porta, M. (ed.). 2014. *A Dictionary of Epidemiology*, 6th ed. New York: Oxford University Press.

Presidential Commission for the Study of Bioethical Issues. 2016. "About the Commission." Accessed September 27. http://bioethics.gov/about.

Tugwell, B. D., L. E. Lee, H. Gillette, E. M. Lorber, K. Hedberg, and P. R. Cieslak. 2004. "Chickenpox Outbreak in a Highly Vaccinated School Population." *Pediatrics* 113 (3): 455–59.

Zhong, L., M. S. Goldberg, Y. T. Gao, and F. Jin. 1999. "A Case-Control Study of Lung Cancer and Environmental Tobacco Smoke Among Nonsmoking Women Living in Shanghai, China." *Cancer Causes & Control* 10 (6): 607–16.

Zoellner, J., J. L. Hill, K. Grier, C. Chau, D. Kopec, B. Price, and C. Dunn. 2013. "Randomized Controlled Trial Targeting Obesity-Related Behaviors: Better Together Healthy Caswell County." *Preventing Chronic Disease* 10: E96.

CHAPTER 7

INFECTIOUS DISEASE EPIDEMIOLOGY

"When you have eliminated the impossible, whatever remains, however improbable, must be the truth."

—Arthur Conan Doyle (1890)

Learning Objectives

After completing this chapter, you should be able to

- discuss the epidemiologic triangle and explain its utility,
- describe the characteristics of infectious disease agents,
- calculate the attack rate for infectious diseases,
- describe the types of epidemic curves and provide an example of each,
- explain the steps involved in a disease outbreak investigation,
- understand the significance of emerging infectious diseases and the factors that contribute to their presence,
- describe the natural progression of disease, and
- discuss the public health interventions for infectious diseases.

communicable disease
An illness that arises through the direct or indirect transmission of an infectious agent or its toxic products from an infected person, animal, or reservoir to a susceptible host.

epidemiologic triangle
A model that helps to explain the causes and origins of infectious disease. Its vertices are host, environment, and agent.

host
A living human or animal that, under natural conditions, provides subsistence or lodgment to an infectious agent.

environment
External conditions, including biological, cultural, physical, social, and other dimensions that influence health.

agent
A factor whose presence, excessive presence, or, in some cases, relative absence is necessary for disease to occur; sometimes called a *pathogen*.

Introduction

Infectious disease epidemiology is an essential branch of epidemiology—one that is relevant to the public on a daily basis. An infectious or **communicable disease** is "an illness due to a specific infectious agent or its toxic products that arises through transmission of such agent or products from an infected person, animal, or reservoir to a susceptible host, either directly or indirectly through an intermediate plant or animal host, vector, or the inanimate environment" (Porta 2014, 51–52). This chapter explores such topics as the factors necessary for disease to occur in a population, the ways disease is transmitted, the research-based process by which disease outbreaks are investigated, and the interventions we use to control the spread of disease. Lastly, the chapter examines the topic of emerging infectious diseases, an ongoing threat to populations in the twenty-first century.

The Epidemiologic Triangle

The **epidemiologic triangle** (see exhibit 7.1) is a model that helps to explain the etiology—that is, the causes and origins—of infectious disease (Friis and Sellers 2014). The triangle has three corners or vertices: host, environment, and agent. The **host** is the living human being or animal that, under natural conditions, affords subsistence or lodgment to an infectious agent (Porta 2014). The **environment** comprises the setting and conditions that are external to the host, and it can include biological, cultural, physical, social, and other dimensions that influence the health status of populations (Porta 2014). The **agent**, or *pathogen*, is a factor—such as a microorganism, chemical substance, or form of radiation—whose "presence, excessive presence, or (in deficiency diseases) relative absence is essential for the occurrence of a disease" (Porta 2014, 5). Disease cannot occur in the absence of any one of the three vertices. For example, if the agent and environment are present but there is no host, disease will not occur.

A host's susceptibility to an agent depends on its defense mechanisms against pathogens. Such defense mechanisms may be specific to particular disease agents, or they may be nonspecific (e.g., tears, saliva, acidic gastric juices, sweat). Immunity may be developed, by either active or passive means, against a particular disease agent. Active immunity occurs when exposure to a pathogen activates the host's immune system to make antibodies; passive immunity results from antibodies received from another person or animal (Friis and Sellers 2014).

The environment is "the sum total of influences that are not part of the host" (Friis and Sellers 2014, 445). It includes physical components such as temperature, humidity, and geologic formations, as well as social conditions such as the attitudes, behaviors, and cultural characteristics of a group. The environment can serve as a reservoir that promotes the survival of agents that transmit infectious disease. Friis and Sellers (2014, 445) state: "The reservoir may be a part of the physical environment or may reside in animals or insects (vectors) or other human beings (human reservoir hosts)."

Exhibit 7.1 Epidemiologic Triangle

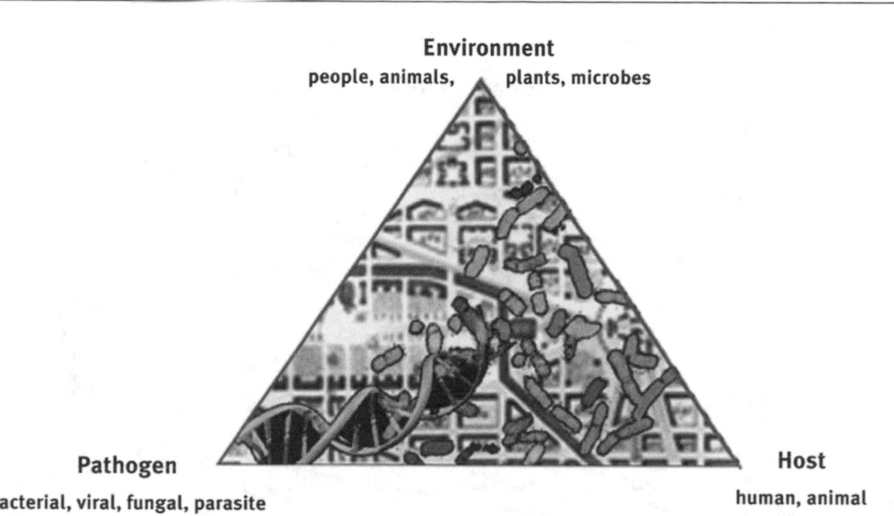

Source: Reprinted from CDC (2015b).

infectivity
A disease agent's capability to enter a host, survive, and multiply.

pathogenicity
The extent to which overt disease occurs in a population infected by a disease agent.

toxigenicity
The capability of an agent to produce a toxin or poison.

resistance
The ability of a disease agent to survive adverse conditions.

virulence
The disease-evoking power of an agent in a particular host.

direct transmission
The direct transfer of an infectious agent to a portal of entry.

Agents can take a variety of forms. Agent types include bacteria (e.g., tuberculosis), viruses (e.g., HIV), fungi (e.g., athlete's foot), protozoa (e.g., malaria), helminths (e.g., intestinal parasites, such as tapeworm), and arthropods (e.g., ticks carrying Lyme disease) (Friis and Sellers 2014). Infectious agents can be described based on their ability to produce disease, the severity of the disease, and the outcome of infection. An agent's capability to enter a host, survive, and multiply is its **infectivity** (Porta 2014). The extent to which overt disease occurs in the population infected by the agent is the agent's **pathogenicity** (Porta 2014). **Toxigenicity** refers to the capability of an agent to produce a toxin or poison (Friis and Sellers 2014). An agent's **resistance** is its ability to survive adverse environmental conditions (Friis and Sellers 2014). The disease-evoking power of an agent in a particular host is its **virulence** (Porta 2014). The case fatality rate indicates the proportion of cases of infection with the agent that are fatal within a given time (Porta 2014).

Infectious Disease Transmission

Infectious agents can be transmitted from a source or reservoir to a person in a variety of ways, both direct and indirect, as illustrated in exhibit 7.2. **Direct transmission** is the "direct and essentially immediate transfer of infectious agents to a receptive portal of entry through which human or animal infection may take place" (Porta 2014, 282). It may occur through direct contact between people (e.g., touching, kissing, biting, sexual intercourse); by the direct projection of droplet spray into the eyes, nose, or mouth; by direct exposure to an agent in soil, compost, or decaying vegetable matter; by animal bite; or by transplacental transmission (Porta 2014).

EXHIBIT 7.2
Chain of Infection

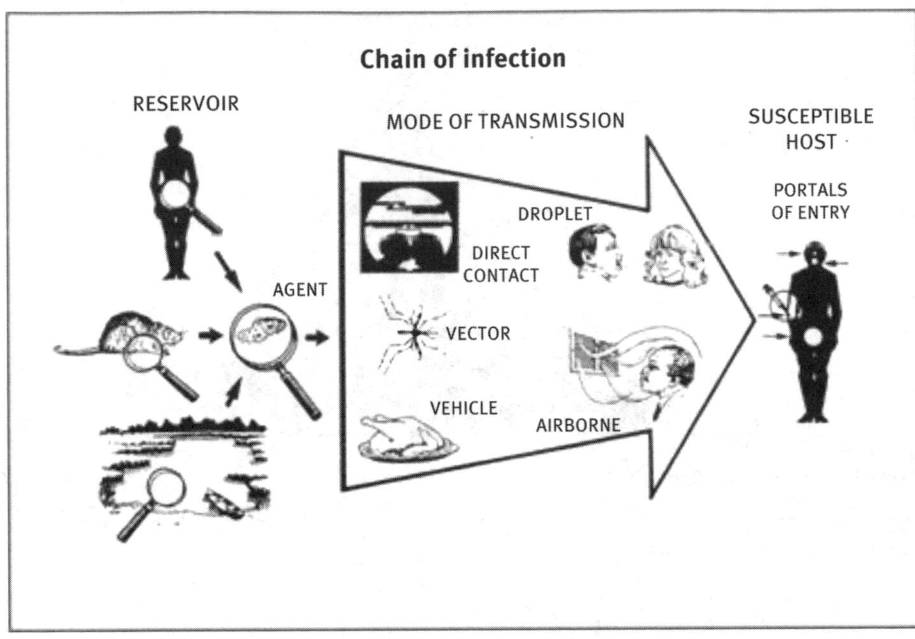

Source: Reprinted from CDC (1992).

indirect transmission The transfer of an infectious agent through an intermediary source.

vehicle-borne transmission Transmission of an infectious agent through contaminated material or objects.

fomite A contaminated object capable of carrying an infection to a person.

vector-borne transmission Transmission of an infectious agent via insect.

inapparent infection An infection that lacks recognizable clinical signs or symptoms.

Indirect transmission occurs through an intermediary source (Friis and Sellers 2014). **Vehicle-borne transmission** occurs through contaminated material or objects. A contaminated object capable of carrying an infection to a person—for instance, a contaminated handkerchief, drinking glass, eating utensil, or surgical instrument—is called a **fomite** (Porta 2014). Vehicle-borne transmission can also occur through food and water; biological products such as blood, serum, plasma, tissues, and organs; or any other substance that introduces an infectious agent to a susceptible host through an appropriate portal of entry (Porta 2014). An agent in some cases might multiply or develop in or on the vehicle prior to transmission. **Vector-borne transmission** can result from the simple carriage of an agent by a crawling or flying insect (Porta 2014). The typical routes of exposure by which infectious agents gain access to the human host include inhalation (through the respiratory tract), ingestion (through the gastrointestinal tract), dermal exposure (through the skin), and ocular exposure (through the eyes) (Friis and Sellers 2014).

When an infectious organism replicates within a host, the incubation period—the time between invasion by the agent and the first sign of disease—is often a certain number of hours, days, or weeks. For instance, the incubation period for measles (rubeola) is usually about 10 days but ranges from 7 to 18, and it takes about 14 days for a rash to appear (Friis and Sellers 2014). In some cases, however, no symptoms become apparent. An **inapparent infection**, also called a *subclinical infection*, involves infection with an

CDC Lesson 2 Section 2

agent but no recognizable clinical signs or symptoms (Porta 2014). Inapparent infection is an important epidemiologic issue because a host who shows no symptoms can still transmit an agent to other susceptible hosts, some of whom may develop severe illness as a result. Infected individuals are more likely to be isolated when the infections are clinically apparent (Friis and Sellers 2014).

Herd immunity occurs when a large percentage of a group or community has immunity to an infectious agent, as a result of either vaccinations or past infections (Friis and Sellers 2014; Porta 2014). Herd immunity can protect a population even when not every single individual has been immunized, because the immune people prevent the spread of disease to the unimmunized (Friis and Sellers 2014).

Epidemiologists use a number of measures to track infectious disease occurrence. **Point prevalence** is the proportion of people in a population who have a particular disease or attribute at a specified point in time (Porta 2014). **Period prevalence** is the proportion of people known to have had the condition at any point during a specified period (Porta 2014). An **attack rate** is used when the occurrence of a disease increases greatly within a population over a short period, often in relation to a specific exposure. It can be used to measure occurrence during acute infectious disease outbreaks (e.g., microbial food-borne illness) and other acute health-related events (e.g., exposures of large groups to toxic agents) (Friis and Sellers 2014). The attack rate is often expressed as a percentage and can be calculated as follows (Friis and Sellers 2014):

$$\text{Attack rate} = \frac{\text{Ill}}{\text{Ill} + \text{Well}} \times 100 \text{ during a given period}$$

Epidemic Curves

An **epidemic curve**, or "epi curve," is a graphic plotting of the distribution of cases during an epidemic (Porta 2014). An epidemic curve shows the pattern in which an outbreak occurs, and it can convey important information about the distribution of cases over time (the time trend), cases that do not follow the usual patterns (outliers), the estimated magnitude of the outbreak, details about the spread of the outbreak, and the pattern of exposure with respect to time (CDC 2016a). The various types of epidemic curves correspond with different types of outbreaks.

A **point source outbreak**, also called a *common source outbreak*, results from the exposure of a group to a noxious influence that is common to the members of the group (Porta 2014). Such an exposure may occur, for instance, when people are gathered for a meal or event. Porta (2014, 94) states: "When the exposure is brief and essentially simultaneous, the resultant cases all develop within one incubation period of the disease." As a result, the epidemic curve for a point source outbreak rises rapidly to a peak and then falls gradually, as shown in the example in exhibit 7.3 (CDC 2016a).

herd immunity
General immunity in a group or community; it occurs when a large percentage of a group or community has immunity to an agent.

point prevalence
The proportion of people who have a particular disease or attribute at a specified point in time.

period prevalence
The proportion of people known to have had a condition at any point during a specified period.

attack rate
A measure of disease occurrence used when a disease increases greatly within a population over a short period.

epidemic curve
A graphic plotting of the distribution of cases during an epidemic; sometimes called an "epi curve."

point source outbreak
A disease outbreak resulting from the exposure of a group to a noxious influence that is common to the members of the group; also called a *common source outbreak*.

Exhibit 7.3
Epidemic Curve for a Point Source Outbreak

Cryptospordiosis Cases Associated with a Child Care Center by Date of Onset in Port Yourtown, Washington, June 1998

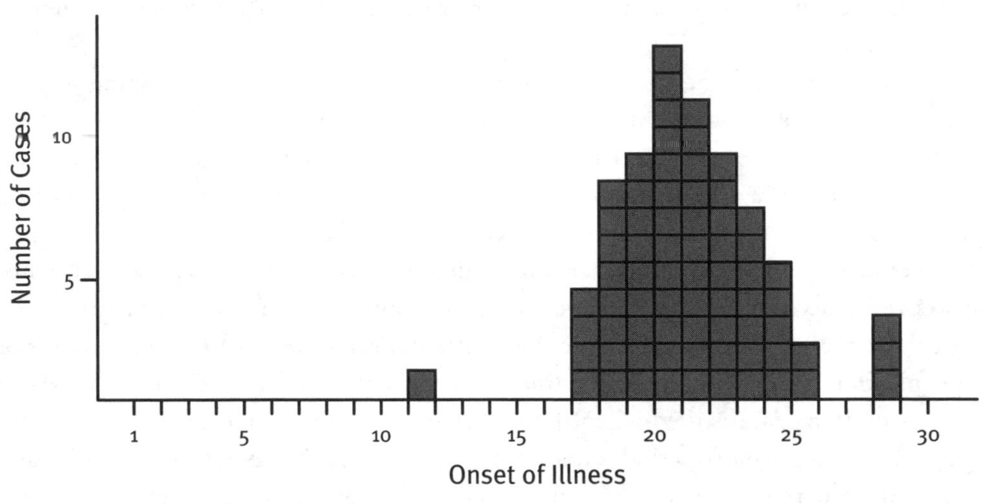

Source: Reprinted from CDC (2016a).

continuous common source outbreak
A disease outbreak in which people are exposed to the same source for a period of days, weeks, or longer.

propagated outbreak
An outbreak in which disease spreads from person to person, without a common source.

In a **continuous common source outbreak**, people are exposed to the same source, but exposure lasts for a period of days, weeks, or longer. In such cases, the epidemic curve rises more gradually and might plateau, as shown in exhibit 7.4 (CDC 2016a).

In a **propagated outbreak**, disease spreads from person to person, without a common source. The resulting epidemic curve will typically show progressively taller peaks, spaced one incubation period apart, as shown in exhibit 7.5 (CDC 2016a).

Disease Outbreak Investigation

The steps in a disease outbreak investigation, as set forth by the Centers for Disease Control and Prevention (CDC), are shown in exhibit 7.6 and described in the paragraphs that follow. The descriptions of the steps—and the specific details provided about the CDC's approach to foodborne outbreaks—highlight the interdisciplinary approach needed to keep populations safe from illness.

Step One: Detect an Outbreak

Timely detection of a disease outbreak can be difficult, especially if cases of disease are distributed over a wide area. Public health surveillance allows for the monitoring of illnesses to determine the "normal" or baseline level of disease in a given area over time. The CDC

Exhibit 7.4
Epidemic Curve for a Continuous Common Source Outbreak

Salmonellosis Cases Exposed to Contaminated Salami by Date of Onset, United States, December 2009–January 2010

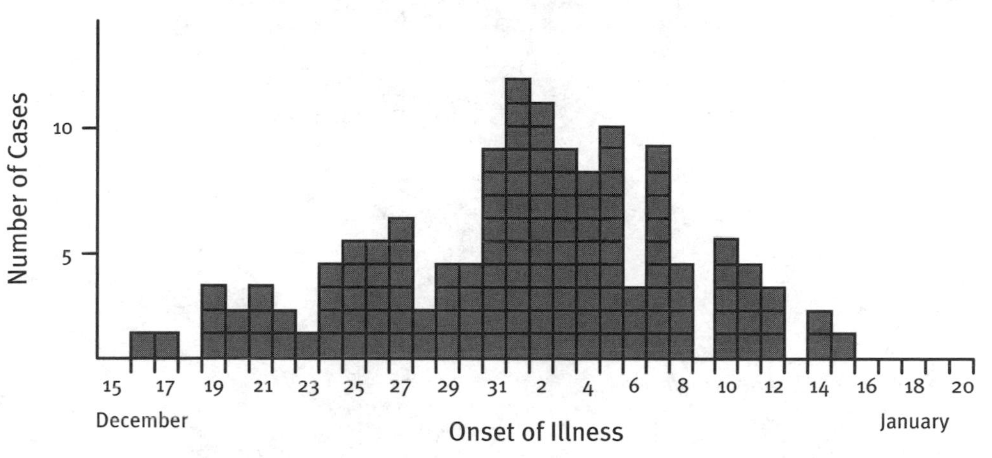

Source: Reprinted from CDC (2016a).

Exhibit 7.5
Epidemic Curve for a Propagated Outbreak

Measles Cases by Date of Onset in Aberdeen, South Dakota, October 15, 1970–January 16, 1971

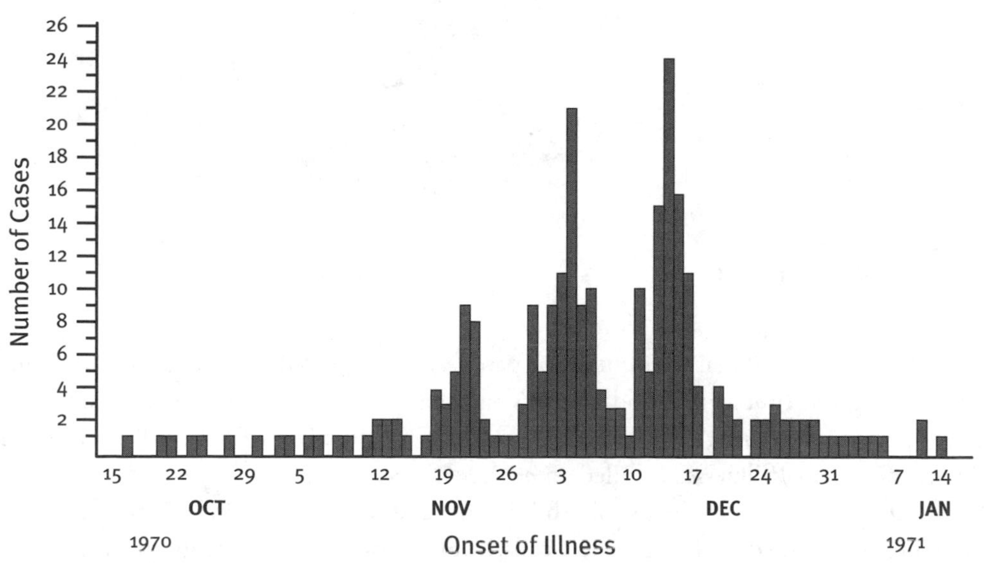

Source: Reprinted from CDC (2016a).

Exhibit 7.6 Steps in a Disease Outbreak Investigation

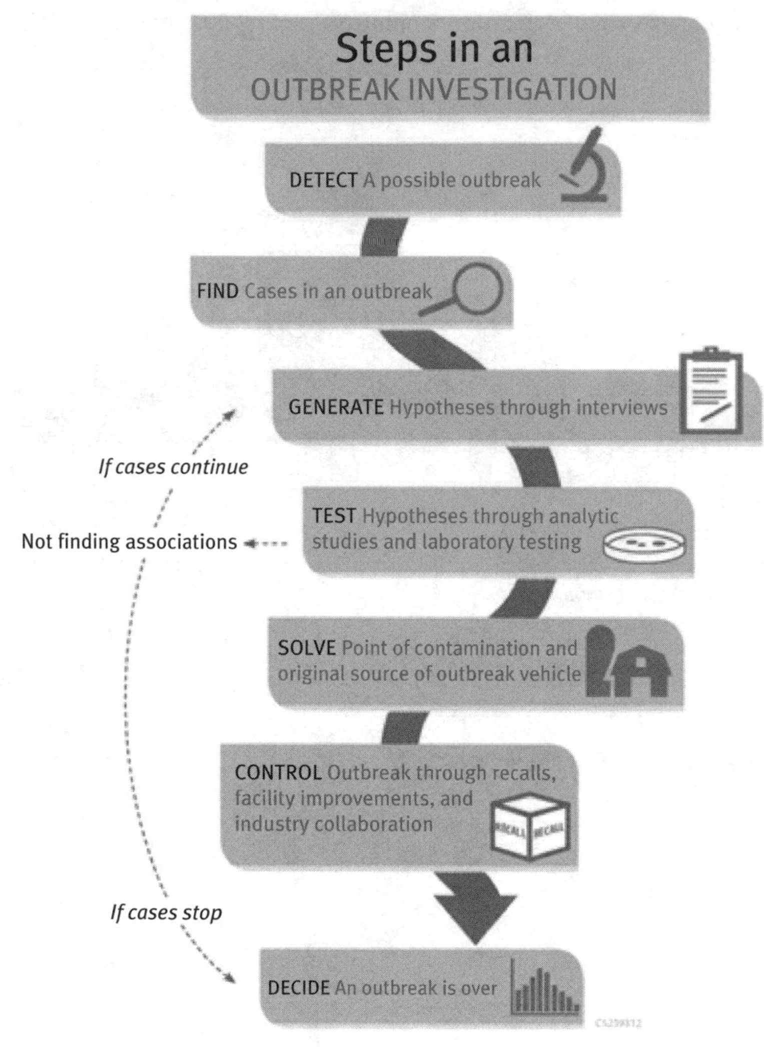

Source: Reprinted from CDC (2015d).

(2015d) explains: "If a larger number of people than expected appear to have the same illness in a given time period and area, it's called a *cluster*. When an investigation shows that ill persons in a cluster have something in common to explain why they all got the same illness, the group of illnesses is called an *outbreak*."

Detection methods include both informal and formal reporting systems. Informal reporting might involve, for instance, calls from members of a community to the local health department to report that several people became sick after eating a group dinner. Formal reporting systems include requirements that doctors and microbiologists report any cases of notifiable diseases detected among their patients. Public health officials who review disease reports might notice that the number of people with a certain illness is higher than expected, or astute clinicians might notice that they are seeing more cases of a particular illness and call the health department directly.

The CDC (2015d) provides additional detail about the processes involved in the detection of foodborne outbreaks:

> For some pathogens, like the bacteria *Salmonella* and *E. coli* O157, public health laboratories do special tests to help detect clusters that might otherwise be missed. When a doctor suspects that a patient has a foodborne illness, he or she sometimes asks the patient to submit a stool sample (or some other type of sample). The doctor's office sends the patient's sample to a clinical laboratory. The clinical laboratory may isolate a certain bacteria and identify it as *Salmonella* or *E. coli* O157, for example. The clinical laboratory tells the doctor's office what the patient has so the doctor can treat the illness, and then sends the bacteria to the state public health laboratory.
>
> The state laboratory does further subtyping tests on the bacteria including serotyping and DNA fingerprinting or pulse-field gel electrophoresis (PFGE). Serotyping identifies the specific strain of bacteria based on markers on the surface of the bacteria. When several strains have the same markers or serotype all at the same time, and there are more with that one serotype than is expected, that's a sign of a possible outbreak. DNA fingerprinting identifies the bacteria's specific genetic pattern or DNA fingerprint. Bacteria can have thousands of different patterns. State laboratories report their DNA results to the PulseNet database.
>
> Coordinated by CDC, PulseNet is the national molecular subtyping network for foodborne disease surveillance. By looking at the PulseNet database, health officials can identify clusters of illnesses caused by bacteria with the same fingerprint at the same time, even if the ill people are spread across many counties or states. This is especially useful when the number of illnesses in any one county or state is not big enough by itself to point to a possible outbreak. It can take 2 or 3 weeks from the day the person became ill to the day that the results of fingerprinting the bacteria are added to the PulseNet database.

Step Two: Find Cases

Once a possible outbreak has been detected, public health officials seek out more cases of the illness in an effort to gain insight into the outbreak's severity, size, timing, and possible causes. Officials use case definitions to determine which ill people will be classified as part of a particular outbreak. A case definition might include features of the illness, a certain pathogen (if known), a time or geographic range, and other criteria. Investigators follow the progression of an outbreak by keeping track of who becomes ill, when they become ill, and where illnesses occur (CDC 2015d).

The CDC (2015d) explains:

> Using the case definition, investigators search for more illnesses related to the outbreak. They do this by:
>
> - Reviewing regular surveillance reports
> - Reviewing laboratory reports to PulseNet
> - Asking local clinical and laboratory professionals to report cases of the particular illness more quickly, as soon as they suspect the diagnosis
> - Reviewing emergency room records for similar illnesses
> - Surveying groups that may have been exposed
> - Asking health officials in surrounding areas to watch for illnesses that might be related

Step Three: Generate Hypotheses

The third step involves developing hypotheses about the cause of disease and the manner of transmission—whether by pathogens in contaminated water, direct contact with someone who is ill, or contact with an infected animal. Hypotheses are continually refined based on information that is collected throughout the investigation (CDC 2015d).

The CDC (2015d) further describes hypothesis generation for foodborne outbreaks:

> When exposure to a food is suspected, the investigators next must consider the large number of foods that may be the source or vehicle of infection. The number of different food items is vast, so the investigation needs to narrow the list to the foods that the ill people actually ate before they got sick, and then further narrow it to the specific foods that many of the ill people remember eating. Health officials interview persons who are ill to find out where and what they ate in the days or weeks before they got sick. These interviews are called "hypothesis-generating interviews."
>
> The time period they ask about depends on the pathogen's incubation period—the time it takes to get sick after eating the contaminated food. This varies for different pathogens. Which foods they ask about depends on what investigators already know about the exposure. If several cases have occurred at a restaurant, hotel, or catered event, for instance, interviews will focus on the menu items prepared, served, or sold there. If there is no obvious place of exposure or subcluster of cases identified,

investigators may use a standardized questionnaire, also known as a "shotgun" questionnaire.

A shotgun questionnaire may include:

- Questions that ask whether a person ate any of a long list of food items
- Open-ended questions that review each meal a person ate in the days before illness began
- Questions about food shopping habits, travel, restaurant dining, and attendance at events where food was served

From the interviews, investigators create a short list of the foods and drinks that many ill persons had in common. Foods that none or very few of the sick people reported eating are considered as less likely to be the source. Investigators then look at other information, such as the results of any food testing, past experience with the suspected pathogen, and the age or ethnicities of ill persons. Based on all the information they gather, the investigators make a hypothesis about the likely source of the outbreak. However, shotgun interviews can only suggest hypotheses that are contained on the questionnaire. This approach may not lead to any refined testable hypothesis. Intensive open-ended interviews can help in this situation.

Coming up with a hypothesis is often challenging and may take time for several reasons. First, interviews of ill persons are highly dependent on their memories. The time from the start of illness to knowing that the ill person was part of an outbreak is typically about 2–3 weeks. Ill persons may not remember in detail what they ate that long ago. Also, when the contaminated food is an ingredient (such as eggs, spices or herbs, or produce in a salsa), the task becomes even harder. People often don't remember or know the ingredients of the foods they ate. These challenges may prevent a hypothesis from quickly appearing. In some cases, ill persons may be interviewed multiple times as new ideas arise about possible sources. It can sometimes be helpful to visit someone's home and look at the foods in their pantry and refrigerator, or to get their permission to review the information from their shopper cards.

A useful method for generating hypotheses in large, multistate outbreaks includes rapid and thorough investigation of restaurant clusters; these cluster investigations are critical to identifying specific food vehicles and provide detailed ingredient content and information on sources of food items for traceback investigations. However, delays inherent in the current system of surveillance for investigation of foodborne disease outbreaks contribute to the time it takes to recognize clusters.

Step Four: Test Hypotheses

Once hypotheses have been generated, they should be tested to see if they are correct. Analytic epidemiologic studies, discussed in chapter 6, are a key part of this step. The CDC (2015d) explains further:

> Case-control studies or cohort studies are the most common type of analytic study conducted so investigators can analyze information collected from ill persons and comparable well persons to see whether ill persons are more likely than people who did not get sick to have eaten a certain food or to report a particular exposure. Controls for a case-control study may be matched on geography to ensure that cases or ill persons and controls or well persons had the same opportunities for exposure to a contaminated food item. . . .
>
> If eating a particular food is reported more often by sick people than by well people, it may be associated with illness. Using statistical tests, the investigators can determine the strength of the association (i.e., how likely it is to have occurred by chance alone), and whether more than one food might be involved. Investigators look at many factors when interpreting results from these studies:
>
> - Frequencies of exposure to a specific food item
> - Strength of the statistical association
> - Dose–response relationships
> - The food's production, preparation, and service
> - The food's distribution
>
> Food testing can provide useful information and help to support a hypothesis. Finding bacteria with the same DNA fingerprint in an unopened package of food and in the stool samples of people in the outbreak can be convincing evidence of a source of illness. However, relying on food testing can also lead to results that are confusing or unhelpful. This is the case for several reasons:
>
> - Food items with a short shelf life, such as produce, are often no longer available by the time the outbreak is known, so they cannot be tested.
> - Even if the actual suspected food is available, the pathogen may be difficult to detect. This is because the pathogen may have decreased in number since the outbreak or other organisms may have overgrown the pathogen as the food started to spoil.
> - The pathogen may have been in only one portion of the food. A sample taken from a portion that was not contaminated will have a negative test result. So, a negative result does not rule out this food as a source of illness or the cause of the outbreak.

- Leftover foods or foods in open containers may have been contaminated after the outbreak or from contact with the food that actually caused the outbreak.
- Some pathogens cannot be detected in food because there is no established test that can detect the pathogen in the suspect food.

Sometimes in testing hypotheses, investigators find no statistical association between the illnesses and any particular food. This is not unusual, even when all the clues clearly point to foodborne transmission. In fact, investigators identify a specific food as the source of illness in about half of the foodborne outbreaks reported to CDC.

Not finding a link between a specific food and illness can happen for several reasons. Public health officials may have learned of the outbreak so long after it occurred that they could not do a full investigation. There may have been competing priorities or not enough staff and other resources to do a full investigation. An initial investigation may not have led to a specific food hypothesis, so no analytic study was done or the initial hypothesis could have been wrong. An analytic study may have been done, but it did not find a specific food exposure because the number of illnesses to analyze was small, because multiple food items were contaminated, or because the food was a "stealth food." Stealth foods are those that people may eat but are unlikely to remember. Examples include garnishes, condiments on sandwiches, and ingredients that are part of a food item (e.g., the filling in a snack cracker). Food testing did not find any pathogen related to the outbreak, or food testing may not have been done at all.

When no statistical association is found, it does not mean that the illness or outbreak was not foodborne. It means only that the source could not be determined. If the outbreak has ended, the source of the outbreak is declared unknown. If people are still getting sick, investigators must keep gathering information and studying results to find the food that is causing the illnesses.

Step Five: Solve the Source of the Outbreak

The testing of hypotheses will often point to a likely source that then must be investigated further. The CDC (2015d) further explains this step as it pertains to foodborne outbreaks:

> If a likely source is identified, investigators may also do an environmental assessment or evaluation to find out how the food was contaminated. The assessment could involve one food facility or several. If the people who got sick ate food prepared in only one kitchen, it is likely the contamination occurred in that kitchen. Investigators interview the people who prepared the food to find out the ingredients used, the steps followed in preparing the food, and the temperatures used to prepare and hold the food. They look at the health practices and training of the workers and at the cleanliness of the

kitchen. They also check the health status of the workers at the time the exposures took place. In a commercial or institutional kitchen, they look at past inspection reports to see if there has been a history of problems.

If an outbreak is linked to a food prepared in a number of different kitchens (like hamburgers from many stores of the same chain) or to a food that was bought from many stores and eaten without further preparation (like peanut butter), it is likely that contamination happened somewhere in the food production chain before the final kitchen. In that case, investigators do a "source traceback" to find out where contamination occurred.

Tracebacks typically start from several ill persons or restaurants to see whether and where the food production chain comes to a common point. Finding this point helps to define where contamination occurred and can help to confirm the hypothesis. Investigators ask about suppliers of the suspect food item for stores, restaurants, or cafeterias where they believe the suspect food was bought or eaten. They then ask food suppliers where they received the suspect food item from, and so on. They study purchase and shipment information to find food items that are most closely associated with the illnesses.

These steps usually involve local or state environmental health specialists. For widespread or severe outbreaks, they often involve state environmental health specialists or other state public health officials and investigators from the Food and Drug Administration (FDA), US Department of Agriculture (USDA), and CDC. Information from the environmental assessment and source traceback suggests ways to control the outbreak and prevent similar outbreaks from happening in the future.

Step Six: Control the Outbreak

Outbreak control measures are essential for protecting the health of communities, and they must be implemented swiftly to prevent additional members of the public from being exposed, becoming ill, and possibly infecting others. Prompt action involves a variety of personal health, safety, and policy considerations. The CDC (2015d) explains:

> Once a food is found to be the source of illness, control measures may be needed right away. If contaminated food stays on store shelves, in restaurant kitchens, or in home pantries, more people may get sick. Outbreak control measures might include requiring specific measures to clean and disinfect food facilities, temporarily closing a restaurant or processing plant, recalling food items, telling the public how to make the food safe or to avoid it completely, or telling consumers to throw away the suspect food from their pantry or refrigerator.
>
> Public health officials may decide on control measures on the basis of strong epidemiological evidence on the disease's origin, spread, and development. They do not need to wait for proof of contamination from the laboratory. This practice can result in

earlier action to protect the public's health. As officials learn more during the investigation, they may change, focus, or expand control measures and advice to the public.

Step Seven: Decide the Outbreak Is Over

The final step in an outbreak investigation occurs when the number of new illnesses returns to normal levels. At this point, investigators determine that the outbreak is over, though observation will typically continue. The CDC (2015d) explains:

> An outbreak ends when the number of new illnesses reported drops back to the number normally expected. The epidemic curve helps investigators see that illnesses are declining. Even when illnesses from the outbreak appear to have stopped, public health officials still continue surveillance for a few weeks to be sure cases don't start to increase again. If that happens, they continue or restart their investigation. It could be that the source was not completely controlled, or that a second contamination involving another food or location is linked to the first outbreak.

A diagram of the CDC's investigation process for foodborne outbreaks is shown in exhibit 7.7.

Exhibit 7.7 Steps in a Foodborne Outbreak Investigation

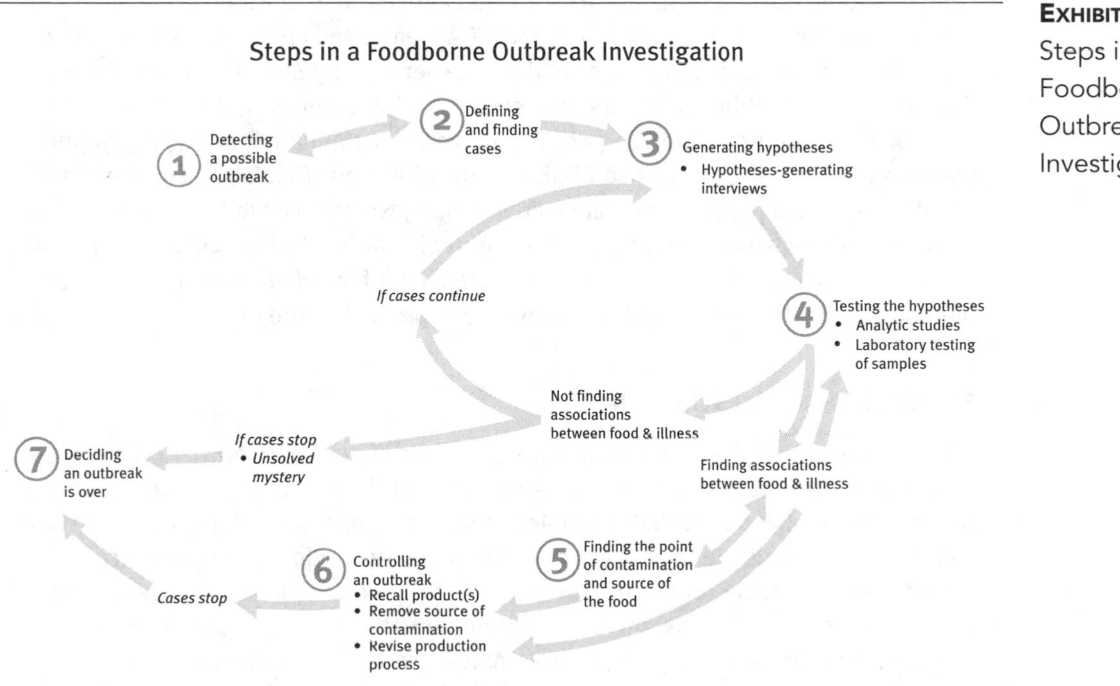

Source: Reprinted from CDC (2015d).

Case Study

Salmonella Outbreak Linked to Cucumbers

The following case study has been reproduced from the CDC (2015e). The report was originally prepared by Kristina M. Angelo, Alvina Chu, Madhu Anand, Thai-An Nguyen, Lyndsay Bottichio, Matthew Wise, Ian Williams, Sharon Seelman, Rebecca Bell, Marianne Fatica, Susan Lance, Deanna Baldwin, Kyle Shannon, Hannah Lee, Elju Trees, Errol Strain, and Laura Gieraltowski. It was published on the CDC's Morbidity and Mortality Weekly Report (MMWR) *website (www.cdc.gov/mmwr) on February 20, 2015.*

OUTBREAK OF *SALMONELLA* NEWPORT INFECTIONS LINKED TO CUCUMBERS—UNITED STATES, 2014

In August 2014, PulseNet, the national molecular subtyping network for foodborne disease surveillance, detected a multistate cluster of *Salmonella enterica* serotype Newport infections with an indistinguishable pulse-field gel electrophoresis (PFGE) pattern (*Xba*I PFGE pattern JJPX01.0061). Outbreaks of illnesses associated with this PFGE pattern have previously been linked to consumption of tomatoes harvested from Virginia's Eastern Shore in the Delmarva region and have not been linked to cucumbers or other produce items (1). To identify the contaminated food and find the source of the contamination, CDC, state and local health and agriculture departments and laboratories, and the Food and Drug Administration (FDA) conducted epidemiologic, traceback, and laboratory investigations. A total of 275 patients in 29 states and the District of Columbia were identified, with illness onsets occurring during May 20–September 30, 2014. Whole genome sequencing (WGS), a highly discriminating subtyping method, was used to further characterize PFGE pattern JJPX01.0061 isolates. Epidemiologic, microbiologic, and product traceback evidence suggests that cucumbers were a source of *Salmonella* Newport infections in this outbreak. The epidemiologic link to a novel outbreak vehicle suggests an environmental reservoir for *Salmonella* in the Delmarva region that should be identified and mitigated to prevent future outbreaks.

EPIDEMIOLOGIC INVESTIGATION

A case was defined as infection with *Salmonella* Newport with PFGE pattern JJPX01.0061 (the outbreak strain) in a person with illness onset occurring during May 20–September 30, 2014. Initial interviews of ill persons conducted by state and local health officials found that travel to the Delmarva region during the incubation period was commonly reported. A structured, focused supplemental questionnaire was developed to collect detailed information on travel and exposure to restaurants, seafood, fruit, and produce, including tomatoes, in the 7 days before illness onset. Exposure frequencies were compared with the 2006–2007 FoodNet Population Survey,

(continued)

in which healthy persons reported foods consumed in the week before interview. Information also was collected on illness subclusters, defined as two or more unrelated ill persons who reported eating at the same restaurant, attending the same event, or shopping at the same grocery store in the week before becoming ill.

A total of 275 cases were reported from 29 states and the District of Columbia (Figure 1). An additional 18 suspected cases not meeting the case definition were excluded from the analysis because they were found to be temporal outliers and unlikely to be related. Illness onset dates ranged from May 25 to September 29, 2014 (Figure 2). Median age of patients was 42 years (range=<1–90 years); 66% (174 of 265) were female. Thirty-four percent (48 of 141) were hospitalized; one death was reported in an elderly man with bacteremia. A total of 101 patients were interviewed using the supplemental questionnaire about exposures in the week before illness onset. This questionnaire focused on leafy greens and tomatoes and contained smaller sections on fruit, vegetables, and seafood common to the Delmarva region. Many patients were unreachable and did not receive the supplemental questionnaire. Sixty-two percent (49 of 79) of respondents reported eating cucumbers in the week before becoming ill. Patients were significantly more likely to report consuming cucumbers compared with respondents in the 2006–2007 FoodNet Population Survey, both for national year-round cucumber consumption (46.9% [p=0.002]) and for cucumber consumption in Maryland during the month of July (54.9% [p=0.04]). The proportion of ill persons who reported eating tomatoes, leafy greens, or any other item on the supplemental questionnaire was not significantly higher than expected compared with findings from the FoodNet Population Survey.

TRACEBACK INVESTIGATION

Officials in Maryland, Delaware, and New York worked with their FDA district offices and FDA and U.S. Department of Agriculture foodborne outbreak rapid response teams to conduct an informational (i.e., nonregulatory) traceback from retail establishments in these states to identify a point of distribution convergence for produce items (i.e., cucumbers, leafy greens, and tomatoes) consumed in nine of 12 subclusters. Each of eight establishments in Maryland and Delaware received cucumbers from a single major distributor. Preliminary traceback from the distributor to several brokers identified a common grower on Maryland's Eastern Shore in the Delmarva region. Traceback from a New York subcluster led to a different distribution chain than in Maryland and Delaware. Officials from the Maryland Department of Agriculture, the Maryland rapid response team, and the FDA Baltimore District Office visited the Maryland farm. Officials collected 48 environmental samples from areas where cucumbers were grown, harvested, and packed. Sediment and manure samples were taken from the farm. No samples yielded *Salmonella*; however, sampling was performed several months after the harvest. Records and interviews indicated that the farm applied poultry litter approximately 120 days before harvest, but it was not available for testing.

(continued)

LABORATORY INVESTIGATION

Twelve distinct illness subclusters were identified across four states, ranging in size from two to six cases. WGS was performed on 58 clinical isolates by state health departments, FDA, and CDC laboratories to further characterize the genetic relatedness of bacteria isolated from patients. Phylogenetic analysis revealed a primary group of highly related clinical isolates from cases in Delaware, Maryland, Ohio, Pennsylvania, and Virginia (median single nucleotide polymorphism distance=26 [97.5% confidence interval=1–37]). An additional group of highly related isolates from patients in New York was also identified, but this group was distinct from the primary phylogenetic group, consistent with the epidemiologic and traceback findings (single nucleotide polymorphism distance between the two phylogenetic groups=102 [97.5% confidence interval=85–114]). CDC's National Antimicrobial Resistance Monitoring System laboratory conducted antibiotic resistance testing on three isolates from ill persons with the outbreak strain. All three were susceptible to all antibiotics tested.

DISCUSSION

The epidemiologic data, traceback investigations, and whole genome sequencing all support the hypothesis that cucumbers were a likely source of *Salmonella* Newport infections in this outbreak. Cucumbers were the only food eaten by patients significantly more often than expected. Traceback investigations performed using invoices from illness subclusters in Maryland and Delaware identified a common grower of cucumbers in the Delmarva region. This is the first multistate outbreak of *Salmonella* Newport implicating a fresh produce item grown in the Delmarva region other than tomatoes. Historically, *Salmonella* Newport outbreaks associated with this PFGE pattern have been linked to red round tomatoes grown on Virginia's Eastern Shore. These outbreaks occurred in 2002 (333 persons), 2005 (72 persons), 2006 (115 persons), and 2007 (65 persons), with an additional suspected outbreak in 2010 (51 persons) (1). A definitive contamination source has not been found, and *Salmonella* Newport has not been isolated directly from any Delmarva region tomatoes. Wildlife have been evaluated as a possible source of contamination, but fecal specimens from deer, turtles, and birds have been negative and do not support the hypothesis that animals are a source (2). Other serotypes of *Salmonella* have been linked to cucumbers; most recently an outbreak of *Salmonella* Saintpaul infections was linked to imported cucumbers from Mexico in 2013 (3).

Investigating illness subclusters can provide critical clues about the source of an outbreak. Informational traceback can support the epidemiologic investigation by quickly assessing the plausibility of one or more vehicles as the source of the outbreak. Informational traceback generally can be completed much more quickly than regulatory traceback, which requires the collection of specific types of records, such as receipts, invoices, and bills of lading, at each step of the distribution chain. In this investigation, the informational traceback quickly provided a critical clue that suggested cucumbers were a likely source in the outbreak.

(continued)

Consultation with independent industry experts early in an outbreak investigation also can provide important clues to help focus the investigation on certain suspected foods. Because of the suspicion that this outbreak was caused by a novel vehicle for this *Salmonella* Newport PFGE pattern, an industry consultation was held on September 11, 2014, with three independent experts from the produce industry to obtain information regarding cucumber harvesting and distribution on the Delmarva region. The consultants provided information regarding crop production and distribution practices that also helped assess the plausibility of cucumbers as an outbreak vehicle.

Advanced molecular detection methods, including WGS, might improve discrimination of subclusters during outbreak investigations. WGS data from the subclusters in this investigation demonstrated a phylogenetic link between clinical isolates from the eight Maryland and Delaware subclusters, in addition to differentiating these clusters from a subcluster in New York. The significance of this differentiation remains unclear at this time but might suggest that some of the illnesses in New York were not related to consumption of cucumbers from the Delmarva region. This is also supported by the informational traceback from the New York establishment, which led to a different distribution chain than those of the Maryland and Delaware establishments.

The findings in this report are subject to at least two limitations. First, no case-control study was performed because illness subclusters were small. Second, not all patients in the subclusters were systematically asked about cucumber consumption.

This outbreak supports the continued evaluation of farm practices by FDA as a part of the development of a Produce Safety Rule. These evaluations include conducting a risk assessment and working with the US Department of Agriculture and other stakeholders. It also includes performing research to strengthen scientific support for determining appropriate intervals between application of raw manure fertilizer and harvest. The Maryland Department of Agriculture plans additional assessments in the Delmarva region before the 2015 planting season to determine whether additional or alternative "best practices" can be implemented.

Given the typical shelf life of cucumbers is 10–14 days, cucumbers from the implicated grower are no longer available for purchase or in person's homes. Consumers and retailers should always follow safe produce handling recommendations. Cucumbers, like all produce, should be washed thoroughly, scrubbed with a clean produce brush before peeling or cutting, and refrigerated as soon as possible to prevent multiplication of bacteria such as *Salmonella*.

ACKNOWLEDGMENTS

William Wolfgang, PhD, David Nicholas, MPH, New York State Department of Health. David Blythe, MD, Maryland Department of Mental Health and Hygiene. Kate Heiman, MPH, Division of Foodborne, Waterborne, and Environmental Diseases, National Center for Emerging and Zoonotic Infectious Diseases, CDC.

(continued)

REFERENCES

1. Bennett SD, Litterell KW, Hill TA, Mahovic M, Behravesh CB. Multistate foodborne disease outbreaks associated with raw tomatoes, United States, 1990–2010: a recurring public health problem. Epidemiol Infect 2014;August 28:1–8 [Epub ahead of print].
2. Gruszynski K, Pao S, Kim C, et al. Evaluating wildlife as a potential source of *Salmonella* serotype Newport (JJPX01.0061) contamination for tomatoes on the Eastern Shore of Virginia. Zoonoses Public Health 2014;61:202–7.
3. CDC. Multistate outbreak of *Salmonella* Saintpaul infections linked to imported cucumbers (final update). Available at http://www.cdc.gov/salmonella/saintpaul-04-13/index.html.

WHAT IS ALREADY KNOWN ON THIS TOPIC?

Salmonella is the most common bacterial cause of foodborne disease in the United States and results in the highest number of hospitalizations and deaths among foodborne pathogens. *Salmonella* Newport has historically been a common cause of tomato-associated outbreaks in the United States. The Virginia Eastern Shore in the Delmarva region has been the site of multiple outbreaks of *Salmonella* Newport infection in recent years.

WHAT IS ADDED BY THIS REPORT?

In August 2014, a multistate cluster of *Salmonella enterica* serotype Newport infections with an indistinguishable pulse-field gel electrophoresis (PFGE) pattern (*Xba*I PFGE pattern JJPX01.0061) was detected, involving 275 patients in 29 states and the District of Columbia with illness onsets occurring during May 20 and September 30. Epidemiologic, product traceback, and laboratory evidence implicated cucumbers. Whole genome sequencing, used to subtype the isolates, and the traceback investigation suggested that some, but not all, of the contaminated cucumbers were from a farm in Maryland. No *Salmonella* was isolated from environmental samples taken at the farm.

WHAT ARE THE IMPLICATIONS FOR PUBLIC HEALTH PRACTICE?

The epidemiologic link to a novel outbreak vehicle from the Delmarva region, cucumbers, suggests an environmental reservoir for *Salmonella* that might also include both the Virginia and Maryland portions of the Delmarva region. Federal, state, and local public health and regulatory authorities should focus on identifying and mitigating this potential environmental reservoir to prevent future outbreaks.

(continued)

FIGURE 1: Number of persons (N = 275) infected with the outbreak strain of *Salmonella* Newport, by state—United States, May 20–September 30, 2014

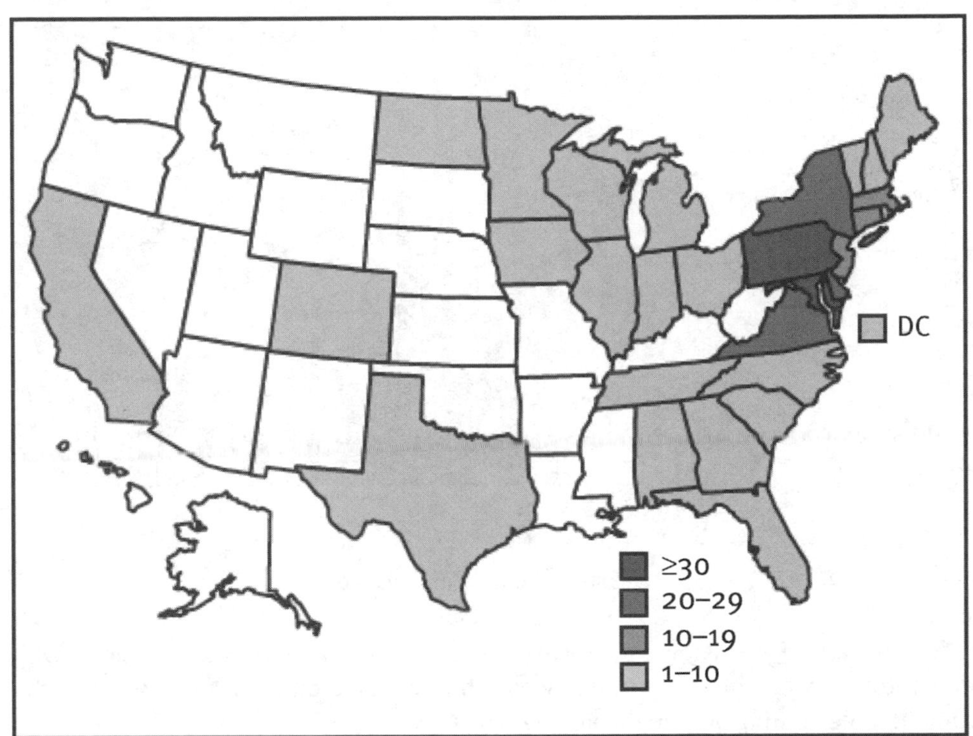

The figure above is a map of the United States showing the number of persons infected with the outbreak strain of *Salmonella* Newport, by state, in the United States during May 20–September 30, 2014. A total of 275 cases were reported from 29 states and the District of Columbia.

(continued)

FIGURE 2: Number of persons (N = 275) infected with the outbreak strain of *Salmonella* Newport, by estimated date of illness onset—United States, May 20–September 30, 2014

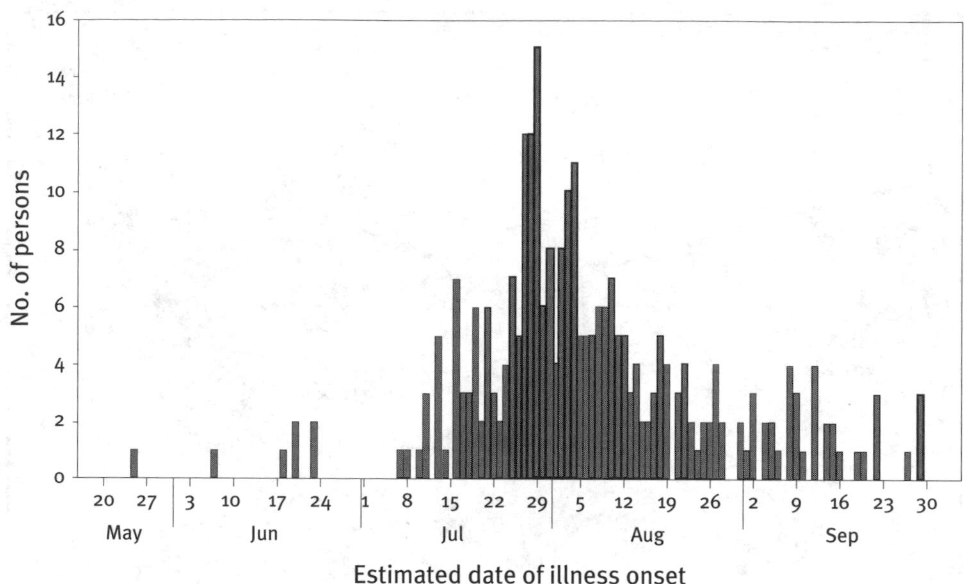

The figure above is a histogram showing the number of persons (N=275) infected with the outbreak strain of *Salmonella* Newport, by estimated date of illness onset, in the United States during May 20–September 30, 2014.

CASE STUDY DISCUSSION QUESTIONS

1. Identify the steps taken to identify the source of contamination.
2. What kind of epidemic curve is illustrated in this case study? Explain.

Emerging Infectious Diseases

One of the key issues facing the public health and healthcare systems this century is the impact of emerging infectious diseases on the health of populations. The CDC (2014) categorizes diseases as "emerging" if their incidence among humans has increased in the last two decades or threatens to increase in the near future. Emerging infectious diseases are not held within national boundaries, and they test our ability to prepare for the unknown. Types of emerging infectious diseases include the following (CDC 2014):

- New infections resulting from changes or evolution of existing organisms
- Known infections spreading to new areas or populations
- Previously unrecognized infections appearing in areas undergoing ecologic transformation
- Old infections reemerging as a result of antimicrobial resistance in known agents or breakdowns in public health measures

Examples of emerging infectious diseases in recent decades have included HIV/AIDS, severe acute respiratory syndrome (SARS), and the 2009 H1N1 influenza pandemic (Morens and Fauci 2013). Emerging vector-borne diseases have included West Nile virus, Lyme disease, and Rocky Mountain spotted fever. Examples of emerging zoonotic diseases—that is, diseases that can be passed between animals and humans—have included hantavirus pulmonary syndrome and rabies (CDC 2013). Factors responsible for the emergence and reemergence of infectious diseases include international trade and travel, microbial adaptation, human susceptibility to infection, inappropriate use of antibiotics contributing to antibiotic resistance, change in climate and ecosystems, poverty, societal inequality, proximity of animal populations to humans, insufficient public health services, war and famine, and a lack of political will to address these issues (Morens and Fauci 2013).

The information made available by the CDC about Bourbon virus, a disease discovered for the first time in 2014, highlights the difficulty and uncertainty in trying to control a newly emerging disease (CDC 2015a):

What is Bourbon virus?
Bourbon virus belongs to a group of viruses called thogotoviruses. Viruses in this group are found all over the world. A few of these viruses can cause people to get sick.

How do people get infected with Bourbon virus?
We do not yet fully know how people become infected with Bourbon virus. However, based on what we know about similar viruses, it is likely that Bourbon virus is spread through tick or other insect bites.

Where have cases of Bourbon virus disease occurred?
As of February 12, 2015, only one case of Bourbon virus disease had been identified in eastern Kansas in late spring 2014. The man who was infected later died. At this time, we do not know if the virus might be found in other areas of the United States.

What are the symptoms of Bourbon virus?
Because there has been only one case identified thus far, scientists are still learning about possible symptoms caused by this new virus. In the one person who was

diagnosed with Bourbon virus disease, symptoms included fever, tiredness, rash, headache, other body aches, nausea, and vomiting. The person also had low blood counts for cells that fight infection and help prevent bleeding.

Who is at risk for infection with Bourbon virus?
People likely become infected with Bourbon virus when they are bitten by a tick or other insect. Therefore, people who do not take steps to protect themselves from tick or insect bites when they work or spend time outside may be more likely to be infected.

How can people reduce the chance of becoming infected with Bourbon virus?
There is no vaccine or drug to prevent or treat Bourbon virus disease. Therefore, preventing bites from ticks and other insects may be the best way to prevent infection. Here are ways to protect yourself from tick and other bug bites when you are outdoors:

- Use insect repellents
- Wear long sleeves and pants
- Avoid bushy and wooded areas
- Perform thorough tick checks after spending time outdoors

Case Study

Zika Virus

The following case study has been reproduced from the CDC (2016b). The report was originally prepared by Emilio Dirlikov, Kyle R. Ryff, Jomil Torres-Aponte, Dana L. Thomas, Janice Perez-Padilla, Jorge Munoz-Jordan, Elba V. Caraballo, Myriam Garcia, Marangely Olivero Segarra, Graciela Malave, Regina M. Simeone, Carrie K. Shapiro-Mendoza, Lourdes Romero Reyes, Francisco Alvarado-Ramy, Angela F. Harris, Aidsa Rivera, Chelsea G. Major, Marrielle Mayshack, Luisa I. Alvarado, Audrey Lenhart, Miguel Valencia-Prado, Steve Waterman, Tyler M. Sharp, and Brenda Rivera-Garcia. It was posted on the CDC's MMWR *website (www.cdc.gov/mmwr) on April 29, 2016.*

UPDATE: ONGOING ZIKA VIRUS TRANSMISSION—PUERTO RICO, NOVEMBER 1, 2015–APRIL 14, 2016

Zika virus is a flavivirus transmitted primarily by *Aedes* species mosquitoes, and symptoms of infection can include rash, fever, arthralgia, and conjunctivitis (1). Zika virus

(continued)

infection during pregnancy is a cause of microcephaly and other severe brain defects (2). Infection has also been associated with Guillain-Barré syndrome (3). In December 2015, Puerto Rico became the first US jurisdiction to report local transmission of Zika virus, with the index patient reporting symptom onset on November 23, 2015 (4). This report provides an update to the epidemiology of and public health response to ongoing Zika virus transmission in Puerto Rico. During November 1, 2015–April 14, 2016, a total of 6,157 specimens from suspected Zika virus–infected patients were evaluated by the Puerto Rico Department of Health (PRDH) and CDC Dengue Branch (which is located in San Juan, Puerto Rico), and 683 (11%) had laboratory evidence of current or recent Zika virus infection by one or more tests: reverse transcription–polymerase chain reaction (RT-PCR) or immunoglobulin M (IgM) enzyme-linked immunosorbent assay (ELISA). Zika virus–infected patients resided in 50 (64%) of 78 municipalities in Puerto Rico. Median age was 34 years (range=35 days–89 years). The most frequently reported signs and symptoms were rash (74%), myalgia (68%), headache (63%), fever (63%), and arthralgia (63%). There were 65 (10%) symptomatic pregnant women who tested positive by RT-PCR or IgM ELISA. A total of 17 (2%) patients required hospitalization, including 5 (1%) patients with suspected Guillain-Barré syndrome. One (<1%) patient died after developing severe thrombocytopenia. The public health response to the outbreak has included increased laboratory capacity to test for Zika virus infection (including blood donor screening), implementation of enhanced surveillance systems, and prevention activities focused on pregnant women. Vector control activities include indoor and outdoor residual spraying and reduction of mosquito breeding environments focused around pregnant women's homes. Residents of and travelers to Puerto Rico should continue to employ mosquito bite avoidance behaviors, take precautions to reduce the risk for sexual transmission (5), and seek medical care for any acute illness with rash or fever.

EPIDEMIOLOGIC SURVEILLANCE

In response to the introduction of Zika virus, PRDH and CDC Dengue Branch incorporated Zika virus case reporting and diagnostic testing into existing dengue and chikungunya virus surveillance systems and developed a laboratory-based Passive Arboviral Diseases Surveillance System. Health providers submit serum specimens to PRDH from patients with a clinical suspicion of Zika, chikungunya, or dengue virus infection using a case report form. Depending on the number of days between onset of illness and specimen collection, specimens are tested for the three arboviruses by a Trioplex RT-PCR assay, for evidence of Zika and dengue virus infection by IgM ELISA, or by both assays (4). Zika virus–infected patients were defined by positive results from either RT-PCR (confirmed) or IgM ELISA with negative dengue virus IgM ELISA (presumptive positive). Zika virus testing has been incorporated into the Sentinel Enhanced Dengue Surveillance System, which tests specimens from all febrile patients treated at either one outpatient clinic or one hospital emergency department in Ponce. Tissue and blood specimens collected during autopsy from patients who died after an acute febrile

(continued)

illness are tested for Zika virus infection through the Enhanced Fatal Acute Febrile Illness Surveillance System. Following CDC interim guidance (6), symptomatic pregnant women are tested using the diagnostic algorithm, and asymptomatic pregnant women are tested for evidence of Zika and dengue virus infection by IgM ELISA. Initiated in February 2016, the Guillain-Barré syndrome Passive Surveillance System allows health providers from across the island to report clinically suspected Guillain-Barré syndrome cases by sending a case report form and serum specimen to PRDH. Specimens from patients with suspected Guillain-Barré syndrome are tested by both RT-PCR and IgM ELISA for all three arboviruses. Diagnostic test results are managed through an Integrated data management system. Results are reported to providers, and aggregate data are available online in a weekly arboviral report.

During November 1, 2015–April 14, 2016, specimens from 6,157 suspected arbovirus-infected patients were evaluated and 683 (11%) were either laboratory-confirmed or presumptive positive for Zika virus infection (Table). Of these 683 Zika virus laboratory confirmed or presumptive patients, 581 (85%) were confirmed by RT-PCR, 73 (11%) were presumptive positive by IgM ELISA, and 29 (4%) were positive by both RT-PCR and IgM ELISA. Dengue, chikungunya, or unspecified flavivirus infection was identified in 110 (2%), 61 (1%), and 32 (<1%) suspected arbovirus-infected patients, respectively. No patients with evidence of coinfection with Zika, dengue, or chikungunya viruses were identified by RT-PCR. Of all identified Zika virus–infected patients, 646 (95%) were reported to the Passive Arboviral Diseases Surveillance System. Thirty-two (5%) Zika virus–infected patients were reported through the Sentinel Enhanced Dengue Surveillance System. Five (1%) suspected cases of Guillain-Barré syndrome reported to the Guillain-Barré syndrome Passive Surveillance System were presumptive positive for Zika virus infection, and two had unspecified flavivirus infection.

Weekly Zika virus disease case counts gradually increased since late November 2015, whereas incidence of dengue and chikungunya cases remained comparatively low (Figure 1). Zika virus–infected patients were reported from 50 (64%) of the 78 total municipalities (Figure 2); 146 (21%) patients were residents of the San Juan metropolitan area. Among all identified Zika virus–infected patients, 436 (64%) were female, and median age was 34 years (range=35 days–89 years). The most frequently reported signs and symptoms were rash (74%), myalgia (68%), headache (63%), fever (63%), and arthralgia (63%). Thrombocytopenia (defined as blood platelets levels <100,000 cells/mm^3) was reported in nine (1%) cases. Sixty-five (10%) symptomatic pregnant women were Zika virus–infected patients. Seventeen (2%) patients required hospitalization, including five (1%) suspected Guillain-Barré syndrome cases. In one (<1%) identified Zika virus–associated case, the patient died of complications related to severe thrombocytopenia.

To ensure the safety of the blood supply, Puerto Rico imported all blood products from the United States during March 5–April 14 (7). On April 2, blood collection resumed with donor screening using a Food and Drug Administration–approved Zika virus investigational nucleic acid detection test (Roche Molecular Systems, Inc.,

(continued)

Pleasanton, California). Emergency blood imports ended on April 15. During April 2–14, nine (<1%) of 1,910 screened donated blood units had positive test results. These units were removed from the blood supply, and testing is pending to confirm presumptive Zika virus infection.

PUBLIC HEALTH RESPONSE

Through the Zika Active Pregnancy Surveillance System, Zika virus–infected pregnant women and their offspring are monitored for adverse maternal, fetal, neonatal, infant, and child health outcomes. Surviving offspring across the island will be referred to the Children with Special Health Care Needs program for developmental surveillance and coordination of specialized services, as needed, up to age 3 years. The Birth Defects Surveillance System will identify newborns with congenital microcephaly, including those born to women infected with Zika virus during pregnancy, and refer all cases to Avanzando Juntos, Puerto Rico's Early Intervention Services System.

With CDC's assistance, PRDH has also implemented comprehensive strategies to prevent Zika virus transmission. Health messaging, including posters and electronic monitors, have been implemented and health education materials are available at various locations, including health care facilities and ports of entry. Community intervention strategies have focused on pregnant women. PRDH has worked closely with Women, Infants, and Children (WIC) clinics, where 90% of Puerto Rican pregnant women received services in 2015 (Dana Miró Medina, WIC Puerto Rico, personal communication, 2016). As of April 13, a total of 13,351 pregnant women participated in Zika virus educational orientations offered by WIC clinics. PRDH and the CDC Foundation financed the purchase and delivery of Zika Prevention Kits, which include locally adapted health information, mosquito repellent, a bed net, larvicidal tablets (tablets placed in water sources where mosquitoes might breed that prevent larvae from maturating into adults), and condoms. In addition, to reduce the risk for unintended pregnancies with adverse fetal outcomes related to Zika virus infection, the response includes increasing the availability of contraceptives (8).

During February–March, an insecticide resistance study of *Aedes aegypti* mosquitoes was conducted to develop vector control strategies, such as truck-mounted, ultra-low volume spraying and indoor and outdoor residual spraying. Mosquitoes from across Puerto Rico were tested using the CDC bottle bioassay to determine insecticide susceptibility, particularly against pyrethroids. Results indicated a high degree of geographical variation with respect to susceptibility to insecticides, and deltamethrin was identified as the most suitable pyrethroid candidate for use in vector control programs (data not shown). Insecticide susceptibility surveillance is ongoing.

A home-based vector control program focused on pregnant women is underway. Women are contacted through WIC clinics, and are offered source reduction services (e.g., removal of water containers that can serve as mosquito breeding sites), larvicide application, and indoor and outdoor residual spraying using deltamethrin. PRDH and

(continued)

CDC have collaborated with the Puerto Rico Department of Housing to incorporate these services into its vector control activities.

DISCUSSION

Zika virus remains a public health challenge in Puerto Rico, and cases are expected to continue to occur throughout 2016. Building upon existing dengue and chikungunya virus surveillance systems, PRDH collaborated with CDC to establish a comprehensive surveillance system to characterize the incidence and epidemiology of Zika virus disease on the island. Expanded laboratory capacity and surveillance provided timely availability of data, allowing for continuous analysis and adapted public health response. Following CDC guidelines, both symptomatic and asymptomatic pregnant women are tested for evidence of Zika virus infection. Information from the Zika Active Pregnancy Surveillance System will be used to raise awareness about the complications associated with Zika virus during pregnancy, encourage prevention through use of mosquito repellent and other methods, and inform health care providers of the additional care needed by women infected with Zika virus during pregnancy, as well as congenitally exposed fetuses and children. In addition, the prevalence of adverse fetal outcomes documented through this system can be compared with baseline rates as further evidence of associations between Zika virus infections and adverse outcomes, such as microcephaly (2).

The finding that women constitute the majority of cases might be attributable to targeted outreach and testing. The most common symptoms among Zika virus disease cases were rash, myalgia, headache, fever, and arthralgia, which are similar to the most common signs and symptoms reported elsewhere in the Americas (9). Although Zika virus–associated deaths are rare (10), the first identified death in Puerto Rico highlights the possibility of severe cases, as well as the need for continued outreach to raise health care providers' awareness of complications that might lead to severe disease or death. To ensure continued blood safety, blood collection resumed with a donor screening program for Zika virus infection, and all units screened positive are removed.

Residents of and travelers to Puerto Rico should continue to employ mosquito bite avoidance behaviors, including using mosquito repellents, wearing long-sleeved shirts and pants, and ensuring homes are properly enclosed (e.g., screening windows and doors, closing windows, and using air conditioning) to avoid bites while indoors. To reduce the risk for sexual transmission, especially to pregnant women, precautions should include consistent and proper use of condoms or abstinence (5). Such measures can also help avoid unintended pregnancies and minimize risk for fetal Zika virus infection (6). Clinicians who suspect Zika virus disease in patients who reside in or have recently returned from areas with ongoing Zika virus transmission should report cases to public health officials.

(continued)

ACKNOWLEDGMENTS

Kathryn Conlon, PhD, National Center for Environmental Health, CDC.

REFERENCES

1. Petersen LR, Jamieson DJ, Powers AM, Honein MA. Zika virus. N Engl J Med 2016;374:1552–63.
2. Rasmussen SA, Jamieson DJ, Honein MA, Petersen LR. Zika virus and birth defects—reviewing the evidence for causality. N Engl J Med 2016. Epub April 13, 2016. http://www.nejm.org/doi/full/10.1056/NEJMsr1604338http://www.ncbi.nlm.nih.gov/entrez/query.fcgi?cmd=Retrieve&db=PubMed&list_uids=27074377&dopt=Abstract
3. Cao-Lormeau VM, Blake A, Mons S, et al. Guillain-Barré syndrome outbreak associated with Zika virus infection in French Polynesia: a case-control study. Lancet 2016;387:1531–9.
4. Thomas DL, Sharp TM, Torres J, et al. Local transmission of Zika virus—Puerto Rico, November 23, 2015-January 28, 2016. MMWR Morb Mortal Wkly Rep 2016;65:154–8.
5. Oster AM, Russell K, Stryker JE, et al. Update: interim guidance for prevention of sexual transmission of Zika virus—United States, 2016. MMWR Morb Mortal Wkly Rep 2016;65:323–5.
6. Petersen EE, Polen KN, Meaney-Delman D, et al. Update: interim guidance for health care providers caring for women of reproductive age with possible Zika virus exposure—United States, 2016. MMWR Morb Mortal Wkly Rep 2016;65:315–22.
7. Vasquez AM, Sapiano MR, Basavaraju SV, Kuehnert MJ, Rivera-Garcia B. Survey of blood collection centers and implementation of guidance for prevention of transfusion-transmitted Zika virus infection—Puerto Rico, 2016. MMWR Morb Mortal Wkly Rep 2016;65:375–8.
8. Tepper NK, Goldberg HI, Bernal MI, et al. Estimating contraceptive needs and increasing access to contraception in response to the Zika virus disease outbreak—Puerto Rico, 2016. MMWR Morb Mortal Wkly Rep 2016;65:311–4.
9. Brasil P, Calvet GA, Siqueira AM, et al. Zika virus outbreak in Rio de Janeiro, Brazil: clinical characterization, epidemiological and virological aspects. PLoS Negl Trop Dis 2016;10:e0004636.
10. Sarmiento-Ospina A, Vásquez-Serna H, Jimenez-Canizales CE, Villamil-Gómez WE, Rodriguez-Morales AJ. Zika virus associated deaths in Colombia. Lancet Infect Dis 2016;16:523–4.

(continued)

TABLE: Demographic characteristics, clinical course, and signs and symptoms of patients* with Zika virus disease (N = 683)—Puerto Rico, November 1, 2015–April 14, 2016

Characteristic	No. of patients (%)
History of recent travel[†]	4 (1)
Female	436 (64)
Pregnant	65 (10)
Hospitalized	17 (2)
Suspected GBS[§]	5 (1)
Thrombocytopenia[¶]	9 (1)
Deaths	1 (<1)
Signs and symptoms**	
Rash	505 (74)
Myalgia	462 (68)
Headache	433 (63)
Fever	429 (63)
Arthralgia	428 (63)
Eye pain	350 (51)
Chills	344 (50)
Sore throat	233 (34)
Petechiae	213 (31)
Conjunctivitis	137 (20)
Nausea/Vomiting	123 (18)
Diarrhea	115 (17)

Abbreviation: GBS = Guillain-Barré syndrome.

* Patients were aged 35 days–89 years (median age = 34 years).

[†] Travel outside of Puerto Rico and the United States in the 14 days before illness onset.

[§] All GBS patients were hospitalized.

[¶] Defined as blood platelets levels <100,000 cells/mm^3.

** Signs and symptoms were reported by the patients' clinician.

(continued)

FIGURE 1: Cases of Zika virus disease (n = 683), dengue (n = 110), and chikungunya (n = 61) by week of onset of patient's illness—Puerto Rico, November 1, 2015–April 14, 2016

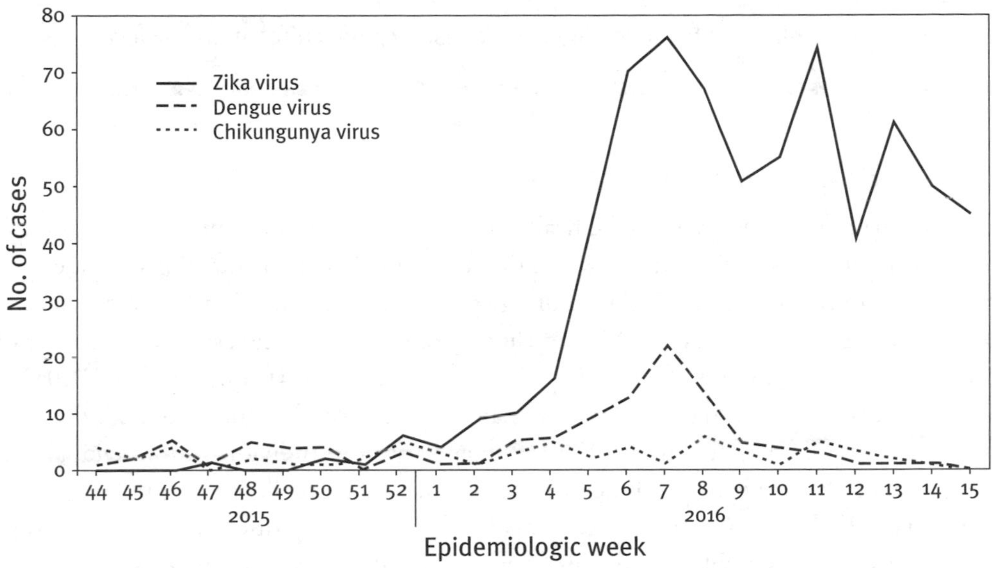

FIGURE 2: Municipality of residence of persons with Zika virus disease (n = 679)*—Puerto Rico, November 1, 2015–April 14, 2016

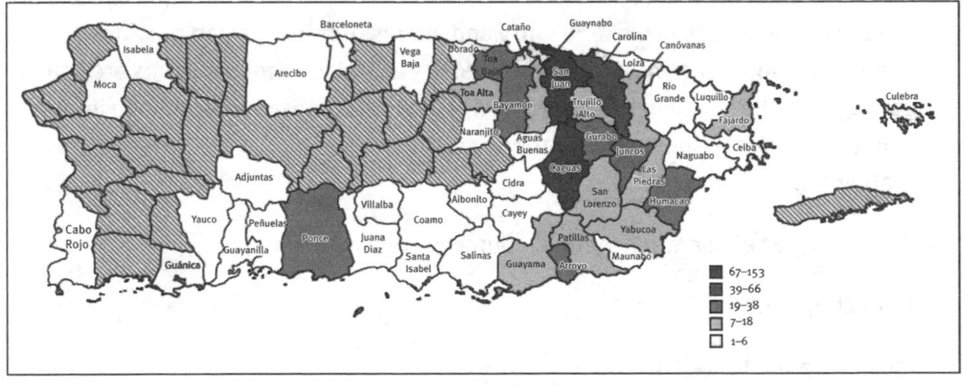

* Four cases were reported with unknown municipality of residence.

(continued)

CASE STUDY DISCUSSION QUESTIONS

1. What is the current understanding of the transmission and prevention of the Zika virus?
2. Explain the public health implications of the research described in the article.

Public Health Interventions

Investment in local and state public health infrastructure is important for educating the population about infectious diseases, conducting surveillance of infectious disease outbreaks, and implementing control measures to prevent further infection. Diseases typically progress in the manner shown in the timeline in exhibit 7.8. A disease's usual manner of progression in the absence of treatment is called its **natural history**. The CDC (2012a) states: "Many, if not most, diseases have a characteristic natural history, although the time frame and specific manifestations of disease may vary from individual to individual and are influenced by preventive and therapeutic measures." The challenge for public health is to intervene and prevent exposure to agents capable of causing disease. And in the event that exposure occurs, public health works with the healthcare system to detect the disease at the earliest possible stage.

natural history
A disease's usual manner of progression in the absence of treatment.

The CDC (2012b) provides additional details about interventions by the public health system at various stages in the progression of a disease to minimize the effects of disease and the development of disability:

> Knowledge of the portals of exit and entry and modes of transmission provides a basis for determining appropriate control measures. In general, control measures are usually directed against the segment in the infection chain that is most susceptible to intervention, unless practical issues dictate otherwise.
>
> Interventions are directed at:
>
> - Controlling or eliminating agent at source of transmission
> - Protecting portals of entry
> - Increasing host's defenses
>
> For some diseases, the most appropriate intervention may be directed at controlling or eliminating the agent at its source. A patient sick with a communicable disease may be treated with antibiotics to eliminate the infection. An asymptomatic but infected person may be treated both to clear the infection and to reduce the risk of transmission to others. In the community, soil may be decontaminated or covered to prevent escape of the agent.

Exhibit 7.8 Timeline for the Natural Progression of Disease

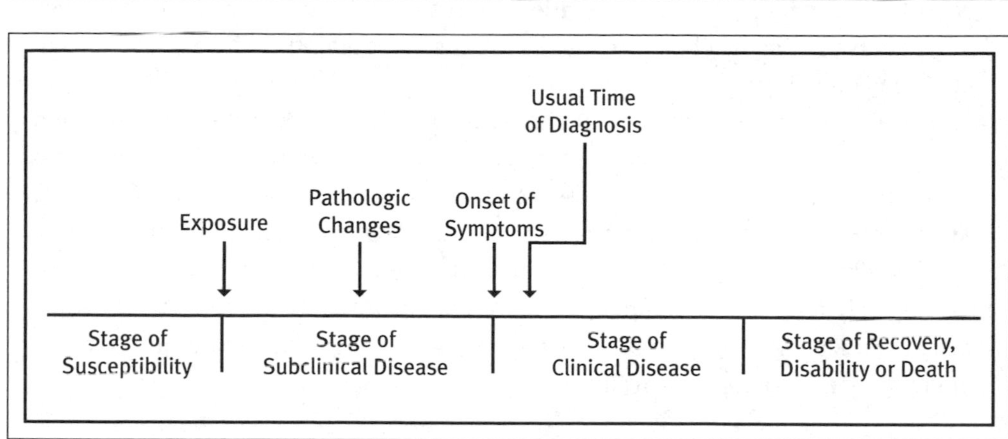

Source: Reprinted from CDC (2012a).

Some interventions are directed at the mode of transmission. Interruption of direct transmission may be accomplished by isolation of someone with infection, or counseling persons to avoid the specific type of contact associated with transmission. Vehicle-borne transmission may be interrupted by elimination or decontamination of the vehicle. To prevent fecal-oral transmission, efforts often focus on rearranging the environment to reduce the risk of contamination in the future and on changing behaviors, such as promoting handwashing. For airborne diseases, strategies may be directed at modifying ventilation or air pressure, and filtering or treating the air. To interrupt vector-borne transmission, measures may be directed toward controlling the vector population, such as spraying to reduce the mosquito population.

Some strategies that protect portals of entry are simple and effective. For example, bed nets are used to protect sleeping persons from being bitten by mosquitoes that may transmit malaria. A dentist's mask and gloves are intended to protect the dentist from a patient's blood, secretions, and droplets, as well to protect the patient from the dentist. Wearing of long pants and sleeves and use of insect repellent are recommended to reduce the risk of Lyme disease and West Nile virus infection, which are transmitted by the bite of ticks and mosquitoes, respectively.

Some interventions aim to increase a host's defenses. Vaccinations promote development of specific antibodies that protect against infection. On the other hand, prophylactic use of antimalarial drugs, recommended for visitors to malaria-endemic areas, does not prevent exposure through mosquito bites, but does prevent infection from taking root.

Finally, some interventions attempt to prevent a pathogen from encountering a susceptible host. The concept of herd immunity suggests that if a high enough proportion of individuals in a population are resistant to an agent, then those few who are susceptible will be protected by the resistant majority, since the pathogen will be unlikely to "find" those few susceptible individuals. The degree of herd immunity necessary to prevent or interrupt an outbreak varies by disease. In theory, herd immunity means that not everyone in a community needs to be resistant (immune) to prevent disease spread and occurrence of an outbreak. In practice, herd immunity has not prevented outbreaks of measles and rubella in populations with immunization levels as high as 85% to 90%. One problem is that, in highly immunized populations, the relatively few susceptible persons are often clustered in subgroups defined by socioeconomic or cultural factors. If the pathogen is introduced into one of these subgroups, an outbreak may occur.

Case Study

Measles Outbreak

The following case study has been reproduced from the CDC (2015c). The report was originally prepared by Jennifer Zipprich, Kathleen Winter, Jill Hacker, Dongxiang Xia, James Watt, and Kathleen Harriman. It was posted on the CDC's MMWR *website (www.cdc.gov/mmwr) on February 13, 2015.*

MEASLES OUTBREAK—CALIFORNIA, DECEMBER 2014–FEBRUARY 2015

On January 5, 2015, the California Department of Public Health (CDPH) was notified about a suspected measles case. The patient was a hospitalized, unvaccinated child, aged 11 years with rash onset on December 28. The only notable travel history during the exposure period was a visit to one of two adjacent Disney theme parks located in Orange County, California. On the same day, CDPH received reports of four additional suspected measles cases in California residents and two in Utah residents, all of whom reported visiting one or both Disney theme parks during December 17–20. By January 7, seven California measles cases had been confirmed, and CDPH issued a press release and an Epidemic Information Exchange (Epi-X) notification to other states regarding this outbreak. Measles transmission is ongoing (Figure).

As of February 11, a total of 125 measles cases with rash occurring during December 28, 2014–February 8, 2015, had been confirmed in US residents connected with this outbreak. Of these, 110 patients were California residents. Thirty-nine (35%) of the California patients visited one or both of the two Disney theme parks during December 17–20, where they are thought to have been exposed to measles, 37 have an unknown exposure source (34%), and 34 (31%) are secondary cases. Among the 34 secondary cases, 26 were household or close contacts, and eight were exposed in a community setting. Five (5%) of the California patients reported being in one or

(continued)

both of the two Disney theme parks during their exposure period outside of December 17–20, but their source of infection is unknown. In addition, 15 cases linked to the two Disney theme parks have been reported in seven other states: Arizona (seven), Colorado (one), Nebraska (one), Oregon (one), Texas (one), Utah (three), and Washington (two), as well as linked cases reported in two neighboring countries, Mexico (one) and Canada (10).

Among the 110 California patients, 49 (45%) were unvaccinated; five (5%) had 1 dose of measles-containing vaccine, seven (6%) had 2 doses, one (1%) had 3 doses, 47 (43%) had unknown or undocumented vaccination status, and one (1%) had immunoglobulin G seropositivity documented, which indicates prior vaccination or measles infection at an undetermined time. Twelve of the unvaccinated patients were infants too young to be vaccinated. Among the 37 remaining vaccine-eligible patients, 28 (76%) were intentionally unvaccinated because of personal beliefs, and one was on an alternative plan for vaccination. Among the 28 intentionally unvaccinated patients, 18 were children (aged <18 years), and 10 were adults. Patients range in age from 6 weeks to 70 years; the median age is 22 years. Among the 84 patients with known hospitalization status, 17 (20%) were hospitalized.

The source of the initial Disney theme park exposure has not been identified. Specimens from 30 California patients were genotyped; all were measles genotype B3, which has caused a large outbreak recently in the Philippines, but has also been detected in at least 14 countries and at least six US states in the last 6 months (1).

Annual attendance at Disney theme parks in California is estimated at 24 million (2), including many international visitors from countries where measles is endemic. The December holiday season coincides with the exposure period of interest. Since 2011, six confirmed measles cases have been reported to CDPH in persons whose notable exposure was to large theme parks that attract international tourists. International travel to countries where measles is endemic is a well-known risk factor for measles, and measles importations continue to occur in the United States; the number of measles cases reported to CDC is updated weekly at http://www.cdc.gov/measles/cases-outbreaks.html. However, US residents also can be exposed to measles in the United States at venues with large numbers of international visitors, such as other tourist attractions and airports. This outbreak illustrates the continued importance of ensuring high measles vaccination coverage in the United States.

ACKNOWLEDGMENTS

California local health jurisdictions. Regina Chase, Giorgio Cosentino, Alex Espinosa, Natasha Espinosa, Ashraf Fadol, Carlos Gonzalez, Kristina Hsieh, Ruth Lopez, Chris Preas, Maria Salas, Diana Singh, Abiy Tadesse, Patricia Stoll, Kim Hansard, Viral and Rickettsial Disease Laboratory, California Department of Public Health. Patrick Ayscue, Brooke Bregman, Cynthia Yen, Anthony Moore, Anna Clayton, Shrimati Datta, Rosie Glenn-Finer, Immunization Branch, California Department of Public Health.

(continued)

REFERENCES

1. CDC. US multi-state measles outbreak, December 2014–January 2015. Atlanta, GA: US Department of Health and Human Services, CDC; 2015. Available at http://emergency.cdc.gov/han/han00376.asp.
2. Themed Entertainment Association, AECOM. Global attractions attendance report. Burbank, CA: Themed Entertainment Association, AECOM; 2014. Available at http://www.aecom.com/deployedfiles/Internet/Capabilities/Economics/_documents/ThemeMuseumIndex_2013.pdf.

FIGURE: Number of confirmed measles cases (N=110),* by date of rash onset—California, December 2014–February 2015

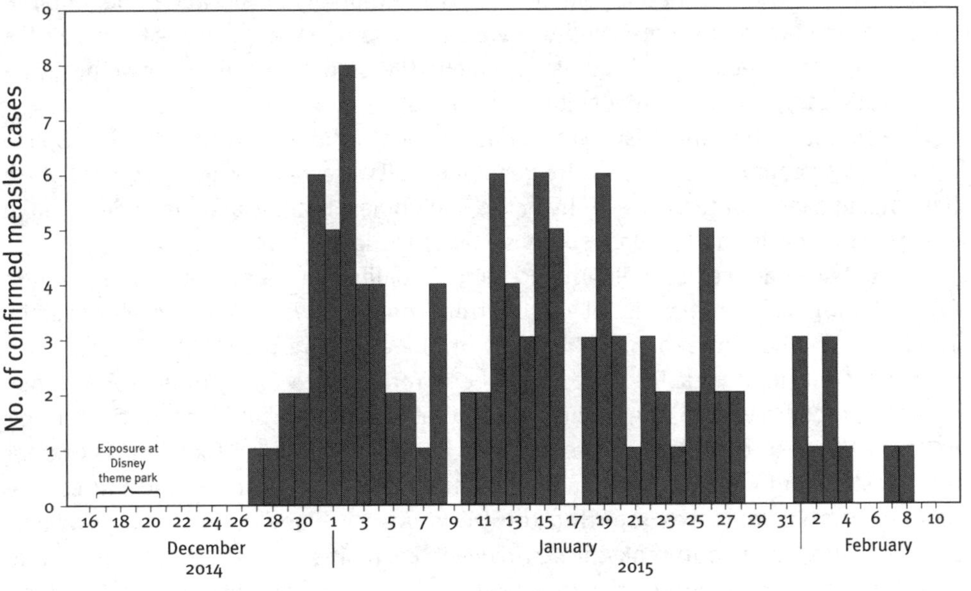

* Reported to the California Department of Public Health as of February 11, 2015.

The figure above is a histogram showing the number of confirmed measles cases (N=110), by date of rash onset in California during December 2014–February 2015.

CASE STUDY DISCUSSION QUESTIONS

1. What is the pathway of measles infection in this case?
2. Discuss the purpose of vaccination and the controversy this case presents.

Key Chapter Points

- The epidemiologic triangle is a model that helps explain the etiology—that is, the causes and origins—of infectious disease. The triangle has three corners or vertices: host, environment, and agent.
- The host is the living human being or animal that, under natural conditions, affords subsistence or lodgment to an infectious agent.
- The environment comprises the setting and conditions that are external to the host; it can serve as a reservoir that promotes the survival of agents that transmit infectious disease.
- The agent, or pathogen, is a factor—such as a microorganism, chemical substance, or form of radiation—whose presence, excessive presence, or, in some cases, relative absence is necessary for disease to occur.
- A host's susceptibility to an agent depends on its defense mechanisms, which may be specific to a particular agent or nonspecific.
- Key characteristics of infectious disease agents include infectivity, pathogenicity, toxigenicity, resistance, virulence, and case-fatality rate.
- Transmission of infectious disease can be either direct (e.g., by direct contact between people) or indirect (e.g., through contact with a contaminated object).
- Vehicle-borne transmission occurs through contaminated material or objects, or fomites. In vector-borne transmission, an agent is carried by a crawling or flying insect.
- Herd immunity occurs when a large percentage of a group or community has immunity to an infectious agent, as a result of either vaccinations or past infections.
- Epidemiologists use various measures to track infectious disease occurrence. Point prevalence indicates the proportion of people in a population who have a particular disease or attribute at a specified point in time. Period prevalence indicates the proportion of people known to have had the condition at any point during a specified period. An attack rate is used when the occurrence of a disease increases greatly within a population over a short period, often in relation to a specific exposure.
- Epidemic curves provide a graphic display of the patterns in which outbreaks occur. The various types of epidemic curves correspond with different types of outbreaks, such as point source outbreaks, continuous common source outbreaks, and propagated outbreaks.
- The steps involved in a disease outbreak investigation are (1) detect an outbreak, (2) find cases, (3) generate hypotheses, (4) test hypotheses, (5) solve the source of the outbreak, (6) control the outbreak, and (7) decide the outbreak is over.

- A disease is categorized as "emerging" if its incidence among humans has increased in the last two decades or threatens to increase in the near future.
- The challenge for public health is to intervene and prevent exposure to agents capable of causing disease. And in the event that exposure occurs, public health works with the healthcare system to detect the disease at the earliest possible stage.

Discussion Questions

1. Explain the significance of the vertices of the epidemiologic triangle.
2. What factors influence the ability of infectious agents to produce disease, the severity of the disease, and the outcome of the infection?
3. Describe the various modes of infectious disease transmission, and provide an example of each.
4. What are some measures of association used in infectious disease outbreaks?
5. What are the types of epidemic curves, and what information can they provide during an outbreak?
6. What are the key steps involved in a disease outbreak investigation?
7. What is the significance of emerging infectious diseases?

References

Centers for Disease Control and Prevention (CDC). 2016a. "Quick-Learn Lesson: Using an Epi Curve to Determine Mode of Spread." Accessed October 11. www.cdc.gov/training/quicklearns/epimode/.

———. 2016b. "Update: Ongoing Zika Virus Transmission—Puerto Rico, November 1, 2015–April 14, 2016." *Morbidity and Mortality Weekly Report*. Published May 6. www.cdc.gov/mmwr/volumes/65/wr/mm6517e2.htm.

———. 2015a. "Division of Vector-borne Diseases: Bourbon Virus." Updated February 19. www.cdc.gov/ncezid/dvbd/bourbon/index.html.

———. 2015b. "Genomes at CDC: Man, Mouse, and Microbe: It's a Genomic World." *Genomics and Health Impact Blog*. Updated January 21. http://blogs.cdc.gov/genomics/2013/05/23/genomes-at-cdc/.

——. 2015c. "Measles Outbreak—California, December 2014–February 2015." *Morbidity and Mortality Weekly Report*. Published February 20. www.cdc.gov/mmwr/preview/mmwrhtml/mm6406a5.htm.

——. 2015d. "Multistate and Nationwide Foodborne Outbreak Investigations: A Step-by-Step Guide." Updated March 24. www.cdc.gov/foodsafety/outbreaks/investigating-outbreaks/investigations/index.html.

——. 2015e. "Outbreak of Salmonella Newport Infections Linked to Cucumbers—United States, 2014." *Morbidity and Mortality Weekly Report*. Published February 20. www.cdc.gov/mmwr/preview/mmwrhtml/mm6406a3.htm.

——. 2014. "EID Journal Background and Goals." *Emerging Infectious Diseases*. Updated May 30. wwwnc.cdc.gov/eid/page/background-goals.

——. 2013. "One Health: Zoonotic Diseases." Updated October 18. www.cdc.gov/onehealth/zoonotic-diseases.html.

——. 2012a. "Principles of Epidemiology in Public Health Practice: An Introduction to Applied Epidemiology and Biostatistics, Lesson 1, Section 9." Self-study course. Updated May 18. www.cdc.gov/ophss/csels/dsepd/ss1978/lesson1/section9.html.

——. 2012b. "Principles of Epidemiology in Public Health Practice: An Introduction to Applied Epidemiology and Biostatistics, Lesson 1, Section 10." Self-study course. Updated May 18. www.cdc.gov/ophss/csels/dsepd/ss1978/lesson1/section10.html.

——. 1992. *Principles of Epidemiology*, 2nd ed. Atlanta , GA: US Department of Health and Human Services.

Doyle, A. C. 1890. *The Sign of the Four.* London: Penguin Classics, 2001.

Friis, R. H., and T. A. Sellers. 2014. *Epidemiology for Public Health Practice*, 5th ed. Burlington, MA: Jones & Bartlett Learning.

Morens, D. M., and A. S. Fauci. 2013. "Emerging Infectious Diseases: Threats to Human Health and Global Stability. *PLOS Pathogens*. Published July 4. http://journals.plos.org/plospathogens/article?id=10.1371/journal.ppat.1003467.

Porta, M. (ed.). 2014. *A Dictionary of Epidemiology*, 6th ed. New York: Oxford University Press.

SECTION 2

DETERMINANTS, ASSESSMENT, AND OUTCOMES

CHAPTER 8

POPULATION HEALTH AND HEALTH DETERMINANTS

"*Population health* is defined as the health outcomes of a group of individuals, including the distribution of such outcomes within the group."

—David Kindig and Greg Stoddart (2003)

Learning Objectives

After completing this chapter, you should be able to

- define *population health*,
- distinguish between public health and population health,
- describe the contributions of Robert G. Evans and Greg L. Stoddart,
- explain the types of health determinants and their significance,
- compare population health outcomes and health outcomes,
- discuss how health determinants affect a population's health, and
- explain how we might measure determinants' impact and propose recommendations based on the information provided.

Population Health Defined

Public health, as discussed in chapter 1, aims to protect and improve the health of communities by promoting healthy lifestyles, conducting research for disease and injury prevention, and detecting and controlling infectious diseases. It focuses on the health of human populations in neighborhoods, census tracts, towns, cities, regions, countries, and the world as a whole. Whereas healthcare focuses on the individual and directs its efforts toward treatment, public health focuses on populations and directs its efforts toward disease prevention and health promotion (CDC Foundation 2016).

In contrast, *population health*, as defined by the Canadian Federal, Provincial, and Territorial Advisory Committee on Population Health, refers to "the health of a population as measured by health status indicators and as influenced by social, economic, and physical environments, personal health practices, individual capacity and coping skills, human biology, early childhood development, and health services" (Public Health Agency of Canada 2013). It "focuses on interrelated conditions and factors that influence the health of populations over the life course, identifies systematic variations in their patterns of occurrence, and applies the resulting knowledge to develop and implement policies and actions to improve the health and well-being of those populations" (Public Health Agency of Canada 2013). Further, Kindig and Stoddart (2003, 381) suggest that *population health as a concept of health* be defined as "the health outcomes of a group of individuals, including the distribution of such outcomes within the group." These populations can be geographic regions, such as nations or communities, or other groups, such as employees, ethnic groups, people with disabilities, or prisoners. Many determinants of health, such as medical care systems and the social and physical environments, have their biological impact largely at a population level (Kindig and Stoddart 2003).

Despite differences in the terms' definitions, population health should not be considered distinct from public health but rather as a complement to it. Population health addresses a wide range of factors—including the physical, cultural, and social environments people are born into, grow up around, and function within throughout their lifetimes (Healthy People 2016)—and considers the outcomes they have for the health of populations.

Health Determinants

health determinant
An event, characteristic, or other factor that brings about change in health.

One of the ways population health aims to improve the health of populations is by reducing the inequities presented by health determinants. Last (2001, 50) defines a **health determinant** as "any factor, whether event, characteristic, or other definable entity, that brings about change in a health condition or other defined characteristic." The World Health Organization (WHO) emphasizes that people's health status is strongly influenced by circumstances and environments: "To a large extent, factors such as where we live, the state of our environment, genetics, our income and education level, and our relationships with friends and family all have considerable impacts on health" (WHO 2016a).

Broadly, the major determinants of health include the social and economic environment; the physical environment; and individual characteristics, lifestyle choices, and behaviors (WHO 2016a). The WHO (2016a) describes the following health determinants specifically:

- *Income and social status.* High income and social status are typically linked with better health. "The greater the gap between the richest and poorest people, the greater the differences in health."
- *Education.* "Low education levels are linked with poor health, more stress, and lower self-confidence."
- *The physical environment.* Clean air and water, adequate shelter, healthy workplaces, and safe communities and roads all contribute to good health. "People in employment are healthier, particularly those who have more control over their working conditions."
- *Social support networks.* Support from families, friends, and communities is usually linked with better health. A culture's beliefs, customs, and traditions can all affect health.
- *Genetics.* "Inheritance plays a part in determining lifespan, healthiness, and the likelihood of developing certain illnesses."
- *Health services.* Access to and use of services that prevent and treat disease influence health.
- *Gender.* Men and women typically deal with different types of diseases at different points as they age.

Such determinants, according to the WHO's (2012) Commission on Social Determinants of Health, account for a majority of diseases and injuries and are a source of health inequities in every country. McGinnis, Williams-Russo, and Knickman (2002, 78) highlight the potential impact of determinants-based health initiatives relative to investments in medical care services:

> Approximately 95 percent of the trillion dollars we spend as a nation on health goes to direct medical care services, while just 5 percent is allocated to populationwide approaches to health improvement. However, some 40 percent of deaths are caused by behavior patterns that could be modified by preventive interventions. (Social

circumstances and environmental exposure also contribute substantially to preventable illness.) It appears, in fact, that a much smaller proportion of preventable mortality in the United States, perhaps 10–15 percent, could be avoided by better availability or quality of medical care.

The Field Model of Health and Well-Being

field model of health and well-being
A model, developed by Evans and Stoddart, suggesting that determinants such as social and physical environment, genetic endowment, prosperity, healthcare access, and individual behavior all factor into the health of a population.

The **field model of health and well-being**, developed by Robert G. Evans and Greg L. Stoddart (1990), proposes that determinants such as the social and physical environment, genetic endowment, prosperity, disease status, healthcare access, and individual behavior all factor into the health of a population. Some of these health determinants are, at least to a certain extent, under individuals' control (e.g., behavior, lifestyle choices), whereas others are not (e.g., genetic inheritance). Furthermore, the health determinants interact as they influence a person's health status. For example, a person's level of economic prosperity will have an influence on her housing (physical environment) and access to nutritious food (physical environment) and healthcare (social environment). The field model's multidimensional approach suggests opportunities for partnerships—such as after-school programs, faith-based programs, and farmer's markets—to help improve a community's health (Caron 2015).

Researchers have maintained that a focus on the multiple determinants of health outcomes, however they are measured, is a hallmark of the field of population health (Kindig and Stoddart 2003; Adler et al. 1999; Keating and Hertzman 1999; Berkman and Kawachi 2000). Kindig and Stoddart (2003, 381) state:

> These determinants include medical care, public health interventions, aspects of the social environment (income, education, employment, social support, culture) and of the physical environment (urban design, clean air and water), genetics, and individual behavior. We note with caution that such a list of categories can lead to a view that they operate independently; population health research is fundamentally concerned about the interactions between them, and we prefer to refer to "patterns" of determinants.

Another key issue that must be considered in population health is the cost-effectiveness of resource allocation to multiple determinants (Kindig and Stoddart 2003). Because the health of populations is complex, with numerous determinants both within our control and outside our control, interventions to improve health are also complex. The interventions must involve multiple stakeholders, resources must be affordable and available, and implementation must address inequities in the community. If an intervention to address health inequality is not effective at a reasonable cost, it will be out of reach for many populations.

The relationship between select health determinants and population health is illustrated in exhibit 8.1. In this simplified diagram, all the arrows lead to the population

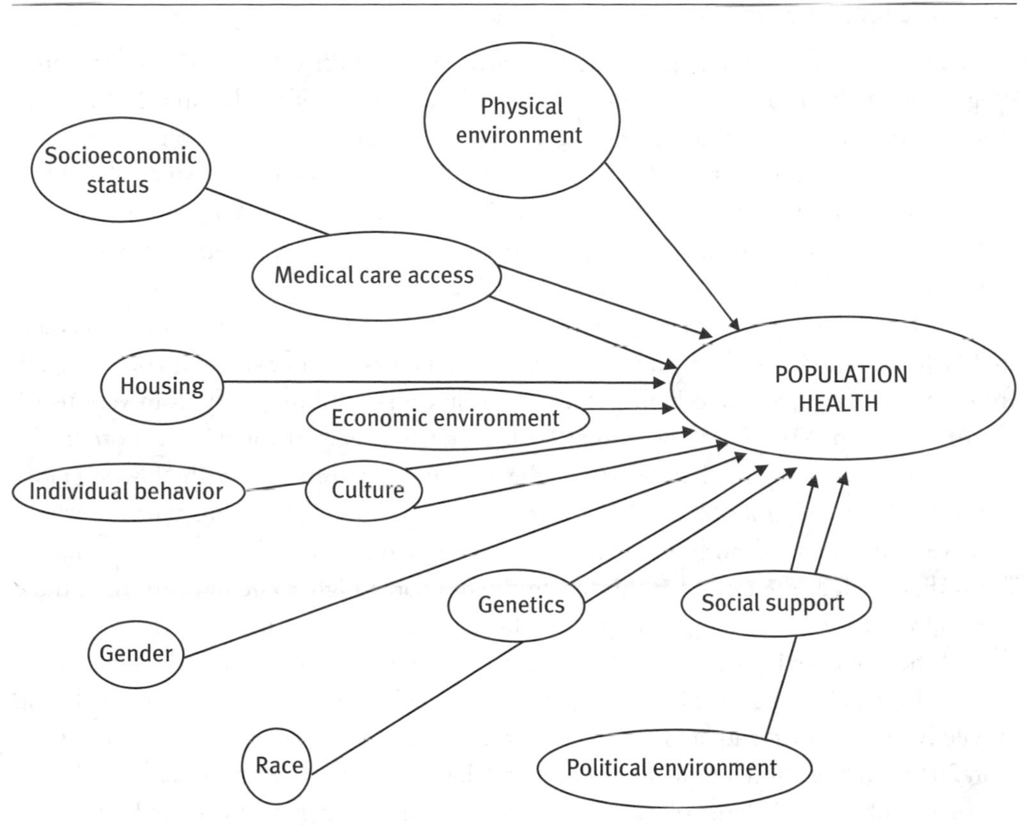

Exhibit 8.1 Relationship Between Health Determinants and Population Health

health outcome. In reality, however, additional connections and interactions occur among the various determinants. These interactions must be considered if an intervention is to be affordable and effective (Kindig and Stoddart 2003).

In summary, the field model calls for an approach to population health that "combines the definition and measurement of health outcomes and their distribution, the patterns of determinants that influence such outcomes, and the policies that influence the optimal balance of determinants" (Kindig and Stoddart 2003, 382). It centers on the following basic principles of population health (Kindig 2010):

- Health outcomes are more than just the absence of disease.
- Health outcomes are produced by complex interactions of multiple determinants (e.g., healthcare, behaviors, genetics, the social and physical environments).
- Because resources are limited, the relative cost-effectiveness of these determinants is key for policy makers.

Social Gradient of Health

social gradient of health
The idea that, in general, people with lower socioeconomic positions have worse health.

A related concept, the **social gradient of health**, was identified by the British epidemiologist Sir Michael Marmot. Marmot was one of the authors of the landmark Whitehall studies, a pair of cohort studies between the 1960s and 1980s that focused on civil servants working in London. Under the British healthcare system, members of the study group had equal access to healthcare. The Whitehall studies thus "set out to investigate the complex relationships among income, work status, psychosocial support, health behaviors, and resulting morbidity and mortality" (Gorman 2012).

The first Whitehall study, known as Whitehall I, followed 17,530 male civil servants from 1967 to 1977. It showed an inverse association between employment grade—ranging from low-level messengers to higher-level administrators—and mortality from various illnesses (Gorman 2012; Marmot et al. 1978). "After ten years of follow-up, those in the highest employment grade had one-third the mortality rate of those in the lowest grade" (Gorman 2012). Marmot (2006, 2083) states: "Among these civil servants, none of whom were destitute, men second from the top of the occupational hierarchy had a higher rate of death than men at the top. Men third from the top had a higher rate of death than those second from the top . . . Why, among men who are not poor in the usual sense of the word, should the risk of dying be intimately related to where they stand in the social hierarchy?"

Whitehall II studied, from 1985 to 1988, a cohort comprising 10,314 male and female British civil servants, and it confirmed some of the key findings of Whitehall I (Gorman 2012). Whitehall II found, for instance, that lower job status was associated with higher prevalence of ischemic heart disease. New findings from Whitehall II centered on gender differences and isolation as possible causes of this relationship. Gorman (2012) explains: "In general, women had greater morbidity than men in all grades of employment. The higher the job status of the man, the more likely he was to be married or cohabitating, but the opposite was true for women." Obesity was found to be more prevalent among people in lower-status jobs. The risk factor that differed most among job categories was smoking.

Gorman (2012) continues: "Perhaps most significantly, the Whitehall II study discovered a firm connection among psychosocial factors, perception about work status and environment, and poor health outcomes." People in lower-status jobs reported less social support, less control, less use of skills, less variety at work, more demanding workloads, and more psychological stress than those in higher-status jobs. All of these factors are associated with increased risk of cardiovascular disease (Gorman 2012).

These findings illustrate the social gradient of health—the idea that, in general, people with lower socioeconomic positions have worse health. The WHO (2016b) explains:

> The poorest of the poor, around the world, have the worst health. Within countries, the evidence shows that in general the lower an individual's socioeconomic position the worse their health. There is a social gradient in health that runs from top to bottom of the socioeconomic spectrum. This is a global phenomenon, seen in low, middle and high income countries. The social gradient in health means that health inequities affect everyone.

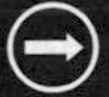

POPULATION HEALTH AND HEALTHCARE

The Institute of Medicine (IOM) has adopted Kindig and Stoddart's (2003, 381) definition of *population health* as "the health outcomes of a group of individuals, including the distribution of such outcomes within the group." In its "Working Definition of Population Health," the IOM (2016) notes that, although multiple health determinants are not specifically mentioned in the definition, the contribution of these determinants (e.g., behavior, genetics, access to healthcare, physical environment) serve as the foundation for health outcomes in a population. The IOM also makes an important point concerning the use of the term *population health* by healthcare organizations: "We recognize that this term is currently being used by some health care organizations to describe the clinical, often chronic disease, outcomes of patients enrolled in a given health plan. Certainly an enrolled patient group can be thought of and managed as a population, but defining population health solely in terms of clinical populations can draw attention away from the critical role that non-clinical factors such as education and income play in producing health."

Population Health Outcomes

Metrics for monitoring population health outcomes differ from those that would be used to assess an individual's health outcomes. Parrish (2010), in the CDC's *Preventing Chronic Disease* journal, writes:

> An ideal population health outcome metric should reflect a population's dynamic state of physical, mental, and social well-being. Positive health outcomes include being alive; functioning well mentally, physically, and socially; and having a sense of well-being. Negative outcomes include death, loss of function, and lack of well-being. In contrast to these health outcomes, diseases and injuries are intermediate factors that influence the likelihood of achieving a state of health.

Based on a review of data for US counties, Parrish (2010) proposes three key metrics for population health outcomes:

1. Life expectancy from birth, or age-adjusted mortality rate
2. Condition-specific changes in life expectancy, or condition-specific or age-specific mortality rates
3. Self-reported level of health, functional status, and experiential status

All of these outcome metrics are of an epidemiological nature, consistent with the ideas presented in the first section of this book. Parrish (2010) further states that, when reported, "outcome metrics should present both the overall level of health of a population and the distribution of health among different geographic, economic, and demographic groups in the population." Hence, his ideas connect with the field model as proposed by Evans and Stoddart (1990). Parrish (2010) also comments on the use of measures of mortality, life expectancy, and premature death: "Although these measures provide information about mortality and longevity, they provide no information about the contribution of specific diseases, injuries, and underlying conditions (for example, water quality, poverty, social isolation, and diet) to death, for which actions might be taken to prolong life." Thus, he advocates considering not only the disease or health status of the population but also the external factors that influence that status. Parrish (2010) states: "The level and distribution of health outcomes in populations result from a complex web of cultural, environmental, political, social, economic, behavioral, and genetic factors. In this causal web, diseases and injuries are intermediate factors, rather than outcomes, that may influence a person's health. Lung cancer, for example, has a substantial effect on physical function and life-span, while first-degree sunburn has little effect." This population-based approach is distinct from the one that would be used in measuring an individual's health outcomes.

Case Study

Where You Live Impacts Your Health

The following story is excerpted from a report by Canada's Federal, Provincial, and Territorial Advisory Committee on Population Health (1999).

Why is Jason in the hospital?
Because he has a bad infection in his leg.
But why does he have an infection?
Because he has a cut on his leg and it got infected.
But why does he have a cut on his leg?
Because he was playing in the junk yard next to his apartment building and there was some sharp, jagged steel there that he fell on.
But why was he playing in a junk yard?
Because his neighbourhood is kind of run down. A lot of kids play there and there is no one to supervise them.
But why does he live in that neighbourhood?
Because his parents can't afford a nicer place to live.
But why can't his parents afford a nicer place to live?

(continued)

Because his Dad is unemployed and his Mom is sick.
But why is his Dad unemployed?
Because he doesn't have much education and he can't find a job.
But why . . . ?

CASE STUDY DISCUSSION QUESTIONS

1. What are the determinants that affect the family's health in this story?
2. Hypothesize as to the root causes of these determinants.
3. Apply the Evans and Stoddart field model of health and well-being to this situation, and discuss your findings.
4. What are the population health outcomes you would use for families in a community like the one described here?

CASE STUDY

CHILDHOOD LEAD POISONING IN A REFUGEE RESETTLEMENT COMMUNITY

This case study focuses on the public health issue of childhood lead poisoning in a refugee resettlement site, and it stems from the lead-related death of a two-year-old child in New Hampshire in 2000. Caron and Serrell (2009) provide background:

The nationwide decline in childhood lead poisoning in recent decades is widely regarded as a public health success story. Lead is a neurotoxin that can lead to impaired speech and hearing, hyperactivity, impairments in learning and memory, and irreversible brain damage. Young children may be extremely vulnerable to its effects due to low body weight, iron deficiency, poor nutritional status, and hand-to-mouth activity. For the past 30 years, epidemiologic studies have found inverse associations between children's intellectual functioning and successively lower blood lead concentrations, thus prompting the Centers for Disease Control and Prevention (CDC) to repeatedly lower its definition of the level of concern. . . . Despite the public health advances associated with removing lead from gasoline and paint, exposure to lead is a persistent hazard for children in many regions of the United States. . . .

New Hampshire has some of the oldest housing stock in the nation, with almost 40% of rental housing and 28% of owner-occupied housing built prior to 1950. Manchester is the largest community in New Hampshire, with a population of approximately 110,000, thus representing an urban microcosm of the childhood lead poisoning problem. About

(continued)

77% of Manchester's housing units were built prior to bans on lead-based paint, and the housing stock in the center city neighborhoods is generally of poor quality. These environmental factors contribute to thousands of point sources for lead exposure.

In addition to these aforementioned environmental health challenges, Manchester also experiences the multifaceted economic and social disparities found in larger cities. . . . The city is a designated refugee resettlement site, and as such is considered the most racially and ethnically diverse community in New Hampshire. Two out of every three refugees that resettled to New Hampshire between 2002 and 2007 reside in Manchester. Furthermore, between 1990 and 2000, the city's Latino immigrant population grew by 126% as compared to 72% for the state. Over 70 different languages are spoken as the primary language by children in the Manchester school system. Hence, language barriers represent another major challenge in addressing the wicked problem of childhood lead poisoning. . . . Although Manchester represents 10% of the state's population, it experiences one-third of all childhood lead poisoning cases in New Hampshire, with the majority of these cases occurring in predominantly center city neighborhoods. In 2007, approximately 25% of the lead-poisoned children in the local health department's caseload were refugees or children of refugees. CDC recommends that all one- and two-year-old children residing in Manchester be tested for lead paint exposure.

The following report, focusing on the incident in New Hampshire in 2000, has been reproduced from the CDC (2001). The report was originally prepared by R. M. Caron, R. DiPentima, C. Alvarado, P. Alexakos, J. Filiano, T. Gilson, J. Greenblatt, G. Robinson, N. Twitchell, L. Speikers, M. A. Abdel-Nasser, H. A. El-Henawy, M. Markowitz, and P. Ashley. It was published on the CDC's Morbidity and Mortality Weekly Report (MMWR) *website (www.cdc.gov/mmwr) on June 8, 2001.*

FATAL PEDIATRIC LEAD POISONING—NEW HAMPSHIRE, 2000

Fatal pediatric lead poisoning is rare in the United States because of multiple public health measures that have reduced blood lead levels (BLLs) in the population. However, the risk for elevated BLLs among children remains high in some neighborhoods and populations, including children living in older housing with deteriorated leaded paint. This report describes the investigation of the first reported death of a child from lead poisoning since 1990 (1). The investigation implicated leaded paint and dust in a home environment as the most likely source of the poisoning. Lead poisoning can be prevented by correcting lead hazards, especially in older housing, and by screening children at risk according to established guidelines (2).

On March 29, 2000, a 2-year-old girl was seen at a community hospital emergency department with a low-grade fever and vomiting of approximately 1 day's duration. The child had been well since arriving in New Hampshire from Egypt with her Sudanese refugee family 3 weeks earlier. Laboratory findings included a microcytic anemia (hemoglobin: 7.6 g/dL; lower limit of normal: 11.5 g/dL) with occasional basophilic stippling

(continued)

of red blood cells. A throat swab streptococcal antigen screening test was positive. She was discharged from the emergency department with prescriptions for an antibiotic and antiemetic to treat presumed strep throat. However, her vomiting worsened, and she was admitted to the same hospital on April 17, and then transferred to a tertiary-care hospital the next day. On April 19, approximately 5 hours after the transfer, she became unresponsive, apneic, and hypotensive. She was intubated and placed on a ventilator. Computerized tomography of the head showed diffuse cerebral edema and dilated ventricles. Later that day, the results of a blood test drawn on April 18 showed a BLL of 391 μg/dL and an erythrocyte protoporphyrin level of 541 μg/dL. Chelation therapy was initiated with intramuscular British antilewisite and intravenous calcium ethylenediaminetetraacetic acid. Despite a decrease in her BLL to 72 μg/dL and treatment for increased intracranial pressure, including surgical ventricular drainage, she remained comatose without spontaneous respirations, brain electrical activity, and intracranial blood flow. She was pronounced brain dead on April 21.

An autopsy found diffuse cerebral edema. A hair sample lead concentration was 31 μg/g in the distal centimeter and 67 μg/g in the proximal centimeter, indicating a large increase in lead exposure during the preceding month. Radiographs of the left knee were equivocal for growth arrest lines that can occur in chronic lead poisoning (3). A bone marrow sample showed no stainable iron, indicating iron deficiency.

On April 19, the Manchester Health Department and New Hampshire Department of Health and Human Services (NHDHHS) initiated an investigation, including interviews and blood lead tests of the patient's family and an inspection of her residence. In addition, to assess a possible contribution of lead exposure from the child's previous residence in Egypt, the Field Epidemiology Training Program of the Egyptian Ministry of Health obtained soil and dust samples from that location.

After living in Egypt for approximately 18 months, on March 9, 2000, the family had moved to Manchester into an apartment constructed before 1920. A wall in a sibling's bedroom had multiple holes from which the patient had been seen removing and ingesting plaster. Two of seven samples of plaster with the adhering surface paint contained lead at levels of 5% and 12%. Peeling paint (35% lead) was present on the balusters and floor (3% lead) of a porch outside the apartment entrance where the patient sometimes had played. She also had played near and looked out of a living room window that occasionally was opened during meal preparation. A wipe sample of dust from the window well showed 6732 μg lead/ft^2, well above the hazardous level of 800 μg/ft^2 (4). NHDHHS ordered the apartment owner to correct the lead hazards identified during the inspection. The patient's family relocated to another dwelling.

BLLs in the mother and three siblings (ages 5, 11, and 15 years) ranged from 4–12 μg/dL. The family did not use or possess nontraditional remedies, food supplements, cosmetics, or ceramic eating or drinking containers acquired abroad. No one in the household was employed or had lead-related hobbies. Measurements of stable lead isotopes (5) in selected environmental samples and the patient's blood showed that the isotopic lead composition of the porch paint and window well dust in the Manchester apartment

(continued)

matched the composition of lead in her blood more closely than did the isotopic composition of other samples, including those from her previous residence in Egypt.

EDITORIAL NOTE:

Lead encephalopathy is a life-threatening complication of lead poisoning that can occur in young children who have very high BLLs (>70–100 μg/dL). Nonspecific symptoms (e.g., lethargy, sporadic vomiting, and constipation) can occur at BLLs >50–70 μg/dL and may precede the abrupt onset of frank encephalopathy characterized by persistent vomiting, ataxia, altered consciousness, coma, and seizures. In this report, the child's anemia with basophilic stippling also suggested lead poisoning. However, symptoms or signs cannot be used to reliably diagnose or exclude lead poisoning; a BLL must be measured whenever lead poisoning is suspected. In young children, BLLs >70 μg/dL or elevated BLLs with symptoms suggesting encephalopathy require prompt inpatient treatment with chelating agents to rapidly reduce BLLs. Providing appropriate intensive care for children with encephalopathy can prevent death, although severe permanent brain damage can occur despite treatment (3).

During the 1950s and 1960s, acute, often fatal, lead encephalopathy was a common cause of pediatric admissions to urban hospitals (6). The subsequent decline in fatal lead poisoning cases is attributable to reduced lead exposure from multiple sources, institution of lead screening programs, and improved treatment of lead poisoning (6). Despite the reduction in severe lead poisoning, in some US counties, >20% of young children tested have BLLs ≥10 μg/dL (7), high enough to adversely affect learning and development (3).

The likely sources of lead poisoning for the child in this report—deteriorated leaded paint and elevated levels of lead-contaminated house dust—are found in an estimated 24 million US dwellings, 4.4 million of which are home to one or more children aged <6 years (US Department of Housing and Urban Development, unpublished data, 2001). Lead hazards are especially common in homes built before 1960 (58%). Although the patient's pica and iron deficiency probably contributed to the severity of her lead poisoning, by increasing ingestion and absorption of lead (3), all children living in homes with lead hazards are at increased risk for developing elevated BLLs (8).

Children who are refugees, adoptees, or recent immigrants may be at increased risk for elevated BLLs, possibly related to lead exposure in their country of origin or to continued use of certain lead-containing traditional remedies or cosmetics. However, such children also are at risk for exposure to leaded paint hazards in older US housing. In addition to ensuring that such children are screened after arrival in the United States, lead poisoning prevention programs and healthcare providers should ensure that families receive timely education about lead hazards. Federal regulations require that property sellers and landlords provide families with information about lead poisoning and about any known lead hazards in a dwelling before its sale or lease. Agencies providing

(continued)

health and social services to refugees and immigrants should become familiar with these regulations and ensure that appropriate information is provided to families in a language they can understand.

REFERENCES

1. CDC. Fatal pediatric poisoning from leaded paint—Wisconsin, 1990. MMWR 1990;40:193–5.
2. CDC. Screening young children for lead poisoning: guidance for state and local public health officials. Atlanta, Georgia: US Department of Health and Human Services, CDC, 1997.
3. CDC. Preventing lead poisoning in young children: a statement by the Centers for Disease Control, October 1991. Atlanta, Georgia: US Department of Health and Human Services, Public Health Service, CDC, 1991.
4. US Department of Housing and Urban Development (HUD). Guidelines for the evaluation and control of lead-based paint hazards in housing. Washington, DC: US Department of Housing and Urban Development, 1995. Available at http://www.hud.gov/lea/learules.html#download. Accessed February 22, 2001.
5. Chaudhary-Webb M, Paschal DC, Elliott WC, et al. ICP-MS determination of lead isotope ratios in whole blood, pottery, and leaded gasoline: lead sources in Mexico City. Atomic Spectroscopy 1998;19:156–63.
6. Lin-Fu JS. Modern history of lead poisoning: a century of discovery and rediscovery. In: Needleman HL, ed. Human lead exposure. Boca Raton, Florida: CRC Press, 1992.
7. CDC. Blood lead levels in young children—United States and selected states, 1996–1999. MMWR 2000;49:1133–7.
8. Lanphear BP, Matte TD, Rogers J, et al. The contribution of lead-contaminated house dust and residential soil to children's blood lead levels: a pooled analysis of 12 epidemiologic studies. Environ Res 1998;79:51–68.

CASE STUDY DISCUSSION QUESTIONS

1. Why is childhood lead poisoning a public health issue?
2. What are the Healthy People 2020 objectives for childhood lead poisoning?
3. Who are the stakeholders in this public health issue?
4. Describe the population most affected by this public health issue, and identify the population health metrics that you think would be most useful in this case. Explain your rationale for the metrics' selection.
5. Describe the community's ecology (i.e., its social, cultural, economic, and political composition), and explain how these factors contribute to this public health issue.

(continued)

6. What health determinants can you identify in this case study? Explain your rationale.
7. Describe the intervention method implemented in this community to address childhood lead poisoning.
8. Propose a feasible public health recommendation, based on addressing the determinants of health, to decrease the incidence of childhood lead poisoning.

Key Chapter Points

- *Population health* can be defined as "the health of a population as measured by health status indicators and as influenced by social, economic, and physical environments, personal health practices, individual capacity and coping skills, human biology, early childhood development, and health services" (Public Health Agency of Canada 2013).
- Kindig and Stoddart (2003, 381) suggest that *population health as a concept of health* be defined as "the health outcomes of a group of individuals, including the distribution of such outcomes within the group." Population health should not be considered distinct from public health but rather as a complement to it.
- Health determinants are factors that bring about change in a health condition or characteristic. In general, the major determinants of health include the social and economic environment; the physical environment; and individual characteristics, lifestyle choices, and behaviors.
- The field model of health and well-being was developed by Robert G. Evans and Greg L. Stoddart. It proposes that determinants such as the social and physical environment, genetic endowment, prosperity, disease status, healthcare access, and individual behavior all factor into the health of a population.
- The field model recognizes that health determinants interact with one another as they influence a person's health status. For example, economic prosperity will influence a person's housing, diet, and access to healthcare.
- The field model emphasized the basic principles that (1) health outcomes are more than just the absence of disease; (2) health outcomes are produced by complex interactions between determinants; and (3) the relative cost-effectiveness of these determinants is critical for policy makers (Kindig 2010).
- The Whitehall studies—a pair of cohort studies focusing on civil servants working in London between the 1960s and 1980s—found that lower employment grade or job status was associated with higher mortality from various diseases.

- Sir Michael Marmot, one of the Whitehall authors, identified the concept of the social gradient of health—the idea that, in general, people with lower socioeconomic positions have worse health.
- Metrics for monitoring population health outcomes differ from those that would be used to assess an individual's health outcomes. Parrish (2010) proposes three key metrics for population health outcomes: (1) life expectancy from birth, or age-adjusted mortality rate; (2) condition-specific changes in life expectancy, or condition-specific or age-specific mortality rates; and (3) self-reported level of health, functional status, and experiential status. He also emphasizes the need to consider not only the disease or health status of the population but also the external factors that influence this status.

Discussion Questions

1. What is population health, and how does it differ from public health?
2. What are health determinants, and how do they contribute to the health status of a population? Provide an example.
3. Discuss the significance of the field model of health and well-being with respect to population health.
4. Describe the key principles of population health.
5. What types of outcome metrics can one use for population health?
6. What is the role of population health in healthcare?

References

Adler, N. E., M. Marmot, B. S. McEwen, and J. Stewart (eds.). 1999. *Socioeconomic Status and Health in Industrial Nations: Social, Psychological, and Biological Pathways*. New York: New York Academy of Sciences.

Berkman, L., and I. Kawachi. 2000. *Social Epidemiology*. New York: Oxford University Press.

Caron, R. M. 2015. *Preparing the Public Health Workforce: Educational Pathways for the Field and the Classroom*. Cham, Switzerland: Springer Publishing.

Caron, R. M., and N. Serrell. 2009. "Community Ecology and Capacity: Keys to Progressing the Environmental Communication of Wicked Problems." *Applied Environmental Education and Communication* 8 (3–4): 195–203.

Centers for Disease Control and Prevention (CDC). 2001. "Fatal Pediatric Lead Poisoning." *Morbidity and Mortality Weekly Report*. Published June 8. www.cdc.gov/mmwr/preview/mmwrhtml/mm5022a1.htm.

Centers for Disease Control and Prevention (CDC) Foundation. 2016. "What Is Public Health?" Accessed October 17. www.cdcfoundation.org/content/what-public-health.

Evans, R.G., and G. L. Stoddart. 1990. "Producing Health, Consuming Health Care." *Social Science and Medicine* 31 (12): 1347–63.

Federal, Provincial, and Territorial Advisory Committee on Population Health. 1999. *Toward a Healthy Future: Second Report on the Health of Canadians*. Minister of Public Works and Government Services Canada. Published September. http://publications.gc.ca/collections/Collection/H39-468-1999E.pdf.

Gorman, S. 2012. "Inequality, Stress, and Health: The Whitehall Studies." *The Pump Handle*. Published October 3. http://scienceblogs.com/thepumphandle/2012/10/03/inequality-stress-and-health-the-whitehall-studies/.

Healthy People. 2016. "Social Determinants of Health." Updated October 13. www.healthypeople.gov/2020/topics-objectives/topic/social-determinants-health.

Institute of Medicine (IOM). 2016. "Working Definition of Population Health." Accessed October 18. www.nationalacademies.org/hmd/~/media/Files/Activity%20Files/PublicHealth/PopulationHealthImprovementRT/Pop%20Health%20RT%20Population%20Health%20Working%20Definition.pdf.

Keating, D. P., and C. Hertzman. 1999. *Developmental Health and the Wealth of Nations: Social, Biological, and Educational Dynamics*. New York: Guilford Press.

Kindig, D. A. 2010. "Is Population Health Finally Coming into its Own?" *Improving Population Health*. Published May 18. www.improvingpopulationhealth.org/blog/2010/05/the-state-of-the-field-of-population-health.html.

Kindig, D., and G. Stoddart. 2003. "What Is Population Health?" *American Journal of Public Health* 93 (3): 380–83.

Last, J. M. (ed.). 2001. *A Dictionary of Epidemiology*, 4th ed. New York: Oxford University Press.

Marmot, M. G. 2006. "Health in an Unequal World." *The Lancet* 368 (9552): 2081–94.

Marmot, M. G., G. Rose, M. Shipley, and P. J. Hamilton. 1978. "Employment Grade and Coronary Heart Disease in British Civil Servants." *Journal of Epidemiology and Community Health* 32 (4): 244–49.

McGinnis, J. M., P. Williams-Russo, and J. R. Knickman. 2002. "The Case for More Active Policy Attention to Health Promotion." *Health Affairs* 21 (2): 78–93.

Parrish, R. G. 2010. "Measuring Population Health Outcomes." *Preventing Chronic Disease*. Published July. www.cdc.gov/pcd/issues/2010/jul/10_0005.htm.

Public Health Agency of Canada. 2013. "What Is the Population Health Approach?" Updated January 15. www.phac-aspc.gc.ca/ph-sp/approach-approche/appr-eng.php.

World Health Organization (WHO). 2016a. "Determinants of Health." Accessed October 17. www.who.int/hia/evidence/doh/en/.

———. 2016b. "Social Determinants of Health: Key Concepts." Accessed October 17. www.who.int/social_determinants/thecommission/finalreport/key_concepts/en/.

———. 2012. *Meeting Report: World Conference on Social Determinants of Health*. Accessed October 17, 2016. www.who.int/sdhconference/resources/Conference_Report.pdf.

CHAPTER 9

COMMUNITY HEALTH ASSESSMENT

"An understanding of the determinants of health and of the nature and extent of community need is a fundamental prerequisite to sound decision-making about health. Accurate information serves the interests both of justice and the efficient use of available resources. Assessment is therefore a core government obligation in public health."

—Institute of Medicine (1988)

Learning Objectives

After completing this chapter, you should be able to

- define *community health assessment* (CHA);
- discuss the CHA process, its strengths, and its limitations;
- describe the types of health data that would be useful for the CHA;
- explain the relationship between the CHA and the community health improvement process (CHIP); and
- understand the CHA's role in improving population health.

Fleming ch. 9

Introduction

Every community is different. Therefore, when assessing community health, one approach does not fit all. This chapter highlights the importance of understanding a community's health status, and it describes a variety of approaches for determining whether a community is healthy or not. Assessing the health of a community is an essential public health service, and assessments provide key information for efforts to manage the health of populations.

A **community health assessment (CHA)**, as defined by the Public Health Accreditation Board (PHAB), is a systematic examination of health status indicators for a population, conducted for the purpose of identifying key problems and assets in a community and assisting with the development of strategies to address the community's health issues (PHAB 2011; Turnock 2009). A CHA is also known as a *community health needs assessment* (CHNA). The assessment involves a variety of tools and processes, but "the essential ingredients are community engagement and collaborative participation" (PHAB 2011, 8). The National Association of County and City Health Officials (NACCHO 2016b) further describes a CHA as follows:

community health assessment (CHA)
A systematic examination of health status indicators for a population, conducted for the purpose of identifying key problems and assets in a community and assisting with the development of strategies to address the community's health issues.

> A community health assessment is a process that uses quantitative and qualitative methods to systematically collect and analyze data to understand health within a specific community. An ideal assessment includes information on risk factors, quality of life, mortality, morbidity, community assets, forces of change, social determinants of health and health inequity, and information on how well the public health system provides essential services. Community health assessment data inform community decision-making, the prioritization of health problems, and the development, implementation, and evaluation of community health improvement plans.

As these definitions make clear, the concept of the CHA is grounded in the core functions of public health—assessment, policy development, and assurance. These core functions interact in such a way that the information gained through assessment will identify health issues and inform the policy development and assurance functions. The ultimate goal of a CHA is to measure how well the public health system assures the health of the population it serves. It assesses the health indicators for the community and evaluates the development and implementation of policies to promote a healthy population (Institute of Medicine 2003; PHAB 2011).

The Community Health Assessment Process

The CHA process incorporates both quantitative and qualitative methods to collect and analyze specific health data within a community. Health data include social determinants of health, mortality and morbidity information, quality-of-life indicators, inequity measures, community assets, and an evaluation of how well the public health system conducts its work. With these data, a CHA can help answer the following questions (Dever 1997; Institute of Medicine 2003; Issel 2004):

- What are the health problems in the community?
- Why do health issues exist in the community?
- What factors create or determine the community's health problems?
- What resources are available to address the health problems?
- What are the community's health needs from a population-based perspective?

The CHA process is carried out by community stakeholders, such as residents, business owners, and nonprofit organizations, in addition to the local public health department (Cibula et al. 2003; Dever 1997; Issel 2004; PHAB 2010). It uses broad networks of data, mobilizes community members, and garners resources to approach public health issues in a comprehensive manner (Issel 2004; PHAB 2010). The key steps in the process are described in the sections that follow.

Describe the Community and Define the Population

Consider what factors would need to be included in a description of the community. Such factors might include, for instance, population size; features of the geography (e.g., urban or rural characteristics); racial, ethnic, gender, and age distribution; socioeconomic status (e.g., education, employment); culture, religion, and history; and the surrounding environment (e.g., politics, economic conditions, housing) (McCoy 2010).

Engage the Community and Understand Their Health Priorities

Members of the community know the issues that most affect their health and quality of life, and they also know the community's habits, customs, attitudes, and social groups (Edberg 2007). Therefore, the community itself must be an active participant in a CHA. NACCHO (2016a) writes: "Successful community health assessments build trust and community ownership of the process through active engagement of organizations and residents. Meaningful engagement involves the community in developing assessment protocols, identifying priorities, and implementing and monitoring community improvement efforts." An additional benefit of community engagement is that community members help bring visibility to CHA and improvement initiatives (Institute of Medicine 2003).

However, developing trust and building collaborative relationships between the community and the local, county, state, or regional health department can take time. Serrell and colleagues (2009) identify four "core values" that are constructive when working in partnership with community members on public health issues: (1) adaptability, (2) consistency, (3) shared authority, and (4) trust. In addition, McCoy (2010) has provided a list of important questions to consider when getting to know the community:

- Who are they?
- Where do they live?
- How do they live?
- What do they do?
- What's important to them?
- Who are the formal and informal leaders?
- What do they know about you?

Identify Key Partners and Stakeholders

A number of factors should be considered when building partnerships with key stakeholders. McCoy (2010) recommends asking the following questions:

- Who will be most affected by the work being conducted?
- Whose voices are rarely heard?
- Who has the most potential to effect change in a positive manner for the community (e.g., community leaders, people with access to resources, decision makers)?

Identify Community Health Indicators and Collect Data

A crucial step in the CHA process involves knowing the data that are available to help identify health issues in the community (McCoy 2010). The data will tell the community's story from a health perspective. When collecting and analyzing the data, carefully consider any issues related to their completeness, timeliness, and quality. You might ask, for instance, what is the cause-specific mortality rate for a particular disease in the community? What are the age-specific mortality rates? How do the mortality rates for the community compare to those of other communities? How do the rates compare to those of the state as a whole? What are the teenage pregnancy and birth rates for the community? Are these rates above or below national benchmarks?

Report the Health Priorities

Based on the analysis of available health data, report to the partners, stakeholders, and community, as a whole, the outcome of the process (McCoy 2010). What are the major health issues affecting the community? Report this information in a format that is respectful of the varying levels of health literacy among community members, as well as the varying preferences for ways of receiving health information (e.g., social media, newspaper, radio, town meeting).

Develop a Community Health Improvement Plan

Once the health priorities have been identified and reported, the partnership needs to develop a feasible plan to improve the health of the community. The plan should specify goals and objectives to be completed within a reasonable timeframe. It should address how resources will be allocated and how the work will take place, and the partners should agree upon the action steps. The plan should also identify performance measures that will indicate whether the actions have been successful (McCoy 2010).

The Community Health Improvement Process

community health improvement process (CHIP)
A broad improvement effort that includes a community health assessment, builds from the assessment's findings, and provides a framework for addressing key health issues.

The **community health improvement process (CHIP)** is a long-term effort that encompasses a CHA, builds from its findings, and provides a framework for addressing key health issues (PHAB 2010). It has the primary goal of improving the health of communities. The CHIP uses CHA data to identify issues, develop and implement strategies for action, and establish accountability to ensure measurable improvement (Durch, Bailey, and Stoto 1997). These aspects of the process are often outlined in the form of a community health improvement plan (which is also sometimes known by the acronym *CHIP*). The community health improvement process looks beyond the performance of a single organization serving a specific segment of the community; instead, it focuses on how the activities of multiple organizations contribute to community health improvement (Durch, Bailey, and Stoto 1997).

Public health experts have developed a variety of CHA and CHIP models that share common elements but differ somewhat in scope or philosophy. Information about several of those models—PRECEDE-PROCEED, Healthy Communities, the Planned Approach to Community Health, the Assessment Protocol for Excellence in Public Health, the CHIP described by Durch and colleagues, and Mobilizing for Action Through Planning and Partnerships (MAPP)—is presented in exhibit 9.1 (NACCHO 2016a). Note that

EXHIBIT 9.1 Community Health Assessment and Community Health Improvement Processes

	Description	Principles	Notes
PRECEDE-PROCEED	A health promotion assessment and planning process in which communities "precede" by defining their desired outcome and conducting an assessment and then "proceed" with intervention and evaluation	Taking time to identify the desired outcome prior to implementing an approach; collaboration; community-based interventions	Usually addresses a single health issue; implements a medical model
Healthy Communities	A health improvement process "owned" by the community	Collective action involving multiple, diverse systems; community ownership; community empowerment; systems change	Influenced MAPP; used in Canada and Europe
Planned Approach to Community Health	Engagement of the community to plan, implement, and evaluate health promotion programs; process includes community health assessment	Data-informed program development; community participation; collaboration; strengthening of local community capacity	Focuses on chronic disease health promotion
Assessment Protocol for Excellence in Public Health (APEXPH)	Tool to help local health departments carry out the core functions of public health	Community involvement; capacity of the local health department	Precursor to MAPP
Community Health Improvement Process	Process with iterative cycles, including identification and prioritization of health issues, analysis, and implementation	Accountability by community collaborators; shared goals; performance measurement	Influenced community health profiles
Mobilizing for Action Through Planning and Partnerships (MAPP)	Strategic planning process "owned" by the community, focusing on improving the health of the community and the local public health system; informed by four assessments	Strategic planning; community collaboration and "ownership"; identification of assets and needs	NACCHO's "gold standard" approach to improving community health

Source: Adapted from NACCHO (2016a).

the processes may include action at a system or agency level, at a local health department level, or even at a specific programmatic level. Some address the underlying factors that affect one or more conditions, while others focus on one specific health condition. Further, some approaches use a socioecological model of health, whereas others use a biomedical model (NACCHO 2016a).

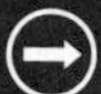

EXERCISE: EXAMPLES OF HIGH-QUALITY CHAs AND CHIPs

A collection of high-quality CHAs and CHIPs are presented on the NACCHO website at www.naccho.org/topics/infrastructure/CHAIP/guidance-and-examples.cfm. Explore the materials at the following links and answer the related discussion questions.

East Central Kansas Public Health Region: CHA/CHIP
http://archived.naccho.org/topics/infrastructure/CHAIP/upload/ECKPHC-CHA_CHIP_2012.pdf

1. Describe the CHA and CHIP processes based on the information provided.
2. Do you agree with the community's rationale for choosing which health issues to work on? Explain.

Alachua County, Florida, Health Department: Community Health Profile
http://archived.naccho.org/topics/infrastructure/CHAIP/upload/Alachua-County-Community-Health-Profile-2012.pdf

1. Review the section titled "Local Public Health System Performance Assessment" (pages 8–10), and describe how that assessment complements the CHA and CHIP.
2. Comment on possible reasons that the "Essential Public Health Services" ranked the way they did for this community. What factors might influence this rank order for a community?

CHA and CHIP Tools

Mobilizing for Action Through Planning and Partnerships

The Mobilizing for Action Through Planning and Partnerships (MAPP) tool is a resource jointly developed by NACCHO and the Centers for Disease Control and Prevention

(CDC). It is a community-driven strategic planning process, facilitated by public health leaders, that helps communities prioritize public health issues, find resources to address them, and ultimately improve the performance of local public health systems (NACCHO 2016c). It centers on a vision of "Communities achieving improved health and quality of life by mobilizing partnerships and taking strategic action." MAPP emphasizes the need for communities to use their resources wisely, take into account their unique circumstances and needs, and form effective partnerships for action. No one approach will fit every community; tailored approaches are more effective.

NACCHO (2016c) lists seven main elements of MAPP:

1. "*MAPP emphasizes a community-driven and community-owned approach.*" The community's strengths, needs, and desires drive the MAPP process, which strengthens community connections and provides access to the community's collective wisdom (NACCHO 2016c).

2. "*MAPP builds on previous experiences and lessons learned.*" MAPP incorporates concepts from previous planning efforts and assessment tools, most notably the Assessment Protocol for Excellence in Public Health (APEXPH) that was released in 1991, but is more progressive in a variety of ways (NACCHO 2016c). See exhibit 9.1 for comparison.

3. "*MAPP uses traditional strategic planning concepts within its model.*" The MAPP model includes such concepts as visioning, an environmental scan, identification of strategic issues, and formulation of strategies (NACCHO 2016c).

4. "*MAPP focuses on the creation and strengthening of the local public health system.*" MAPP defines *local public health systems* as the "human, informational, financial, and organizational resources, including public, private, and voluntary organizations and individuals, that contribute to the public's health"—a definition from the Institute of Medicine's *Improving Health in the Community* (Durch, Bailey, and Stoto 1997). The MAPP tool aims to bring these diverse elements together to carry out public health activities in a collaborative effort (NACCHO 2016c).

5. "*MAPP creates governmental public health leadership.*" MAPP helps create a greater recognition of the roles governmental entities (e.g., local health departments, boards of health, environmental agencies) play in their communities (NACCHO 2016c).

6. "*MAPP uses the essential public health services to define public health activities.*" The essential public health services (EPHS) discussed in

chapter 1, as well as other public health practice concepts, are incorporated into MAPP, helping to link it with other public health initiatives (NACCHO 2016c).

7. "*MAPP brings four assessments together to drive the development of a community strategic plan.*" The four assessments are the Community Themes and Strengths Assessment, which focuses on themes of interest to the community, quality-of-life perceptions, and community assets; the Local Public Health System Assessment, which measures the ability of the local public health system to carry out essential services; the Community Health Status Assessment, which analyzes data about health status, quality of life, and risk factors; and the Forces of Change Assessment, which identifies forces that affect or will affect the community or local public health system (NACCHO 2016c).

Community Tool Box

The Community Tool Box is an online resource developed by the Work Group for Community Health and Development at the University of Kansas, along with collaborating partners. It offers a variety of educational modules and other tools in support of its mission to "promote community health and development by connecting people, ideas, and resources" (Community Tool Box 2016). "The vision behind the Community Tool Box is that people—locally and globally—are better prepared to work together to change conditions that affect their lives."

County Health Rankings & Roadmaps

The County Health Rankings & Roadmaps program, previously discussed in chapter 4, is a collaboration between the Robert Wood Johnson Foundation and the University of Wisconsin Population Health Institute. The program provides a variety of data—including information about education, employment, income, obesity, and quality of air and water—to help answer the question, "How healthy is your community?" The Rankings provide a "snapshot of how health is influenced by where we live, learn, work and play," and the Roadmaps offer guidance and strategies for moving from education to action (County Health Rankings & Roadmaps 2016).

The program's goals include building awareness of the various factors that influence health; providing a reliable, sustainable source of local data to help communities find opportunities to improve health; engaging and activating local leaders from various sectors to create change; and empowering community leaders working to improve health (County Health Rankings & Roadmaps 2016).

Healthy People 2020 MAP-IT

Healthy People 2020, previously discussed in chapter 1, is an initiative of the US Department of Health and Human Services that helps guide health promotion and disease prevention efforts. An important part of the initiative is the Mobilize, Assess, Plan, Implement, Track (MAP-IT) tool, which helps the public health system plan and evaluate interventions aimed at achieving the Healthy People objectives. The MAP-IT tool operates under the premise that no two public health interventions are exactly alike, because no two communities are exactly alike (Healthy People 2016).

The Healthy People (2016) website provides guidance for each of MAP-IT's components:

Mobilize
Questions to ask and answer:

- What is the vision and mission of the coalition?
- Why do I want to bring people together?
- Who should be represented?
- Who are the potential partners (organizations and businesses) in my community?

Start by mobilizing key individuals and organizations into a coalition. Look for partners who have a stake in creating healthy communities and who will contribute to the process. Aim for broad representation.

Next, identify roles for partners and assign responsibilities. This will help to keep partners engaged in the coalition. For example, partners can:

- Facilitate community input through meetings, events, or advisory groups.
- Develop and present education and training programs.
- Lead fundraising and policy initiatives.
- Provide technical assistance in planning or evaluation.

Assess
Questions to ask and answer:

- Who is affected and how?
- What resources do we have?
- What resources do we need?

Assess both needs and assets (resources) in your community. This will help you get a sense of what you can do, versus what you would *like* to do.

Work together as a coalition to set priorities. What do community members and key stakeholders see as the most important issues? Consider feasibility, effectiveness, and measurability as you determine your priorities.

Start collecting state and local data to paint a realistic picture of community needs. The data you collect during the assessment phase will serve as baseline data. Baseline data provide information you gather before you start a program or intervention. They allow you to track your progress.

Plan

Questions to ask and answer:

- What is our goal?
- What do we need to do to reach our goal? Who will do it?
- How will we know when we have reached our goal?

A good plan includes clear objectives and concrete steps to achieve them. The objectives you set will be specific to your issue or community; they do not have to be exactly the same as the ones in Healthy People 2020.

Consider your intervention points. Where can you create change?

Think about how you will measure your progress. How will you know if you are successful?

When setting objectives, remember to state exactly what is to be achieved. What is expected to change, by how much, and by when? Make your objectives challenging, yet realistic.

Remember: Objectives need a target. A target is the desired amount of change (reflected by a number or percentage). A target needs a baseline (where you are now—your first data point).

Implement

Questions to ask and answer:

- Are we following our plan?
- What can we do better?

First, create a detailed workplan that lays out concrete action steps, identifies who is responsible for completing them, and sets a timeline and/or deadlines. Make sure all partners are on board with the workplan.

Next, consider identifying a single point of contact to manage the process and ensure that things get done. Be sure to share responsibilities across coalition members. Do not forget to periodically:

- Bring in new partners for a boost of energy and fresh ideas.
- Check in with existing partners often to see if they have suggestions or concerns.

Get the word out: develop a communication plan. Convene kick-off events, activities, and community meetings to showcase your accomplishments (and partners).

Track

Questions to ask and answer:

- Are we evaluating our work?
- Did we follow the plan?
- What did we change?
- Did we reach our goal?

Plan regular evaluations to measure and track your progress over time. Consider partnering with a local university or state center for health statistics to help with data tracking. Some things to think about when you are evaluating data over time:

- *Data quality*: Be sure to check for standardization of data collection, analysis, and structure of questions.
- *Limitations of self-reported data*: When you are relying on self-reported data (such as exercise frequency or income), be aware of self-reporting bias.
- *Data validity and reliability*: Watch out for revisions of survey questions and/or the development of new data collection systems. This could affect the validity of your responses over time. (Enlist a statistician to help with validity and reliability testing.)
- *Data availability*: Data collection efforts are not always performed on a regular basis.

Do not forget to share your progress—and successes—with your community. If you see a positive trend in data, issue a press release or announcement.

National Public Health Performance Standards

The CDC's National Public Health Performance Standards (NPHPS) provide a tool with which to assess the performance of the public health system and related governing bodies.

The NPHPS framework assists with identifying areas for improvement in the system, building stronger partnerships, and ensuring proper management of public health issues. Its tools are used to identify partners and community members in the public health system; engage those partners in health assessment and improvement planning; and promote improvement in agencies, systems, and communities (CDC 2016). The CDC (2016) identifies four key concepts that helped frame and inform the NPHPS:

- The ten essential public health services
- Focus on the overall public health system
- Focus on optimal performance rather than on minimum expectations
- Support for a process of continuous quality improvement

The standards incorporate three assessments: the State Public Health System Assessment Instrument, which focuses on state public health agencies and other partners at the state level; the Local Public Health System Assessment Instrument, which assesses the local public health system and entities that contribute to public health services in a community; and the Public Health Governing Entity Assessment Instrument, which focuses on governing bodies (e.g., boards of health, councils, or county commissioners) accountable for public health at the local level (CDC 2016).

Issues in Data Collection and Analysis for Community Health

The process of improving the health of a community starts with understanding the public health issues affecting the population and identifying those for which a feasible intervention can be implemented in a timely manner. Earlier in this chapter, we examined the steps of the CHA process. But once the community has been defined in terms of demographics, how do we know if the public health issues that were identified are indeed problematic? One way is by comparing the community's data with data from other areas that can serve as benchmarks. Common benchmarks include similar or nearby communities; state and national experiences; and state and national targets and goals (Tutko 2013).

quantitative data
Data that can be counted or expressed numerically.

Types of Data

qualitative data
Data provided in a verbal or narrative form.

Often, two types of data are collected about communities: **quantitative data**, which can be counted or expressed numerically, and **qualitative data**, which are provided in a verbal or narrative form. Quantitative data might include, for instance, vital records data, numbers of physician office and emergency room visits, Behavioral Risk Factor Surveillance System findings, and US Census figures. Qualitative data might include information obtained via key informant interviews, open-ended survey questions, or focus groups. Both types of data present certain advantages. Quantitative data can quickly summarize events and allow for easy comparison with benchmarks. Qualitative data, meanwhile, can offer explanations behind the quantitative data—in other words, the "hows" and "whys" behind the numbers—and allow for investigation of matters for which quantitative data are not available. In addition, the collection of quantitative data can lead to increased buy-in from stakeholders who have been directly asked about their experiences and opinions.

Data can also be classified as either primary or secondary. **Primary data** are collected by investigators for their own specific purpose, whereas **secondary data** have already been collected by someone else but can be used by other investigators for their own purposes. For example, quantitative primary data might come from an observation survey of seatbelt usage, and qualitative primary data might come from personal interviews about why respondents do or do not wear seatbelts. Quantitative secondary data might be obtained from a hospital discharge data set, and qualitative secondary data might include healthcare provider notes in an electronic medical record (Turko 2013).

primary data
Data collected by investigators for their own specific purpose.

secondary data
Data that have already been collected by others.

Obstacles to Data Collection

Accessing data for the assessment of community health can be challenging. Some data of interest might not be collected at the required geographic level, or even collected at all. Other data might be out of date or unable to be released because of confidentiality concerns. Another issue involves the privacy of individuals who represent rare or unusual events. For instance, if only a very small number of cases of a condition exist in a community, the reporting of health data might enable others to identify those individuals. To prevent personal identification in such cases, local and state health departments and other agencies will often suppress the reporting of events if they number fewer than, say, five cases.

The Community Benefit Standard and Population Health

In 1969, the US Internal Revenue Service (IRS) set forth the **community benefit standard**, which enables eligible nonprofit hospitals to maintain a tax-exempt status and receive federal funding for services provided to the poor in their communities (Miller 2009). To qualify under the community benefit standard, a nonprofit hospital must meet the following requirements (Miller 2009):

- It must have a board made up of community members.
- Qualified physicians in the area must have medical privileges at the hospital.

community benefit standard
A set of requirements for nonprofit hospitals in the United States seeking tax-exempt status and federal funding for services provided to the poor.

- It must have an emergency department.
- It must admit all types of patients without discrimination.
- Funding must be directed to benefit the patients served by the hospital.

The community benefit standard relates to community health assessments in a number of ways. First, the Affordable Care Act (ACA) of 2010 included provisions to more closely tie the community benefit standard to community health, and these provisions require hospitals to conduct CHAs and develop CHIPs (IRS 2016; Turner and Evashwick 2014). In addition, the IRS, in monitoring compliance with the standard, has recognized that hospitals can benefit their communities not only by providing charitable care but also by providing community-oriented health promotion efforts (Turner and Evashwick 2014). Furthermore, the Public Health Accreditation Board has developed national accreditation guidelines for local and state public health departments, and these guidelines also include a CHA requirement (PHAB 2015). As a result of these and other developments, a significant sector of the public health system will be assessing community health.

In conducting assessments and developing feasible interventions, the public health system should recall the Evans and Stoddart field model of health and well-being (discussed in chapter 8), which emphasizes the wide range of determinants contributing to a community's health status. Turner and Evashwick (2014, 159) highlight the complex nature of the work:

> No single entity in a community can take full credit for "preventing a disease," because too many relevant factors are beyond the control of any single organization. This means that health-related organizations serving any target population must work together to impact the health status of that population, and no single entity can measure the impact of its activities without acknowledging the potential impact, positive or negative, of other entities affecting the same target population. Collaboration on needs assessment, interventions, and impact measurement become essential.

Stoto (2013) summarizes, "Population health is fundamentally about measuring health outcomes and their upstream determinants and using these measures to coordinate the efforts of public health agencies, the healthcare delivery system, and many other entities in the community to improve health." He concludes: "Managing a shared responsibility, however, is challenging; given the many factors that influence health, no single entity can be held accountable for health outcomes."

Key Chapter Points

- A community health assessment (CHA) is a systematic examination of health status indicators for a population. It is conducted for the purpose of identifying key problems and assets in a community and assisting with the development of strategies to address the community's health issues. The concept of the CHA is grounded in the core functions of public health—assessment, policy development, and assurance.
- The steps involved in the CHA include the following: (1) describe the community and define the population; (2) engage the community and understand their health priorities; (3) identify key partners and stakeholders; (4) identify community health indicators and collect data; (5) report the health priorities; and (6) develop a community health improvement plan.
- The CHA is part of a broader community health improvement process (CHIP). The CHIP uses CHA data to identify issues, develop and implement strategies for action, and establish accountability to ensure measurable improvement.
- Public health experts have developed a variety of CHA and CHIP models that share common elements but differ somewhat in scope or philosophy.
- The Mobilizing for Action Through Planning and Partnerships (MAPP) tool was jointly developed by the National Association of County and City Health Officials (NACCHO) and the Centers for Disease Control and Prevention (CDC). It provides a strategic planning process to help communities prioritize public health issues, find resources to address them, and ultimately improve the performance of local public health systems.
- NACCHO (2016c) describes the key elements of MAPP: It is community-driven and community-owned, builds on previous experiences and lessons learned, uses traditional strategic planning concepts, focuses on the creation and strengthening of the local public health system, creates governmental public health leadership, incorporates the essential public health services, and brings four assessments together to drive the development of a strategic plan.
- The Community Tool Box is an online resource developed by the Work Group for Community Health and Development at the University of Kansas, along with collaborating partners. It offers a variety of educational modules and other tools.
- The County Health Rankings & Roadmaps program is a collaboration between the Robert Wood Johnson Foundation and the University of Wisconsin Population Health Institute. Its goals include building awareness of the factors that influence health; providing a reliable, sustainable source of local data for communities; and engaging and empowering community leaders to improve health.

- The Mobilize, Assess, Plan, Implement, Track (MAP-IT) tool helps the public health system plan and evaluate interventions aimed at achieving the objectives of the US government's Healthy People initiative.
- The CDC's National Public Health Performance Standards (NPHPS) provide a tool with which to assess the performance of the public health system and related governing bodies. They incorporate three assessments: the State Public Health System Assessment Instrument, the Local Public Health System Assessment Instrument, and the Public Health Governing Entity Assessment Instrument.
- Quantitative data can be counted or expressed numerically, whereas qualitative data are provided in a verbal or narrative form. Both types of data present certain advantages. For example, quantitative data can summarize events and allow for comparison to benchmarks, whereas qualitative data can offer useful explanations.
- Accessing data for the assessment of community health can be challenging. Some data of interest might not be collected at the required geographic level, or even collected at all. Other data might be out of date or unable to be released because of confidentiality concerns.
- The community benefit standard, set forth by the US Internal Revenue Service (IRS), enables nonprofit hospitals, if they meet certain requirements, to maintain a tax-exempt status and receive federal funding for services provided to the poor in their communities.
- The Affordable Care Act (ACA) of 2010 included provisions to more closely tie the community benefit standard to community health, and these provisions require hospitals to conduct CHAs and develop CHIPs. In addition, the Public Health Accreditation Board (PHAB) has developed national accreditation guidelines for local and state public health departments, and these guidelines include a CHA requirement.

Discussion Questions

1. What is a community health assessment? Briefly describe the CHA process.
2. How are CHAs and CHIPs useful in improving the health of communities?
3. Describe two tools used to conduct a CHIP.
4. What types of data are useful in a CHA?
5. What is the community benefit standard?
6. How can the community benefit standard be useful in improving population health?

7. Using a diagram, show the relationship between community health and the systems that deliver healthcare.
8. What are the similarities and differences between MAPP and MAP-IT?

References

Centers for Disease Control and Prevention (CDC). 2016. *National Public Health Performance Standards: Strengthening Systems, Improving the Public's Health*. Accessed October 21. www.cdc.gov/nphpsp/documents/nphpsp-factsheet.pdf.

Cibula, D. A., L. F. Novick, C. B. Morrow, and S. M. Sutphen. 2003. "Community Health Assessment." *American Journal of Preventive Medicine* 24 (4 Suppl.): 118–23.

Community Tool Box. 2016. "About the Community Tool Box." Accessed October 21. http://ctb.ku.edu/en/about-the-tool-box.

County Health Rankings & Roadmaps. 2016. "About." Accessed September 16. www.countyhealthrankings.org/about-project.

Dever, G. E. A. 1997. *Improving Outcomes in Public Health Practice: Strategy and Methods*. Gaithersburg, MD: Aspen Publishers.

Durch, J. S., L. A. Bailey, and M. A. Stoto. 1997. *Improving Health in the Community: A Role for Performance Monitoring*. Washington, DC: National Academies Press.

Edberg, M. 2007. *Essentials of Health Behavior: Social and Behavioral Theory in Public Health*. Sudbury, MA: Jones & Bartlett.

Healthy People. 2016. "MAP-IT: A Guide to Using Healthy People 2020 in Your Community." Accessed October 21. www.healthypeople.gov/2020/tools-and-resources/Program-Planning.

Institute of Medicine. 2003. *The Future of the Public's Health in the 21st Century*. Washington, DC: National Academies Press.

———. 1988. *The Future of Public Health*. Washington, DC: National Academies Press.

Internal Revenue Service (IRS). 2016. "New Requirements for 501(c)(3) Hospitals Under the Affordable Care Act." Updated July 29. www.irs.gov/charities-non-profits/charitable-organizations/new-requirements-for-501c3-hospitals-under-the-affordable-care-act.

Issel, L. M. 2004. *Health Program Planning and Evaluation: A Practical, Systematic Approach for Community Health*. Sudbury, MA: Jones & Bartlett.

McCoy, K. 2010. *Multi-State Learning Collaborative—III, Learning Session 1*. Slide presentation at the Minnesota Department of Health, St. Paul, MN, March 25.

Miller, S. T. 2009. "Charitable Hospitals: Modern Trends, Obligations, and Challenges." Internal Revenue Service. Published January 9. www.irs.gov/pub/irs-tege/miller_speech_011209.pdf.

National Association of County and City Health Officials (NACCHO). 2016a. "Community Health Assessment and Improvement Processes." Accessed October 20. http://archived.naccho.org/topics/infrastructure/CHAIP/upload/CHA-and-CHIP-Processes-JJE.pdf.

——. 2016b. "Definitions of Community Health Assessment (CHA) and Community Health Improvement Plans (CHIPs)." Accessed October 19. http://archived.naccho.org/topics/infrastructure/community-health-assessment-and-improvement-planning/upload/Definitions.pdf.

——. 2016c. "MAPP Basics: Introduction to the MAPP Process." Accessed October 20. www.naccho.org/topics/infrastructure/mapp/framework/mappbasics.cfm.

Public Health Accreditation Board (PHAB). 2015. *Guide to National Public Health Department Initial Accreditation*. Published June. www.phaboard.org/wp-content/uploads/Guide-to-Accreditation-final_LR2.pdf.

——. 2011. *Acronyms and Glossary of Terms: Version 1.0*. Published September. www.phaboard.org/wp-content/uploads/PHAB-Acronyms-and-Glossary-of-Terms-Version-1.02.pdf.

——. 2010. *PHAB E-Newsletter, Issue #27*. Published September. http://conta.cc/iGPOVA.

Serrell, N., R. M. Caron, B. Fleishmann, and E. D. Robbins. 2009. "An Academic-Community Outreach Partnership: Building Relationships and Capacity to Address Childhood Lead

Poisoning." *Progress in Community Health Partnerships: Research, Education, and Action* 3 (1): 53–59.

Stoto, M. 2013. "Community Health Needs Assessments—An Opportunity to Bring Public Health and the Healthcare Delivery System Together to Improve Population Health." *Improving Population Health.* Published April 16. www.improvingpopulationhealth.org/blog/2013/04/community-health-needs-assessments-an-opportunity-to-bring-public-health-and-the-healthcare-delivery.html.

Turner, J. S., and C. Evashwick. 2014. "Population, Community, and Public Health: Measuring the Benefits." *Advances in Health Care Management* 16: 151–69.

Turnock, B. J. 2009. *Public Health: What It Is and How It Works*, 4th ed. Burlington, MA: Jones & Bartlett Learning.

Tutko, H. 2013. Guest lecture in HMP 501, Epidemiology and Community Medicine, at the University of New Hampshire.

CHAPTER 10

MANAGERIAL EPIDEMIOLOGY: A PRIMER

"Knowledge of health and disease in a population is as important to the healthcare executive as it is to the public health officer."

—Peter J. Fos and David J. Fine (2005)

Learning Objectives

After completing this chapter, you should be able to

- define *managerial epidemiology*,
- describe the role of managerial epidemiology in healthcare,
- explain how a healthcare administrator would use managerial epidemiology to make decisions,
- discuss the population health approach with respect to health services management, and
- explain the population health care management model.

Introduction

Managerial epidemiology can be defined simply as "the study of the application of epidemiologic concepts and principles to the practice of management" (Fleming 2015, 1), or as the "application of the tools and principles of epidemiology to the decision-making process" within healthcare settings (Fleming 2013, 148). Managerial epidemiology is comprehensive in its approach, and it uses information from communities and healthcare settings to improve health outcomes for populations. This chapter begins by examining the role of managerial epidemiology in the healthcare system; it then addresses the population health approach with respect to the healthcare management model.

managerial epidemiology
The application of epidemiologic tools and principles to decision-making processes and the practice of management in healthcare settings.

Managerial Epidemiology and the Healthcare System

Fleming (2013, 148) argues that management (i.e., planning, controlling, staffing, financing) of the healthcare system can benefit from the tools provided by the field of epidemiology, and he points out the difficulty of developing a strategic plan without incorporating epidemiologic estimates: "For example, strategic planning and needs assessment must consider the present and future burden of disease (measured by what epidemiologists call 'prevalence') and the burden of risk factors, which can translate into subsequent disease, by a factor that epidemiologists call 'relative risk.'" He further states that "the tools of epidemiology provide critical information for managers and planners seeking to predict future demand for services amid the current insurance markets." Fos and Fine (2005, xix) support Fleming's argument on the utility of managerial epidemiology, pointing out that contemporary applications in healthcare management can involve "monitoring the quality and effectiveness of clinical services, strategic and program planning, marketing, and managing insurance and managed care."

Like the community health assessment (discussed in the previous chapter), the managerial epidemiology approach defines the population and strives to understand the demographics and trends with respect to the living environment (i.e., the physical, socioeconomic, and political environment). Next, it evaluates the population's healthcare needs based on the people's knowledge, attitudes, and beliefs concerning health and health issues, as well as on the accessibility of healthcare services. In addition, it considers how healthcare providers are influenced to manage patients' care needs.

Epidemiologic data can be quite useful in highlighting community needs. Think about the data sources previously discussed in this book, and then consider which ones might be helpful in painting an epidemiologic picture of "need" in a community. Birth data for adolescent mothers, for instance, might reflect needs relating to comprehensive health education. Behavioral Risk Factor Surveillance System data for the community can reveal issues with how the population perceives its own health. Absenteeism from work or school might suggest high stress levels or the beginning of an infectious disease outbreak.

Finally, borrowing from operations research, one might use hospital data to better understand why members of the population go to the emergency room or to ambulatory care centers. Effective identification of needs in the community can help the public health and healthcare systems allocate sufficient resources, develop appropriate interventions, and evaluate the actions taken.

Oleske (2001) proposes that healthcare managers must consider the population size served by healthcare providers; the distribution of health needs in the population; the genesis and consequences of health problems; the way the healthcare system and its organizational characteristics affect the health status of the people; techniques for monitoring performance of the health system, organizations, and programs; the need for restructuring in response to a changing environment; and the development and evaluation of public policy affecting healthcare delivery. She challenges healthcare managers to answer the following questions using an epidemiologic framework (Oleske 2001, 21):

1. Who is the population served?
   a. How is this population defined?
   b. What are the major size and demographic trends in this population?
   c. From what distances do individuals travel to receive health care?
2. What are the population's health care needs?
   a. How can these needs be measured?
   b. What is the prevalence of risk factors?
   c. What is the burden of disease and other problems?
3. What health services are feasible for addressing the population's health care needs?
   a. What are barriers the population can experience when attempting to access health care services?
   b. What are the capabilities of the organization/system relative to the size and needs of the population (personnel, equipment, facilities)?
   c. How do the services of the local health system link to national or regional policy goals or initiatives?
   d. What environmental influences affect health services delivery (payment conditions, provisions, market competition, trends affecting preferred delivery mode/setting)?
4. What is the population's health status?
   a. How will the health status be measured at the present and over time?

Oleske (2001, 22) concludes: "To improve the health status of a population, one needs to understand the population characteristics, the distribution and level of need, factors affecting the use of health care services, and the implications on the system if the desired level of health status is not achieved."

A Population Health Approach

A population health approach can help health administrators apply managerial epidemiology to their work. First, let's revisit the population health approach, as described by the Public Health Agency of Canada (2013):

> *Population health* refers to the health of a population as measured by health status indicators and as influenced by social, economic, and physical environments, personal health practices, individual capacity and coping skills, human biology, early childhood development, and health services. As an approach, population health focuses on the interrelated conditions and factors that influence the health of populations over the life course, identifies systematic variations in their patterns of occurrence, and applies the resulting knowledge to develop and implement policies and actions to improve the health and well-being of those populations.

Recall that the "patient" of public health is not the individual but rather the population. Thus, actions to improve health are directed at the population level and not at the individual level. This approach requires the public health system to identify inequalities in the health status of population groups and to address those inequalities. The Public Health Agency of Canada (2013) continues:

> An underlying assumption of a population health approach is that reductions in health inequities require reductions in material and social inequities. The outcomes or benefits of a population health approach, therefore, extend beyond improved population health outcomes to include a sustainable and integrated health system, increased national growth and productivity, and strengthened social cohesion and citizen engagement.

The population health approach requires a change in the ways that public health and healthcare systems do business. Implementation can be challenging and is resource intensive.

How to Implement a Population Health Approach

The Canadian approach to population health is a model for any community striving to improve the health of its population. The Public Health Agency of Canada (2013) explains:

> In 1989, the Canadian Institute for Advanced Research (CIAR) introduced the population health concept, proposing that individual determinants of health do not act in isolation. It is the complex interaction among determinants that can have a far more significant effect on health. For example, unemployment can lead to social isolation and poverty, which in turn influences one's psychological health and coping skills.

Together, these factors can then lead to poor health. As we learn more about how these interactions affect health, we'll better understand why and how policies and different health approaches affect the health of a population. We'll also better understand why some groups within populations are healthier than others in spite of the fact that all Canadians have access to the health care system.

Based on work from the Public Health Agency of Canada (2013), we can identify several actions that are key to the implementation of a population health approach:

- *Invest upstream.* When considering what keeps a population healthy or sick, focus should be directed at the root causes. That way, direct interventions will have the greatest potential to positively affect the health status of the population.
- *Make evidence-based decisions.* Decision making should be grounded in current research. As communities are examined, new information can improve our understanding of how various factors act as determinants of health and how the effectiveness of interventions can be maximized.
- *Implement multiple strategies.* Consider not only the social determinants of health but also the economic, environmental, and political factors. Also, consider what agency or organization will implement the strategies and how they will be evaluated.
- *Collaborate.* Public health is interdisciplinary and collaborative in its approach, and the same philosophy applies when developing a population health framework. The public health and healthcare sectors must integrate for a population health approach to be successfully implemented.
- *Engage citizens.* Members of the community must play a meaningful role in the population health approach, just as they must in the community health assessment and community health improvement processes described previously. Community members live with the health issues affecting the population and can contribute essential qualitative information.
- *Increase accountability for health outcomes.* Improved health outcomes are the goal of a population health approach. Evaluating processes, impacts, and outcomes and communicating this information to stakeholders are key components of the approach.

The American Medical Association (AMA 2002) published a number of population health principles for clinical settings in *Paradigms for Clinical Practice: A Primer on Population-Based Medicine.* Dever (2006, 101) highlights the following key elements from the primer:

- A *holistic view* to treat the patient's unique characteristics and also the societal influences on the patient
- A *systems approach* to coordinate and integrate the delivery of care by using multidisciplinary teams and multiorganizational arrangements for referral
- An *epidemiological foundation* to improve objectivity in clinical and policy decision making
- An *anthropologic view* to understand the patient's perspective of his/her health
- *Distributive justice* to recognize and reduce the unequal distributions of illness, disease, disability, and death across different groups

Dever (2006, 101) states that "incorporating these principles into medical care and health services management can facilitate the process to optimize health." Health services managers who do so "will ensure that their planning and management approach will be responsive to the populations in the communities and to the individuals in their clinics" (Dever 2006, 102).

Population Health Care Management Model

Transitioning to a population health care management model will require a change in orientation and the development of new management skills. Fos and Fine (2005) write:

> The "reformed" health care executive will directly interact with the community and its health insurance vehicles in the planning of medical services to be delivered, including allocation of human and material resources to preventive, curative, restorative, and rehabilitative services. The executive's duties include the design of medical interventions and the monitoring and evaluation of medical services and programs. Clinical outcome measurement and comparison will become a major source of information for management decision making. Population health care design and planning will gain importance in the evolving integrated delivery systems of the future.

The population health care management model focuses chiefly on the health of the population and the containment of costs. Fos and Fine (2005, 10) explain: "In the population health care management model, the management objectives change to include the reduction in volume of services utilized, shift of utilization to lower-cost settings, achievement of clinical improvement by focusing on the health status of the population, integration of healthcare services, organization of providers into networks, and evaluation and documentation of quality."

Using this model, managerial epidemiology "incorporates the business aspects of health care that monitor demand, delivery, clinical outcome measurement, resource allocation, strategic analysis, program planning, and managed care" (Caron 2010, 1549). In the wake of the Affordable Care Act, with the number of people in the US healthcare system growing dramatically, the ability to provide equitable care while containing costs and ultimately reducing the demand for healthcare is crucial. Managerial epidemiology will allow for healthcare administrators to align "social and economic objectives so that the improvement of population health is the prime metric of success" (Caron 2010, 1549).

Case Study

A Community with Two Hospitals

The community of Greater Manchester, New Hampshire, is primarily served by two hospitals: Catholic Medical Center (CMC) and Elliot Hospital. This case provides information about the two hospitals and a community health assessment for Greater Manchester. Once you have read the materials, answer the discussion questions.

CATHOLIC MEDICAL CENTER

The following is an excerpt from the CMC (2016b) website:

> In today's turbulent healthcare environment, we . . . need to focus on evolving from volume-based (payments based on the number of patients we see) to value-based (payments based on the quality of care we provide to patients) and we are proud of our progress to-date. We are participating in the Anthem Patient Centered Primary Care (PC2) program, Cigna shared savings, and the top 10 in the country for quality—NH Accountable Care Organization. CMC is a proud member of Granite Health—a partnership of five independent New Hampshire charitable community health systems (Catholic Medical Center, Concord Hospital, LRGHealthcare, Southern New Hampshire Health System, and Wentworth-Douglass Hospital) leading the transformation of health care delivery in the communities they serve. . . . Granite Health members are committed to sharing resources to provide better, more seamless and less expensive care for their patients.
>
> CMC has also been focused on growing and enhancing our services. We have a Patient Transfer Center that large hospital systems are looking to model. We continue to expand our cardiac, vascular, and bariatric (weight loss) services throughout the state and announced our Telestroke and Teleneurologist program that complements our hospital-based neurologist (neurohospitalist) and award-winning Gold Plus stroke program. We are proud of our continued collaborative spirit with critical access hospitals throughout the state to focus on improving the quality of care available to their patients and the communities they serve.

(continued)

The CMC (2016a) mission statement is as follows: "The heart of Catholic Medical Center is to provide health, healing, and hope in a manner that offers innovative high-quality services, compassion, and respect for the human dignity of every individual who seeks or needs our care as part of Christ's healing ministry through the Catholic Church."

ELLIOT HOSPITAL

The Elliot Hospital (2016) website offers the following description:

> Elliot Health System (EHS) is the largest provider of comprehensive healthcare services in Southern New Hampshire. The cornerstone of EHS is Elliot Hospital, a 296-bed acute care facility located in Manchester (New Hampshire's largest city). Established in 1890, Elliot Hospital offers Southern New Hampshire communities caring, compassionate, and professional patient service regardless of race, religion, national origin, gender, age, disability, marital status, sexual preference, or ability to pay.
>
> EHS is home to Manchester's designated Regional Trauma Center, Urgent Care Centers, a Level 3 Newborn Intensive Care Unit, Elliot Physician Network, Elliot Specialists, Elliot Regional Cancer Center, Elliot Senior Health Center, Visiting Nurse Association of Manchester and Southern New Hampshire, Elliot 1-Day Surgery Center, Elliot at River's Edge, and Elliot Pediatrics.

The EHS mission statement is as follows:

> Elliot Health System strives to:
>
> INSPIRE wellness
> HEAL our patients
> SERVE with compassion in every interaction.

GREATER MANCHESTER COMMUNITY HEALTH NEEDS ASSESSMENT

The following are excerpts from a community health needs assessment (CHNA) for Greater Manchester from June 2013. It was conducted jointly by CMC and EHS (2013), with assistance from the City of Manchester Health Department.

Community

> The 2013 Community Health Needs Assessment focused on the Health Service Area (HSA) of Greater Manchester, a market which is primarily served by Catholic Medical Center and Elliot Hospital. The Manchester HSA is home to approximately 180,000 residents and is comprised of the towns of Auburn, Bedford, Candia, Deerfield, Goffstown, Hooksett, New Boston, as well as the City of Manchester. These towns are located in three different counties (Hillsborough, Rockingham, and Merrimack) within the State of New Hampshire with 60% of the residents of the HSA living within the City of Manchester. (CMC and EHS 2013, 4)

(continued)

Demographics

The population of the Manchester HSA is changing; not only is it aging, it is becoming increasingly multicultural with residents reflecting a variety of nationalities, languages, ethnic traditions, religious beliefs, and ideologies.

The City of Manchester is home to 60% of the residents of the HSA and, in alignment with the State of New Hampshire, the population of the Manchester HSA is aging. The 65+population within the HSA is projected to realize an 18% growth through 2018, and many other towns within the HSA will experience over 30% growth in the 65+age group. . . . The City of Manchester's pediatric population is projected to realize an increase of about 2% in children ages 0–17. (CMC and EHS 2013, 5)

Access to Health Care

Residents in the City of Manchester are much more likely not to have health care coverage than the rest of the State of New Hampshire. Residents earning less than $25,000 are more than twice as likely to not have health coverage as the rest of the city and almost three times as likely to not have coverage as the rest of the state. People who do not have health care coverage need to pay the entire costs for care themselves. The statistics are almost exactly the same for not being able to see a doctor because of cost. Residents earning less than $25,000 are more than twice as likely to not see a doctor because of cost than the rest of the city and almost three times as likely as the rest of the state. . . . Such barriers to accessing health services attribute to: unmet health needs, delays in receiving appropriate care, inability to get preventive services, as well as preventable hospitalizations. (CMC and EHS 2013, 38–39)

Health Issues

The CHNA workgroup reviewed the data collected, the surveys, key leader interviews, and focus group minutes and after much discussion has identified the following needs to be addressed in the community:

- Behavioral health issues: mental health services and access, substance abuse—specifically illicit drug use and tobacco use
- Obesity: diabetes, poor eating habits, lack of physical activity
- Aging issues: stroke, Alzheimer's, pneumonia, transportation, medication coordination, caregiver support, inadequate out-of-home care
- Chronic disease: heart disease, cancer, COPD
- Ambulatory care sensitive conditions—marker for lack of adequate preventive care: need care coordination
- Barriers to access of health care services related to poverty: lack of insurance, cost, transportation, lack of information on how to access care and what services are available if uninsured, language, lack of a medical home

(continued)

- Teen pregnancy
- STDs: specifically chlamydia
- Dental services/access: specifically for adults
- Asthma
- Violence and crime: neglect and abuse, safe neighborhoods, suicide, youth crime (CMC and EHS 2013, 50–51)

Suggestions and Issues Raised by Community Members and Survey Respondents

- More mental health providers
- Coping skills for mentally ill
- Additional substance abuse services
- Coordination across agencies to promote better services and programs
- Collaborate as a community with other like organizations and support each other—so all groups can share with people
- More shelters
- More homeless housing
- Open a free/low-cost dental care facility
- Low-cost dental clinics
- Better dental care for Medicare/Medicaid people without insurance
- Health providers giving inadequate time/attention to patients
- Increase healthcare options for low-income/uninsured people
- Expand medication bridge programs to help more people get access to patient assistance programs
- Improved access for affordable health insurance to low-income/nondisabled
- People should have enough food and access to more food pantries
- More assistance for the elderly
- Volunteers to visit nursing home residents
- More gyms geared toward 65+ population
- Improve housing conditions and options—hold landlords accountable for deplorable conditions, decrease wait list time
- Clean out the lead-painted old multifamily units, especially the ones with poor heating systems
- Clean up the run-down areas . . .
- Low-cost weight management programs outside of bariatric surgery
- Make Manchester a smoke-free city

(continued)

- Affordable public transportation
- Transportation for appointments
- Increase funding for schools
- Work for change in American beliefs and attitudes regarding how health is valued and what it means to be healthy (CMC and EHS 2013, 64)

CASE STUDY DISCUSSION QUESTIONS

1. Describe the services provided by the two hospitals in the Greater Manchester community.
2. Considering that two hospitals serve a population of approximately 180,000 people, would you expect the population of this hospital service area to be healthier than other communities in New Hampshire? Explain your rationale.
3. Review the community needs assessment and the suggestions from community members. Propose a way that the hospitals might work together to implement a population health approach to address two of the identified needs.
4. Identify four health determinants that might be contributing to poor health for the community.
5. Research the amount of charitable care provided to the community from the two hospitals, and comment on the type of community benefit activities these hospitals provide.

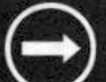

EXERCISE: A HEALTHY COMMUNITY?

Introduction

The city of Portsmouth, New Hampshire, is part of the Greater Portsmouth Public Health Region, and it is located in Rockingham County. In this exercise, you will examine Portsmouth's epidemiologic indicators and healthcare services—essentially, conducting a mini-CHA—and generally assess whether Portsmouth is a healthy community.

For this exercise, you will use the following set of indicators for Portsmouth:

- Population breakdown by race for 2006–2010 (using the racial categories of white/Caucasian, black or African American, American Indian or Alaska Native, Asian or Pacific Islander, and "other races")
- Percentage of children younger than 18 years old living with families at or below the federal poverty level for 2006–2010

(continued)

- Age-adjusted heart disease death rate (per 100,000 population) for 2008
- Percentage of the population 18 years or older at a healthy weight for 2009–2010
- Percentage of low-birthweight births in 2008

You will use this health indicator set to compare Portsmouth with three benchmarks: the state of New Hampshire, the United States as a whole, and the Healthy People 2020 targets (if available for the indicator in question).

Part 1: Identify and Describe Data Sources

1. Access the New Hampshire Health Data Inventory (NH HDI) at www.nhhealthdata.org and view the introductory tutorial presented on the site.
2. Using the NH HDI, identify the data sources for the five indicators, both for Portsmouth and for the three benchmarks. For national benchmark data, the NH HDI will point you to respective national data sources; for the Healthy People 2020 targets, go to www.healthypeople.gov/2020/default.
3. Once you have located your anticipated data sources, prepare a table to describe them. The format of the table and one sample entry (to demonstrate the level of detail expected) are shown here:

Data Source Name	Data Source Description	Data Steward (Organization Name)	Latest Data Year Available	Geographic Aggregation	Indicators Supported
Youth Risk Behavior Surveillance System	A school-based survey implemented annually in all states that assesses risk behaviors among high school students	NH data stewarded by the New Hampshire Dept. of Education	2007	1. City of Manchester 2. NH state	Percent of high school students who smoked in 2007

Note: When you write the description of a data source, use your own words. Also, the "Geographic Aggregation" column should indicate all the geographic levels of data aggregation (e.g., city, public health region, county, state, nation) that your team will be using in this mini-CHA.

(continued)

Part 2: Find and Record Indicator Data

1. Locate the indicator data for Portsmouth and the three benchmarks. Data for the indicators can be retrieved using the following resources:

   - The New Hampshire Health Web-Based Reporting and Query System (NH HealthWRQS) website (www.nhhealthwrqs.org)
   - The NH HDI website (www.nhhealthdata.org), which links to data not available through NH HealthWRQS
   - The Healthy People 2020 website (www.healthypeople.gov/2020/default.aspx)

2. Record the indicator data in a Microsoft Excel workbook. The data for each indicator should be listed on a separate workbook page.

Note:

- *In some cases, data for a specific community may not be available on the NH HealthWRQS website. In such cases, substitute another community that is close to the Portsmouth community. For example, data might be unavailable at the city level but available at the public health region level. For this exercise, you are not expected to complete data requests or obtain "secure access use" privileges through NH HealthWRQS.*
- *Unless otherwise indicated, disease and injury rates should be age-adjusted to the 2000 national population and expressed as a rate per 100,000 people (e.g., 250 deaths per 100,000 persons). In the rare event that a rate is expressed as "per 10,000 persons," convert the rate to "per 100,000 people" by adding a zero to the numerator. (A rate of 34 hospitalizations per 10,000 people, for instance, would become 340 hospitalizations per 100,000 people.)*
- *Typically, Healthy People 2020 will have several target measures (e.g., death rates, hospitalization rates) within a topic area. Review them carefully to pick the target that matches your indicator definition.*
- *Some data sources vary in their definition of the United States (for instance, they may provide data for the 50 states plus DC, or for the 50 states plus DC and territories). For this exercise, use data for the 50 states plus DC.*

Part 3: Create Data Displays and Interpret Data Findings

Using the chart-making functionality in Excel, create a data display of Portsmouth's indicator data compared to the benchmarks. Then describe the key "takeaway"

(continued)

message the display reveals. The data display types appropriate for the various indicators are listed here:

Indicator Type	Data Display Type
Age and race distributions	Pie chart
Income, poverty, education indicators	Table
Disease and injury death/hospitalization rates	Bar chart
Behavioral risk factors (e.g., smoking, weight)	Column chart
Maternal and child health (e.g., low-birthweight babies, infant mortality rate)	Column chart

Each data display should meet the following requirements:

1. A chart title must be centered above the data display.
2. A list of data sources and years must be provided at the bottom of the display.
3. Pertinent data notes must be provided. For instance, if a rate is age-adjusted, the population to which it is adjusted should be documented. Similarly, if data for your community are not available and an alternate community definition is used, an explanation should be provided (e.g., "Data were not available for Manchester, so the above display uses data for Hillsborough County, the county in which Manchester is located.").
4. For bar and column charts, the *y* axis must be labeled with the appropriate unit of measurement for the indicator (e.g., "deaths per 100,000").
5. For tables, bar charts, and column charts, the top line should show your target community's indicator result. For pie charts, the first pie chart should show the results for the target community, and separate pie charts should represent the benchmarks.
6. The display should include a succinct and easily understood sentence that describes to residents of the community the key "takeaway" message.

Part 4: Use a Population Health Approach

1. For the health outcomes of each indicator examined for Portsmouth, identify the appropriate health services available in the community and the organizations that are best equipped to address these health issues.

(continued)

2. Identify community collaborations that can address these health issues.
3. Identify any health outcome information. (For instance, is there a particular health outcome that is more prevalent than another?)

Source: Adapted from a pilot project conducted by the New Hampshire Institute for Health Policy and Practice and the University of New Hampshire Department of Health Management and Policy, with funding from the University of New Hampshire Office of the Provost. Exercise developed by Rosemary M. Caron and Holly Tutko, 2011; used in HMP 501 Epidemiology and Community Medicine course.

Case Study

Diabetes and Hospital Readmissions

The following is the abstract from a study by Jiang and colleagues (2005, 1561) titled "Racial/Ethnic Disparities in Potentially Preventable Readmissions: The Case of Diabetes":

> *Objectives.* Considerable differences in prevalence of diabetes and management of the disease exist among racial/ethnic groups. We examined the relationship between race/ethnicity and hospital readmissions for diabetes-related conditions.
>
> *Methods.* Non-maternal adult patients with Medicare, Medicaid, or private insurance coverage hospitalized for diabetes-related conditions in 5 states were identified from the 1999 State Inpatient Databases of the Healthcare Cost and Utilization Project. Racial/ethnic differences in the likelihood of readmission were estimated by logistic regression with adjustment for patient demographic, clinical, and socioeconomic characteristics and hospital attributes.
>
> *Results.* The risk-adjusted likelihood of 180-day readmission was significantly lower for non-Hispanic whites than for Hispanics across all 3 payers or for non-Hispanic blacks among Medicare enrollees. Within each payer, Hispanics from low-income communities had the highest risk of readmission. Among Medicare beneficiaries, blacks and Hispanics had higher percentages of readmission for acute complications and microvascular disease, while whites had higher percentages of readmission for macrovascular conditions.
>
> *Conclusions.* Racial/ethnic disparities are more evident in 180-day than in 30-day readmission rates, and greatest among the Medicare population. Readmission diagnoses vary by race/ethnicity, with blacks and Hispanics at higher risk for those complications more likely preventable with effective post-discharge care.

(continued)

CASE STUDY DISCUSSION QUESTIONS

1. How would you explain the differences in hospital readmission rates for Hispanics, blacks, and whites?
2. Explain why "racial/ethnic disparities are more evident in 180-day than in 30-day readmission rates"?
3. What services could the local public health system provide to reduce the readmission rate for a preventable health condition?

Key Chapter Points

- Managerial epidemiology is the application of epidemiologic tools and principles to decision-making processes and the practice of management in healthcare settings.
- Fleming (2013) argues that management (i.e., planning, controlling, staffing, financing) of the healthcare system can benefit from the tools provided by the field of epidemiology, and he highlights the importance of epidemiologic estimates in developing strategic plans.
- Oleske (2001) proposes that healthcare managers must consider the population size served by healthcare providers; the distribution of health needs in the population; the genesis and consequences of health problems; the way the healthcare system and its characteristics affect people's health status; techniques for monitoring performance of the health system, organizations, and programs; the need for restructuring in response to a changing environment; and the development and evaluation of public policy affecting healthcare delivery.
- "As an approach, population health focuses on the interrelated conditions and factors that influence the health of populations over the life course, identifies systematic variations in their patterns of occurrence, and applies the resulting knowledge to develop and implement policies and actions to improve the health and well-being of those populations" (Public Health Agency of Canada 2013).
- The "patient" of public health is not the individual but rather the population. Thus, actions to improve health are directed at the population level and not at the individual level. This approach requires the public health system to identify inequalities in the health status of population groups and to address those inequalities.

- Actions key to the implementation of a population health approach include investing upstream, making evidence-based decisions, implementing multiple strategies, collaborating, engaging citizens, and increasing accountability for health outcomes.
- "In the population health care management model, the management objectives change to include the reduction in volume of services utilized, shift of utilization to lower-cost settings, achievement of clinical improvement by focusing on the health status of the population, integration of healthcare services, organization of providers into networks, and evaluation and documentation of quality" (Fos and Fine 2005, 10).

Discussion Questions

1. What is managerial epidemiology?
2. Explain the population health approach.
3. Describe the population health care management model.
4. How might a healthcare administrator use managerial epidemiology to make decisions?
5. Diagram the relationship between managerial epidemiologic functions and the objectives of epidemiology.

References

American Medical Association (AMA). 2002. *Paradigms for Clinical Practice: A Primer on Population-Based Medicine*. Chicago: American Medical Association.

Caron, R. M. 2010. "Managerial Epidemiology Is the Best Evaluation Tool for Our New Health Care System." *Academic Medicine* 85 (10): 1549.

Catholic Medical Center (CMC). 2016a. "Our Mission, Vision, & Values." Accessed October 25. www.catholicmedicalcenter.org/about-us/our-mission.aspx.

———. 2016b. "President's Message." Accessed October 25. www.catholicmedicalcenter.org/about-us/our-ceo-and-board-of-directors.aspx.

Catholic Medical Center (CMC) and Elliot Health System (EHS). 2013. *The Greater Manchester Community Health Needs Assessment, June 2013*. Published June. www.catholicmedicalcenter.org/uploads/2013%20CHNA%20FINAL%207-10-13.pdf.

Dever, G. E. A. 2006. *Managerial Epidemiology: Practice, Methods, and Concepts*. Sudbury, MA: Jones & Bartlett.

Elliot Hospital. 2016. "About the Elliot." Accessed October 25. http://elliothospital.org/website/about-us.php.

Fleming, S. T. 2015. *Managerial Epidemiology: Concepts and Cases*, 3rd ed. Chicago: Health Administration Press.

———. 2013. "Managerial Epidemiology: It's About Time!" *Journal of Primary Care & Community Health* 4 (2): 148–49.

Fos, P. J., and D. J. Fine. 2005. *Managerial Epidemiology for Health Care Organizations*, 2nd ed. San Francisco: Jossey-Bass.

Jiang, H. J., R. Andrews, D. Stryer, and B. Friedman. 2005. "Racial/Ethnic Disparities in Potentially Preventable Readmissions: The Case of Diabetes." *American Journal of Public Health* 95 (9): 1561–67.

Oleske, D. M. (ed.). 2001. *Epidemiology and the Delivery of Health Care Services*, 2nd ed. New York: Kluwer Academic / Plenum Publishers.

Public Health Agency of Canada. 2013. "What Is the Population Health Approach." Updated January 15. www.phac-aspc.gc.ca/ph-sp/approach-approche/appr-eng.php.

CHAPTER 11

POPULATION HEALTH IMPROVEMENT

"The roundtable's vision is of a strong, healthful, and productive society which cultivates human capital and equal opportunity. This vision rests on the recognition that outcomes such as improved life expectancy, quality of life, and health for all are shaped by interdependent social, economic, environmental, genetic, behavioral, and health care factors, and will require robust national and community-based policies and dependable resources to achieve it."

—National Academies of Sciences, Engineering, and Medicine (2016b)
Roundtable on Population Health Improvement

Learning Objectives

After completing this chapter, you should be able to

- define *population health improvement,*
- identify four approaches to improving population health,
- describe the role of quality improvement in population health, and
- explain the plan-do-check-act cycle.

Introduction

The National Academy of Medicine (NAM), formerly the Institute of Medicine, regularly convenes a Roundtable on Population Health Improvement, at which leaders in public health, healthcare, business, education, and other fields gather to "catalyze urgently needed action toward a stronger, more healthful, and more productive society" (National Academies of Sciences, Engineering, and Medicine 2016b). NAM has adopted Kindig and Stoddart's (2003, 381) definition of *population health*: "the health outcomes of a group of individuals, including the distribution of such outcomes within the group." NAM notes that, although the interaction of multiple health determinants is not specifically mentioned in the definition, such determinants (e.g., behaviors, genetics, access to healthcare, the physical environment) provide the foundation for the health outcomes in a population (National Academies of Sciences, Engineering, and Medicine 2016b).

The NAM roundtable engages leaders, experts, and other stakeholders around three main goals: "(1) supporting fruitful interaction between primary care and public health, (2) strengthening governmental public health, and (3) exploring community action in transforming the conditions that influence the public's health" (National Academies of Sciences, Engineering, and Medicine 2016a). Those same goals are central to the population health improvement approaches described in this chapter.

Approaches to Improving Population Health

This section describes four approaches to improving population health: (1) the community health needs assessment, as required under the Affordable Care Act; (2) the Public Health Foundation's population health driver program; (3) public health and healthcare system collaboration; and (4) the Health in All Policies approach.

Community Health Needs Assessment

The Affordable Care Act (ACA) of 2010 requires that nonprofit hospitals conduct community health needs assessments (CHNAs), which are essentially the same as the community health assessments (CHAs) described previously. The purpose of the CHNAs is not only to assess the health needs of the communities the hospitals serve but also to implement strategies to address those needs (Rosenbaum 2013; Stoto 2013). The CHNA mandate complements the community benefit standard and the Public Health Accreditation Board's CHA and CHIP requirements for public health departments (both discussed in chapter 9).

Stoto (2013) proposes that the ACA requirement has the potential to improve population health outcomes by encouraging collaboration and aligning the efforts and resources of the public health system, the healthcare sector, and other community organizations. Stoto and Smith (2015, 1) explain: "Collecting data and measuring results consistently on a short list of indicators at the community level and across all participating organizations not only ensures that efforts remain aligned but also enables the participants to hold each other accountable and learn from each other's successes and failures." They continue: "Given the many factors that influence health, no single entity can be held accountable for health outcomes, and neither hospitals nor health departments want to publish indicators that they cannot influence by their activities" (Stoto and Smith 2015, 2).

Stoto and Smith (2015) propose a two-pronged approach: First, a community health profile—essentially, a CHNA or CHA—should establish priorities; second, stakeholders should work toward agreed-upon health outcomes for the community and share the accountability for meeting the identified goals. Establishing the community health profile involves many of the concepts already discussed in this book: measures of health determinants, access to healthcare, and health behaviors; observation of trends (e.g., increases, decreases, or no change); and comparison with benchmarks (e.g., national data, state data). "As long as the focus of these activities is aligned with an evidence-based overall community health improvement strategy in which hospitals, health departments, and other organizations contribute according to their interests and strengths, these indicators can include process measures and be tailored to the target populations that each of these entities serve" (Stoto and Smith 2015, 11).

EXERCISE: HEALTHY MONADNOCK

The following is an excerpt from the website of Healthy Monadnock (2017), a community engagement initiative in New Hampshire:

> Healthy Monadnock is a community engagement initiative designed to foster and sustain a positive culture of health throughout Cheshire County and the Monadnock region . . . . Founded and developed by the Cheshire Medical Center / Dartmouth-Hitchcock Keene in 2007, Healthy Monadnock's action plans are being guided in the community by the Healthiest Community Advisory Board, a group of 30 individuals representing schools, organizations, coalitions and businesses. Currently, the City of Keene, the Keene School District and five area coalitions are implementing action strategies designed to improve quality of life and prevent the leading causes of death for everyone.

The city of Keene, New Hampshire, in the heart of the Monadnock region, developed a *Comprehensive Master Plan* that outlines the community's efforts to work toward its laudable goal.

(continued)

For this exercise, explore the Keene plan (available at www.ci.keene.nh.us/departments/planning/keene-comprehensive-master-plan), and then answer the following questions:

1. Examine the section of the Keene plan titled "Community Snapshot." How is the community changing with respect to population, health, housing, and land use?
2. Review the section titled "The Plan," and describe Keene's plan for community health and wellness.
3. What stakeholders are involved in addressing the issue of community health and wellness?
4. What is the role of Keene State College in improving the health of the community?
5. Select another topic in the section labeled "The Plan," and describe how it is connected to improving the health of the community.
6. Navigate to the section titled "The Six Vision Focus Areas." Do you agree with this list? Should efforts be made in a related or unrelated area? Explain your rationale.
7. How is Keene's plan being implemented?
8. Specifically describe how the Keene community will know whether it has improved the health of the population.

Population Health Driver Diagram Framework

Another approach to population health improvement is the **population health driver diagram** framework developed by the Public Health Foundation (PHF). The diagram, shown in exhibit 11.1, helps align the efforts of public health and healthcare organizations to better "tackle challenges at the crossroads" of those two sectors (Bialek, Moran, and Kirshy 2015, 1). Bialek, Moran, and Kirshy (2015, 2) explain:

population health driver diagram
A tool for aligning the efforts of public health and healthcare organizations to address health issues. The diagram links key health aims with broad primary drivers and more specific secondary drivers.

> A population health driver diagram identifies primary and secondary drivers of an identified community health objective and serves as a framework for determining and aligning actions that can be taken within a community for achieving the objective. This framework offers not only a starting point for discussion but also flexibility for identifying and addressing unique community characteristics, assets, and needs. It helps create an atmosphere of cooperation by enabling each participant working to address the specific community health objective the opportunity to identify and articulate roles already being played by that individual's organization and to develop an understanding

> of how what he or she is doing fits in with other community organizations. In addition, this framework can be used to determine other actions that can be taken individually and collectively to positively impact the particular community health objective.

The PHF (2015) summarizes: "A population health driver diagram can be used collaboratively by public health, health care, and other partners to identify the potential primary and secondary drivers that can help to achieve an identified community health objective." The diagram can serve as a starting point for discussion among stakeholders, and it can promote an atmosphere of cooperation by enabling all participants to identify their roles in addressing a health challenge.

> *"Public health and health care organizations are more effective when they combine their efforts to address a community population health issue than when they work separately and competitively"*
>
> —Bialek, Moran, and Kirshy (2015)

Exhibit 11.1
Population Health Driver Diagram

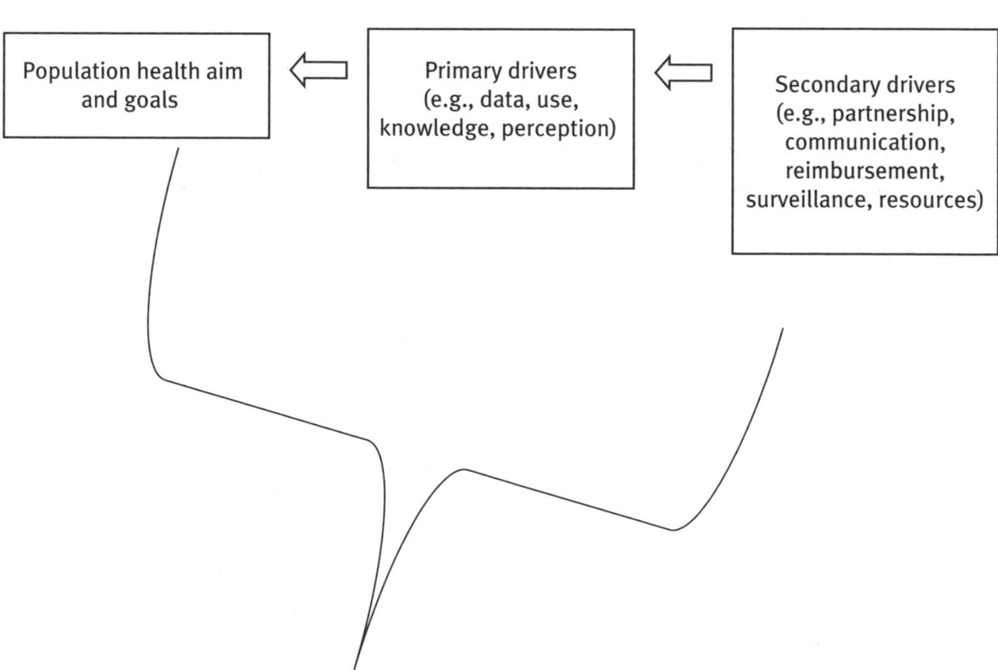

Source: Adapted from Bialek, Moran, and Kirshy (2015).

The population health driver diagram uses a "tree diagram" structure. The left side provides a general "aim statement," broadly identifying the issue being addressed, and a list of goals related to that aim. In the center of the diagram are the primary drivers, a set of key factors for achieving the goals. The primary drivers are broad in scope, and they can be explored and broken down into a set of secondary drivers, which appear to the right side of the diagram. The secondary drivers are more specific and precise, and they provide a basis from which targeted interventions can be developed (PHF 2015).

Bialek, Moran, and Kirshy (2015) describe the PHF's application of the population health driver framework to the issue of improving the use of antibiotics. Through a "Public Health Antibiotic Stewardship Driver Diagram," health departments and hospitals in three separate states worked together to identify primary and secondary drivers and to develop interventions that could be applied by the various stakeholders. The primary drivers identified by the public health and healthcare systems included the following (Bialek, Moran, and Kirshy 2015):

- Appropriate use of antibiotics
- Data monitoring
- Knowledge and awareness of proper antibiotic use

The secondary drivers were as follows:

- Information about which antibiotics are most effective
- Identification of prevalent diseases in the community
- Incentives for proper antibiotic use
- Appropriate policies for work and school settings
- Use of community-specific resistance data to inform proper antibiotic selection
- Intervention plans for specific target audiences (e.g., patients, providers, insurers)

Community-specific interventions were developed at each site. "Although the specific accomplishments of each site differed, implementation of protocols to tackle antibiotic use and the spread of antibiotic-resistant disease, as well as the education of physicians, nurses, pharmacists, child care workers, and others about the appropriate and inappropriate use of antibiotics, were pillars of achievement common among the pilots" (Bialek, Moran, and Kirshy 2015, 2).

EXERCISE: CREATE A POPULATION HEALTH DRIVER DIAGRAM FOR ADOLESCENT SMOKING

Go to the Public Health Foundation website and access the resource titled "Developing a Population Health Driver Diagram" (www.phf.org/resourcestools/Pages/Developing_a_Population_Health_Driver_Diagram.aspx). Download and read the document provided, and then develop your own population health driver diagram for preventing the smoking of tobacco among the adolescent population.

Public Health and Healthcare System Collaboration

A key focus across many population health improvement approaches is the need for collaboration among public health and healthcare entities. Many entities (whether complying with Affordable Care Act provisions, the community benefit standard for tax exemptions, or Public Health Accreditation Board requirements) must assess the health of the communities in which they provide services; as they do so, they should coordinate their assessments to avoid duplication and to maximize resources (Montero, Lupi, and Jarris 2015).

Significant and sustained improvement in a population's health requires "clear direction, commitment, and effective collaboration" between many entities that provide care or engage in improvement efforts (Montero, Lupi, and Jarris 2015, 1). Montero, Lupi, and Jarris (2015, 2) further point out the risks that emerge when hospitals carry out their assessments in isolation:

> While most hospitals genuinely want to improve the health of the communities they serve, without meaningful community participation, some hospitals could perform CHNAs and CHIPs in a manner that only minimally satisfies federal requirements. Without review, a hospital could also possibly steer CHNAs and CHIPs to prioritize preferred clinical programs and interventions. In addition, without crucial information from health agencies and communities, hospitals could inadvertently underrepresent vulnerable populations in their CHNA processes. To counter these risks, local and state public health officials can vigorously educate and engage their communities and assertively seek partnerships with local hospitals' top leadership to share data, assessment methodologies, and evidence-based interventions, and connect hospitals with existing community coalitions. Given the opportunities presented by the fundamental health system changes underway across the country, governmental public health should join forces with hospitals by playing a leading role in this aspect of the community health improvement process.

Such integration and collaboration efforts should focus not only on clinical services but also on community-based prevention efforts (Montero, Lupi, and Jarris 2015).

Health in All Policies (HiAP)

Health in All Policies (HiAP) is a collaborative approach to improving population health by incorporating health considerations into decision making across various sectors and policy areas (Rudolph et al. 2013a). The World Health Organization (2013, 2) explains HiAP as follows:

Health in All Policies (HiAP)
A collaborative approach to improving population health by incorporating health considerations into decision making across various sectors and policy areas.

> Health in All Policies is an approach to public policies across sectors that systematically takes into account the health implications of decisions, seeks synergies, and avoids harmful health impacts, in order to improve population health and health equity. A Health in All Policies approach is founded on health-related rights and obligations. It improves accountability of policymakers for health impacts at all levels of policymaking. It includes an emphasis on the consequences of public policies on health systems, determinants of health, and well-being.

HiAP emphasizes a collaborative approach to issues that fall under the purview of public health but also affect other sectors—for instance, efforts to fluoridate tap water, restrict tobacco use in public spaces, improve sanitation, prevent drunk driving, or require the use of seatbelts or child car seats. Rudolph and colleagues (2013b, 2) explain: "Health in All Policies takes project-by-project collaboration further by formalizing structures and mechanisms to incorporate a health, equity, and sustainability lens across the whole of government." They continue:

> Medical services, while vitally important, play a lesser role in overall population health improvement than the social determinants of health—the environments in which people live, work, learn, and play. Economic status, educational attainment, structural racism, and neighborhood characteristics are critical determinants of health and health inequities. Improvements in a community's economic, physical, social, and service environments can help ensure opportunities for health and support healthy behaviors. However, health agencies rarely have the mandate, authority, or organizational capacity to make the policy, systems, and environmental changes that can promote healthy living through healthy environments. That responsibility falls to housing, transportation, education, air quality, parks, criminal justice, agriculture, energy, and employment agencies, among others.
>
> Solutions to these complex and urgent problems will require collaborative efforts across many sectors at the local, state, regional, and federal levels, including government agencies, businesses, and community-based organizations. Collaboration across

sectors can also promote efficiency by identifying opportunities to share resources and reduce redundancies, thus potentially decreasing costs and improving performance and outcomes in a time of great pressure on government resources. (Rudolph et al. 2013b)

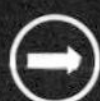

EXERCISE: HEALTH IN ALL POLICIES

Access the peer-reviewed article "Health in All Policies for Big Cities," by Wernham and Teutsch (2015), at www.ncbi.nlm.nih.gov/pmc/articles/PMC4243805/. Read the article, and answer the following questions:

1. Describe how HiAP can be used to develop healthy populations. What are some specific examples?
2. Select one of the cities discussed in the article, and research additional information to update the case.
3. What tools are useful when engaging in the HiAP approach?

quality improvement (QI)
The continuous use of deliberate processes to improve efficiency, effectiveness, outcomes, and other aspects of performance.

plan-do-check-act (PDCA) cycle
A process consisting of four phases (*plan*, *do*, *check*, and *act*) for developing, implementing, testing, and refining quality-improvement activities.

Population Health and Quality Improvement

Quality improvement (QI) in public health involves the use of defined and deliberate processes to improve the activities of responding to community needs and improving population health. It represents "a continuous and ongoing effort to achieve measurable improvements in the efficiency, effectiveness, performance, accountability, outcomes, and other indicators of quality in services or processes which achieve equity and improve the health of the community" (NACCHO 2016). One of the most important QI processes is the **plan-do-check-act (PDCA) cycle**, illustrated in exhibit 11.2.

Gorenflo and Moran (2015) outline the phases of the PDCA process as follows:

- *Plan.* The focus of this phase is to investigate the current situation, understand the nature of the problem to be solved, and develop potential solutions that can be tested. It involves six steps: (1) Identify and prioritize the issue to be addressed; (2) describe the goal, the target audience, and the measure for determining your effectiveness; (3) describe the current approach to the issue, and identify areas for improvement; (4) collect both baseline data and trend data on the issue; (5) identify factors contributing to the problem; and (6) develop an action plan.

- *Do.* This phase involves the implementation of the action plan; the collection of data; and the documentation of problems, observations, and lessons learned.
- *Check.* The third phase focuses on analyzing the effect of the intervention.
- *Act.* The fourth phase involves acting upon what was learned—typically either adopting the intervention, modifying it, or abandoning it and returning to the "plan" phase.

The steps in the PDCA process are reminiscent of the core functions of public health, as discussed earlier in the book: assessment, policy development, and assurance.

Exhibit 11.2
The Plan-Do-Check-Act Cycle

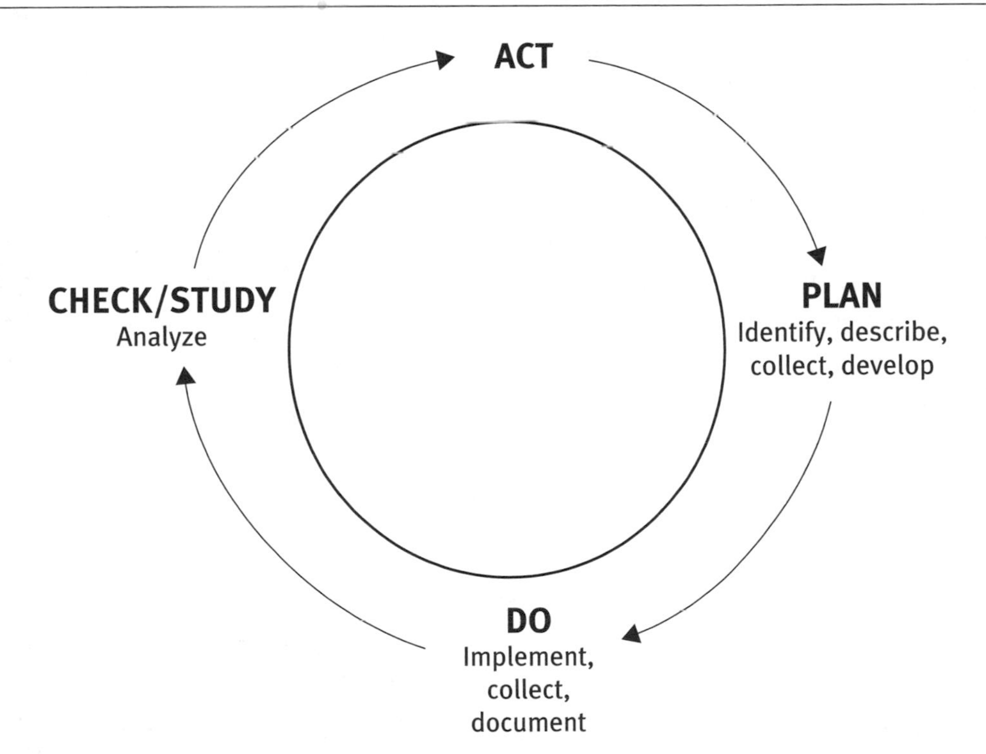

Source: Adapted from Gorenflo and Moran (2015).

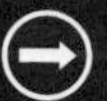

EXERCISE: EXAMINING QUALITY IMPROVEMENT INITIATIVES

Access the Public Health Foundation's (2016) summary page for the QI project titled "From Good to Great: Using QI to Standardize Prescription for Health" (available at www.phf.org/resourcestools/Pages/From_Good_to_Great_Using_QI_to_Standardize_Prescription_for_Health.aspx). Read the article, and answer the following questions:

1. What is the key issue being addressed for this population?
2. Describe the QI goals and processes that were implemented.
3. How does the program work?
4. What have been the results of this QI process?
5. Describe the partners involved.
6. Do you think this project is reproducible in other communities? Explain your reasoning. Consider the barriers that would need to be overcome and the resources required to initiate a similar program in another community.

Now access the Public Health Foundation's (2014) summary page for the QI project titled "Maine CDC: Working with Healthcare to Address Antibiotic Resistant Disease" (available at www.phf.org/resourcestools/Pages/Public_Health_and_Healthcare_Collaborate_to_Reduce_Maines_Antibiotic_Resistant_Infections.aspx). Read the article, and answer the following questions:

1. What is the key issue being addressed for this population?
2. Consider the interventions described in the article. What drivers are they addressing?
3. How was QI implemented in addressing this issue?
4. Describe the partners involved.
5. Do you think this project is reproducible in other communities? Explain your reasoning. Consider the barriers that would need to be overcome and the resources required to initiate a similar program in another community.

Key Chapter Points

- The National Academy of Medicine's Roundtable on Population Health Improvement engages leaders, experts, and other stakeholders to improve interaction between healthcare and public health, to strengthen governmental public health, and to consider community actions to affect the conditions that influence the public's health. These concepts are central to a number of approaches to population health improvement.
- The Affordable Care Act (ACA) requires nonprofit hospitals to conduct community health needs assessments (CHNAs), which are essentially the same as the community health assessments (CHAs) described previously. The purpose of the CHNAs is not only to assess the health needs of the communities the hospitals serve but also to implement strategies to address those needs.
- The population health driver diagram framework, developed by the Public Health Foundation, helps align the efforts of public health and healthcare organizations to better address the challenges facing both sectors. The diagram links a given health issue with broad primary drivers and more specific secondary drivers, providing a basis from which targeted interventions can be developed.
- Significant and sustained improvement in a population's health requires direction, commitment, and collaboration between many entities that provide care or engage in improvement efforts.
- Health in All Policies (HiAP) is a collaborative approach to population health improvement that seeks to incorporate health considerations into decision making across various sectors and policy areas.
- Quality improvement (QI) in public health involves the use of defined and deliberate processes to improve the activities of responding to community needs and improving population health.
- The plan-do-check-act cycle is a process, consisting of four phases, for developing, implementing, testing, and refining quality-improvement activities.

Discussion Questions

1. Define *population health improvement*.
2. What are four approaches to improving population health?
3. Identify two potential barriers to a collaborative approach among public health and healthcare organizations.

4. What is the role of quality improvement in population health?
5. Explain the plan-do-check-act cycle.

References

Bialek, R., J. Moran, and M. Kirshy. 2015. *Using a Population Health Driver Diagram to Support Health Care and Public Health Collaboration*. National Academy of Sciences. Published February 4. https://nam.edu/wp-content/uploads/2015/06/DriverDiagramCollaboration1.pdf.

Gorenflo, G., and J. W. Moran. 2015. "The ABCs of PDCA." Accessed June 8. www.phf.org/resourcestools/Pages/The_ABCs_of_PDCA.aspx.

Healthy Monadnock. 2017. "Becoming the Nation's Healthiest Community." Accessed January 12. https://healthymonadnock.org/.

Kindig, D., and G. Stoddart. 2003. "What Is Population Health?" *American Journal of Public Health* 93 (3): 380–83.

Montero, J. T., M. V. Lupi, and P. E. Jarris. 2015. *Improved Population Health Through More Dynamic Public Health and Health Care System Collaboration*. National Academy of Sciences. Published February 6. https://nam.edu/wp-content/uploads/2015/06/DynamicPHHCCollaboration.pdf.

National Academies of Sciences, Engineering, and Medicine. 2016a. "Activity: Roundtable on Population Health Improvement." Updated October 19. http://nationalacademies.org/HMD/Activities/PublicHealth/PopulationHealthImprovementRT.aspx.

———. 2016b. "Vision, Mission, and Definition of the Roundtable on Population Health Improvement." Updated April 22. www.nationalacademies.org/hmd/Activities/PublicHealth/PopulationHealthImprovementRT/VisionMission.

National Association of County and City Health Officials (NACCHO). 2016. "Quality Improvement." Accessed October 31. www.naccho.org/topics/infrastructure/accreditation/quality.cfm.

Public Health Foundation (PHF). 2016. "From Good to Great: Using QI to Standardize Prescription for Health." Accessed October 31. www.phf.org/resourcestools/Pages/From_Good_to_Great_Using_QI_to_Standardize_Prescription_for_Health.aspx.

——. 2015. "Developing a Population Health Driver Diagram." Accessed June 9. www.phf.org/resourcestools/Pages/Developing_a_Population_Health_Driver_Diagram.aspx.

——. 2014. "Maine CDC: Working with Healthcare to Address Antibiotic Resistant Disease." Published February. www.phf.org/resourcestools/Pages/Public_Health_and_Healthcare_Collaborate_to_Reduce_Maines_Antibiotic_Resistant_Infections.aspx.

Rosenbaum, S. 2013. "Update: Treasury/IRS Proposed Rule on Community Benefit Obligations of Nonprofit Hospitals." HealthReformGPS. Published April 17. www.healthreformgps.org/resources/update-treasuryirs-proposed-rule-on-community-benefit-obligations-of-nonprofit-hospitals/.

Rudolph, L., J. Caplan, K. Ben-Moshe, and L. Dillon. 2013a. *Health in All Policies: A Guide for State and Local Governments*. American Public Health Association and Public Health Institute. Accessed October 31, 2016. www.apha.org/~/media/files/pdf/factsheets/health_inall_policies_guide_169pages.ashx.

Rudolph, L., J. Caplan, C. Mitchell, K. Ben-Moshe, and L. Dillon. 2013b. *Health in All Policies: Improving Health Through Intersectoral Collaboration*. Public Health Institute. Published September 18. www.phi.org/uploads/application/files/q79jnmxq5krx9qiu5j6gzdnl6g9s41l65co2ir1kzolvmx67to.pdf.

Stoto, M. 2013. "Population Health in the Affordable Care Act Era." *AcademyHealth*. Accessed June 8, 2015. www.academyhealth.org/files/AH_2013%20Population%20Health%20final.pdf.

Stoto, M. A., and C. R. Smith. 2015. "Community Health Needs Assessments? Aligning the Interests of Public Health and the Health Care Delivery System to Improve Population Health." National Academy of Sciences. Published April 9. https://nam.edu/perspectives-2015-community-health-needs-assessments-aligning-the-interests-of-public-health-and-the-health-care-delivery-system-to-improve-population-health/.

Wernham, A., and S. M. Teutsch. 2015. "Health in All Policies for Big Cities." *Journal of Public Health Management and Practice* 21 (Suppl. 1): S56–S65.

World Health Organization. 2013. "Health in All Policies—Framework for Country Action." Published May 9. www.healthpromotion2013.org/images/130509_HiAP_Framework_for_Country_Action_Draft.pdf.

SECTION 3

POPULATION HEALTH MANAGEMENT

CHAPTER 12

PRINCIPLES OF POPULATION HEALTH MANAGEMENT

"Although primary care and public health share a goal of promoting the health and well-being of all people, these two disciplines historically have operated independently of one another. Problems that stem from this separation have long been recognized, but new opportunities are emerging for bringing the sectors together in ways that will yield substantial and lasting improvements in the health of individuals, communities, and populations."

—Institute of Medicine (2012)

Learning Objectives

After completing this chapter, you should be able to

- define *population health management*,
- identify three principles and skills key to the management of population health,
- explain three population health management approaches, and
- describe two challenges of implementing population health management.

Introduction

As noted in the quote that opens this chapter, the public health and healthcare systems have traditionally worked in relative isolation from each other. The focus of healthcare, or primary care, is treating patients via medical services; the focus of public health, meanwhile, is preventing disease and promoting health via collective community efforts. The management of population health, however, requires these two systems to integrate their work with the aim of ensuring a healthy population. Public health and healthcare have a great deal to learn from each other, but they must overcome challenges in adopting a new business model.

In 2012, a committee of the Institute of Medicine (IOM)—now the National Academy of Medicine—noted that "it is not possible to prescribe a specific model or template for how integration (of primary care and public health) should look" because "the types of interactions between the two sectors are so varied and dependent on local circumstances" (IOM 2012, 1–2). However, the IOM (2012) did identify a few "core principles" that should be included in integration efforts:

- The common goal of improving population health
- A focus on identifying and addressing the community's needs
- Leadership commitment to bridging disciplines, programs, and jurisdictions
- Analysis of data in a collaborative manner with stakeholders

Furthermore, the IOM (2012, 2) argued not for a complete merger of the two systems, but rather for varying "degrees of integration"—ranging from "mutual awareness" to "cooperation" to "collaboration" to "partnership"—appropriate to each community. Mutual awareness enables the healthcare and public health systems to be informed of the issues the other is addressing. Cooperation allows for the sharing of human and financial resources. Collaboration enables the systems to work in a combined effort, though it requires the development of trust and mutual respect (which can take time). Finally, partnership helps the systems work toward a shared, common goal.

population health management (PHM) The application of management strategies to improve the delivery of healthcare for populations, with an emphasis on achieving the highest quality at the lowest cost.

Understanding Population Health Management

Population health management (PHM) is a complex and sometimes vague concept, as evidenced by the variety of themes that will be returned in a literature search on the term. However, the term has become widely used in healthcare and public health, and it represents a worthwhile approach for the delivery of care in a rapidly changing system.

PHM involves changes in the organization and management of healthcare delivery systems to make them more clinically effective, more cost-effective, and safer (Burton 2013). It refers to "the proactive application of strategies and interventions to defined cohorts of individuals across the continuum of healthcare delivery in an effort to maintain and/or improve the health of the individuals within the cohort at the lowest necessary cost" (Burton 2013, 2). The integration of healthcare and public health systems is necessary for its success.

Whereas the term *population health* focuses more broadly on the determinants of health for a population, PHM emphasizes the delivery of healthcare for populations with the highest quality and lowest cost. However, Lewis (2014) notes that the intersection between the two terms can become blurred in certain instances:

> Consider, for example, the comprehensive care designs that serve the needs of your most complex, high-risk, and costly patients. The identification, understanding, and segmentation of your population; the redesign of services for that population; and the delivery of those services at scale require organizations to understand and address the broader social, environmental, and behavioral determinants of health in order to achieve better outcomes, improve the care experience, and control total cost.

Research indicates that healthcare accounts for approximately 20 percent of a population's health; health behaviors account for 30 percent, socioeconomic factors for 40 percent, and the physical environment for 10 percent (Magnan et al. 2012). Therefore, successful PHM must consider not only the management of lifestyle, disease, critical care, and disability; it must also consider the Health in All Policies approach (discussed in chapter 11) and supportive community initiatives focused on disease prevention and health promotion (Halfon and Conway 2013; McAlearney 2003).

Population Health Management and the Triple Aim

PHM's emphasis on collaborative effort is consistent with the **Triple Aim** framework developed by the Institute for Healthcare Improvement (IHI). The Triple Aim represents an approach to optimizing health system performance by emphasizing three dimensions: "improving the patient experience of care (including quality and satisfaction), improving the health of populations, and reducing the per capita cost of healthcare" (IHI 2016). None of the three factors of the Triple Aim can exist in isolation, or else the attempted improvement will fail. As the US healthcare system undergoes substantial reform and a shift from fee-for-service payment to value-based models, PHM works in concert with the Triple Aim to improve the health experience for populations across multiple dimensions.

Triple Aim
A framework for optimizing health system performance by emphasizing three dimensions: improving the patient experience, improving the health of populations, and reducing cost per capita; developed by the Institute for Healthcare Improvement.

> *"There is a growing realization that the successful health and health care systems of the future will be those that can simultaneously deliver excellent quality of care, at optimized costs, while improving the health of their population. This is known as the IHI Triple Aim."*
>
> —Institute for Healthcare Improvement (2016)

Core Measures for Population Health Management

The IOM (2015, 2–3) developed the following "core measure set" of 15 indicators that healthcare and public health systems should track to determine how well they are managing the health of populations:

1. Life expectancy
2. Well-being
3. Overweight and obesity
4. Addictive behavior
5. Unintended pregnancies
6. Healthy communities
7. Preventive services
8. Access to care
9. Patient safety
10. Evidence-based care
11. Care that matches patient goals
12. Personal spending burden
13. Population spending burden
14. Individual engagement
15. Community engagement

In selecting these indicators, the IOM (2015, 2) first considered "importance for health, likelihood to contribute to progress, understandability, technical integrity, potential to have broader system impact, and utility at multiple levels." In refining the list, the IOM

(2015, 2) aimed to ensure that the measures, taken together, "have systemic reach, are outcomes-oriented, are meaningful at the personal level, are representative of concerns facing the US healthcare system, and have use at many levels." The resulting list highlights the overlap between population health and PHM.

Population Health Management Approaches

A number of approaches can help put PHM principles into effective practice. They include "hot-spotting," "cold-spotting," health coaching, patient-centered medical homes, accountable care organizations, health exchanges, and telemedicine.

Hot-Spotting and Cold-Spotting

Analysis of healthcare data often reveals high utilization of healthcare services by a relatively small percentage of the population—typically people living with a chronic disease (e.g., heart disease, mental illness, diabetes, cancer) who experience poor coordination of care among their healthcare providers. **Hot-spotting** is a PHM practice that seeks to identify populations that are accessing the healthcare system excessively, and it can indicate "red flag" problems with the management of people's diseases and conditions. Hot-spotting is closely related to the assessment function of public health in that it identifies areas of need and helps in the development of interventions to meet those needs. By providing enhanced services to patient groups who need them the most, hot-spotting can promote wellness, reduce the burden of chronic illness, and deliver value to populations (Birk 2013; Westfall 2013).

hot-spotting
A population health management approach that involves identifying population groups with particular areas of need and developing interventions to address those needs.

Related to hot-spotting is another PHM approach known as **cold-spotting**. Westfall (2013, 239) explains:

cold-spotting
A population health management approach that involves identifying population groups who lack access to healthcare or other community supports that influence health.

> Today, identifying individual patients with high utilization of health care is relatively easy given the vast improvements in health information technology, electronic health records, and all-payor databases. However, is the super-utilizer the real problem? Do they have some medical defect or general disregard for their community? Are hot spots the problem? Or is the problem really "cold spots," communities in which the social determinants of health, support, and access to primary care have broken down?

Westfall (2013) concludes that cold spots call for "a community approach, linking public health and primary care in explicit partnerships that address the needs of the individual and build an environment and community that supports healthy living" (Westfall 2013, 240).

Health Coaching

health coaching
An effort to engage people to modify their behaviors and address their health risks.

Health coaching is a PHM approach that involves engaging the people to modify their behaviors and address their health risks, and it is a common feature of wellness programs developed by employers looking to reduce health insurance costs for their employee base. WebMD Health Services (2010, 2, 4) explains:

> Health coaching focuses not only on helping high-risk individuals improve health, but also helps moderate-risk individuals to lower their risks and those who are healthy to stay that way. Health coaching, with its proactive approach, helps people before they "become a claim"—rather than waiting until they require medical intervention. In contrast to programs that focus on managing a specific disease or condition, a whole-person model of health coaching addresses all of an individual's risk factors . . .
>
> A whole-person coaching approach guides each participant to focus first on the changes that he or she is ready to make, rather than comply with a set of behaviors he or she is not contemplating practicing. . . . To meet plan goals, the coach helps guide participants to find their own motivation, break through their barriers, cultivate the support that they need, and reward themselves when goals are achieved.

Patient-Centered Medical Homes

patient-centered medical home (PCMH)
A model for changing the way primary care is organized and delivered, based on the principles of physician-led practice, whole-person orientation, integrated and coordinated care, focus on quality and safety, and access.

The **patient-centered medical home (PCMH)** is a model for changing the way primary care is organized and delivered (Agency for Healthcare Research and Quality 2016). Central to the model is a set of joint principles, developed by the American Academy of Family Physicians (AAFP), the American College of Physicians, the American Academy of Pediatrics, and the American Osteopathic Association. The AAFP (2016b) describes the principles as follows:

- *Physician-led practice*: Patients have access to a personal physician who leads the care team within a medical practice.
- *Whole-person orientation*: The care team provides comprehensive care, including acute care, chronic care, preventive services, and end-of-life care, at all stages of life.
- *Integrated and coordinated care*: Practices take steps to ensure that patients receive the care and services they need from the medical neighborhood, in a culturally and linguistically appropriate manner.
- *Focus on quality and safety*: Practices use the quality improvement process and evidence-based medicine to continually improve patient outcomes.
- *Access*: Practices commit to enhancing patients' access to care.

The PCMH model applies a proactive, team-based approach to care that focuses on prevention, early intervention, and close partnerships with patients (AAFP 2016a). At the core of the model is a focus on PHM. The PCMH requires that the patient be viewed both as an individual and as a member of a population. According to the AAFP (2016a), this emphasis on PHM supports the use of health data stored in patient registries to identify patients who need evidence-based chronic or preventive care; the provision of planned care, outreach, and patient self-management support; improved monitoring of patient progress, identification of care plans, and management of care plans through prompts in electronic health records; and the ability to monitor practice performance by comparing patient data with national guidelines and internal benchmarks.

Accountable Care Organizations

An **accountable care organization (ACO)** is a collaboration of healthcare professionals—including doctors, hospitals, and other providers—that works to provide coordinated, high-quality care to Medicare patients. The Centers for Medicare & Medicaid Services (2015) explains the benefits of this voluntary collaboration: "The goal of coordinated care is to ensure that patients, especially the chronically ill, get the right care at the right time, while avoiding unnecessary duplication of services and preventing medical errors. When an ACO succeeds both in delivering high-quality care and spending health care dollars more wisely, it will share in the savings it achieves for the Medicare program."

accountable care organization (ACO)
A collaboration of healthcare professionals—including doctors, hospitals, and other providers—that works to provide coordinated, high-quality care to Medicare patients.

Turcan (2015) emphasizes that the success of an ACO depends on its systematic effort to keep the patient population as healthy as possible and to mitigate chronic disease—in other words, success depends on PHM. With effective PHM, an ACO can avoid unnecessary hospitalizations, prevent emergency department visits, reduce the need for expensive tests and procedures, and bring about better patient outcomes. Turcan (2015) points out: "Of course, many factors in population health are not under the control of healthcare providers. That's why an effective PHM strategy depends partly on the ACO's ability to engage patients in managing their own care and modifying their health behavior." The PHM focus on preventive and chronic care represents a shift from the traditional acute care environment. To accomplish this shift, the ACO must coordinate care across a range of healthcare settings and, if necessary, monitor patients and interact with them between scheduled visits.

Turcan (2015) explains:

> Where most of today's healthcare is episodic, PHM is continuous. What this means is that ACO providers must proactively reach out to patients who need preventive and chronic care and bring them in for follow-up. They must transform their systems for communicating with patients. They must expand patient access to providers. And they must design a range of non-visit interventions for very sick patients, those who have less severe chronic diseases, and healthy people who need preventive care.

Health Exchanges

health exchange
A marketplace that helps individuals, families, and small businesses view, compare, and purchase health insurance plans that meet government standards.

One of the key elements of US healthcare reform under the Affordable Care Act was the creation of health insurance marketplaces, or **health exchanges**. Exchanges available in each state help individuals, families, and small businesses view, compare, and purchase health insurance plans that meet federal government standards. Middle- and low-income families are eligible for federal subsidies to cover some of the costs of coverage (US Department of Health and Human Services 2015). As a result, individuals of lower socioeconomic status have improved access to health insurance and to nonemergent care services.

The health exchanges provide a good example of the healthcare and public health systems working together. Hoffman (2013) explains:

> Every plan sold on an exchange must meet minimum coverage requirements called "essential health benefits," which the exchange establishes by selecting a benchmark plan currently offered in the state. These benefits must include elements such as preventive care, prescription drugs, maternity and newborn care, and mental health services, and states must ensure that plans cover enough providers to make it possible for patients to actually see a doctor in their area.

Health exchanges not only aim to increase the number of people who have health coverage; they also provide an opportunity to educate the population about health issues and the availability and importance of primary care. Often, people who have been uninsured or who have little interaction with the healthcare system have lacked information about chronic conditions, coverage options, and basic preventive health issues like nutrition and safety (Hoffman 2013). The exchanges can contribute to increased understanding of these key issues. Ultimately, data on access, intervention, and outcomes will help us determine whether the exchanges have achieved their aims.

Telemedicine

telemedicine
The exchange of information via electronic communications (e.g., e-mail, two-way video, remote monitoring) for the purpose of improving a patient's health status.

Another development in healthcare with significant PHM opportunities is the emergence of **telemedicine**. The American Telemedicine Association (2015) defines *telemedicine* as "the use of medical information exchanged from one site to another via electronic communications to improve a patient's clinical health status." It involves a variety of applications and services incorporating e-mail, smartphones, remote monitoring, two-way video, and other telecommunications technologies. The American Telemedicine Association (2015) notes that "telemedicine is not a separate medical specialty"; instead, "products and services related to telemedicine are often part of a larger investment by healthcare institutions in either information technology or the delivery of clinical care." The use of telemedicine is growing as people become more aware of the advantages it brings, such as improved access for both patients and providers, lower costs of healthcare delivery, quality of care equal to that found in on-site services, and savings of time and (potentially) money for patients (American Telemedicine Association 2015).

Challenges to Population Health Management

Implementation of PHM approaches can be hampered by a variety of challenges associated with identifying high-risk populations; developing, implementing, and monitoring care plans; and communicating with patients and communities (Sirois 2015). For healthcare providers specifically, notable barriers can include reluctance by physicians to engage in a new way of doing business, concerns about changes in physician compensation, issues about the expenses associated with a new management paradigm, and aversion to risk (*HIT Consultant* 2015). Overcoming these challenges typically requires the education, engagement, and interaction of key stakeholders; the prioritization of technical infrastructure to support information exchange and analytics; and a commitment to process improvement (Sirois 2015).

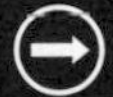

EXERCISES

Integration Success Stories

Read the following cases from the Association of State and Territorial Health Officials:

- "Boot Camp Translation: A Method for Building a Community of Solution in Rural Colorado" (available via www.astho.org/PCPHCollaborative/Success-Stories/Cancer/)
- "Maine's Patient-Centered Medical Home Launch" (available via www.astho.org/PCPHCollaborative/Success-Stories/Patient-Centered-Medical-Home/)

For both cases, answer the following questions:

1. What is the issue being addressed?
2. What is the purpose of the work?
3. Who are the stakeholders involved?

(continued)

4. What additional stakeholders might be helpful or might benefit from the project?
5. Discuss a limitation that was encountered while doing the work.
6. Describe the current state of the work.
7. How does the project illustrate the PHM concepts discussed in this chapter?

Health Leads

Explore the Health Leads website (https://healthleadsusa.org/), and answer the following questions:

1. What is the organization's vision?
2. How do Health Leads programs work?
3. Explain how Health Leads operates according to specific PHM and system integration principles discussed in this chapter.
4. Research a specific Health Leads project. Describe the project, outcome, and role of Health Leads.

Identifying an Example in Healthcare

Find an example of a healthcare system that is implementing the principles of PHM. Prepare a one-page executive summary covering the utility and outcomes of PHM in the system's work.

Key Chapter Points

- The focus of healthcare is treating patients via medical services; the focus of public health is preventing disease and promoting health via collective community efforts. The management of population health requires these two systems to integrate their work with the aim of ensuring a healthy population.
- The Institute of Medicine (2012) identified some core principles for the integration between healthcare and public health: a common goal of improving population health; a focus on identifying and addressing community needs; commitment to bridging disciplines, programs, and jurisdictions; and analysis of data in a collaborative manner.

- Population health management (PHM) is "the proactive application of strategies and interventions to defined cohorts of individuals across the continuum of healthcare delivery in an effort to maintain and/or improve the health of the individuals within the cohort at the lowest necessary cost" (Burton 2013, 2).
- Whereas the term *population health* focuses more broadly on the determinants of health for a population, PHM emphasizes the delivery of healthcare for populations with the highest quality and lowest cost.
- The Triple Aim, developed by the Institute for Healthcare Improvement, emphasizes three dimensions for optimizing health system performance: improving the patient's experience of care, improving the health of populations, and reducing the per capita cost of healthcare (IHI 2016). PHM is consistent with the Triple Aim framework.
- Hot-spotting is a PHM practice that involves identifying particular areas of need in defined population groups and developing interventions to address those needs.
- Cold-spotting involves identifying population groups who lack access to healthcare or other community supports that influence health.
- Health coaching involves engaging the people to modify their behaviors and address their health risks. It is a common feature of wellness programs developed by employers.
- The patient-centered medical home (PCMH) is a model for changing the way primary care is organized and delivered. It is based on the principles of physician-led practice, whole-person orientation, integrated and coordinated care, focus on quality and safety, and access (AAFP 2016b).
- Accountable care organizations (ACOs) are voluntary collaborations of healthcare professionals—including doctors, hospitals, and other providers—that work to provide coordinated, high-quality care to Medicare patients.
- As a result of the Affordable Care Act, health exchanges, or health insurance marketplaces, were made available in each US state to help individuals, families, and small businesses purchase health insurance plans. Middle- and low-income families are eligible for federal subsidies to cover some of the costs of coverage. The exchanges not only aim to increase the number of people with health coverage; they also provide an opportunity to educate people about health issues and the availability and importance of primary care.
- Telemedicine is "the use of medical information exchanged from one site to another via electronic communications to improve a patient's clinical health status" (American Telemedicine Association 2015). It involves a variety of applications and services incorporating e-mail, smartphones, remote monitoring, two-way video, and other telecommunications technologies.

Discussion Questions

1. What is population health management?
2. What are three principles or skills necessary for the management of population health?
3. Describe three PHM approaches.
4. What are some of the advantages and limitations of the PHM approaches described in this chapter?
5. Describe two challenges commonly encountered when implementing PHM approaches. What are some strategies for overcoming these challenges?

References

Agency for Healthcare Research and Quality. 2016. "Defining the PCMH." Accessed November 2. https://pcmh.ahrq.gov/page/defining-pcmh.

American Academy of Family Physicians (AAFP). 2016a. "High Impact Changes for Practice Transformation." Accessed November 2. www.aafp.org/practice-management/transformation/pcmh/high-impact.html.

———. 2016b. "The Patient-Centered Medical Home (PCMH)." Accessed November 2. www.aafp.org/practice-management/transformation/pcmh.html.

American Telemedicine Association. 2015. "About." Accessed June 29. www.americantelemed.org/about-telemedicine/what-is-telemedicine#.VZLfuUavwmo.

Birk, S. 2013. "Population Health: Strategies That Deliver Value and Results." *Healthcare Executive* July/August, 10–18.

Burton, D. A. 2013. *Population Health Management: Implementing a Strategy for Success.* Health Catalyst. Accessed November 1, 2016. www.healthcatalyst.com/wp-content/uploads/2013/07/WhitePaper_PopulationHealthManagement.pdf.

Centers for Medicare & Medicaid Services (CMS). 2015. "Accountable Care Organizations." Updated January 6. www.cms.gov/Medicare/Medicare-Fee-for-Service-Payment/ACO/index.html.

Halfon, N., and P. H. Conway. 2013. "The Opportunities and Challenges of a Lifelong Health System." *New England Journal of Medicine* 368 (17): 1569–71.

HIT Consultant. 2015. "Top 4 Population Health Management Challenges." Published February 18. http://hitconsultant.net/2015/02/18/top-4-population-health-management-challenges/.

Hoffman, S. 2013. "Health Insurance Exchanges and Population Health: Key Elements in Expanding Access and Preventive Care." Leonard Davis Institute of Health Economics. Published February. http://ldihealtheconomist.com/he000057.shtml.

Institute for Healthcare Improvement (IHI). 2016. "Triple Aim for Populations." Accessed November 1. www.ihi.org/Topics/TripleAim/Pages/Overview.aspx.

Institute of Medicine (IOM). 2015. *Vital Signs: Core Metrics for Health and Health Care Progress.* Published April. http://nationalacademies.org/hmd/~/media/Files/Report%20Files/2015/Vital_Signs/VitalSigns_RB.pdf.

———. 2012. *Primary Care and Public Health: Exploring Integration to Improve Population Health.* Published March. www.nationalacademies.org/hmd/~/media/Files/Report%20Files/2012/Primary-Care-and-Public-Health/Primary%20Care%20and%20Public%20Health_Revised%20RB_FINAL.pdf.

Lewis, N. 2014. "Populations, Population Health, and the Evolution of Population Management: Making Sense of the Terminology in US Health Care Today." Institute for Healthcare Improvement. Published March 19. www.ihi.org/communities/blogs/_layouts/ihi/community/blog/itemview.aspx?List=81ca4a47-4ccd-4e9e-89d9-14d88ec59e8d&ID=50.

Magnan, S., E. Fisher, D. Kindig, G. Isham, D. Wood, M. Eustis, C. Backstrom, and S. Leitz. 2012. "Achieving Accountability for Health and Health Care." *Minnesota Medicine* 95 (11): 37–39.

McAlearney, A. S. 2003. *Population Health Management: Strategies to Improve Outcomes.* Chicago: Health Administration Press.

Sirois, M. 2015. "The Population Health Management Conundrum: Overcoming Challenges to Sustainable PHM Strategies." *Becker's Hospital Review.* Published June 16. www.beckershospitalreview.com/population-health/the-population-health-management-conundrum-overcoming-challenges-to-sustainable-phm-strategies.html.

Turcan, D. 2015. "Population Health Management: The Life Blood of ACOs." *Healthcare Executive Insight*. Accessed June 22. http://healthcare-executive-insight.advanceweb.com/ACO-Resource-Center/Web-Extras/Online-Extras/Population-Health-Management-The-Lifeblood-of-ACOs.aspx.

US Department of Health and Human Services. 2015. "Key Features of the Affordable Care Act by Year." Accessed November 2, 2016. www.hhs.gov/healthcare/facts-and-features/key-features-of-aca-by-year/index.html.

WebMD Health Services. 2010. "The Value of Health Coaching in Population Health Management." Accessed November 2, 2016. http://christinatarantola.com/wp-content/uploads/2014/01/white-paper-the-value-of-health-coaching-in-population-health-management.pdf.

Westfall, J. M. 2013. "Cold-Spotting: Linking Primary Care and Public Health to Create Communities of Solution." *Journal of the American Board of Family Medicine* 26 (3): 239–40.

CHAPTER 13

A DATA-DRIVEN APPROACH

"America's healthcare system is neither healthy, caring, nor a system."

—Walter Cronkite (1990)

Learning Objectives

After completing this chapter, you should be able to

- understand the need for a data-driven approach to managing the health of populations,
- describe key elements of a data-driven approach to population health management,
- identify the strengths and weaknesses of those approaches, and
- describe the key categories of big data.

Introduction

According to the Centers for Disease Control and Prevention (CDC), chronic conditions such as heart disease, stroke, cancer, diabetes, obesity, and arthritis are among "the most common, costly, and preventable of all health problems," and they are in large part a result of our lifestyles (CDC 2016a). Much of the illness, suffering, and early death related to these conditions results from changeable health risk behaviors, such as lack of exercise, poor nutrition, tobacco use, and excessive alcohol consumption. The CDC (2016a) reports: "In the United States, chronic diseases and conditions and the health risk behaviors that cause them account for most health care costs."

This chapter's opening quote from Walter Cronkite describes the contradictions and shortcomings of the US healthcare system, and these shortcomings are compounded by issues rooted in people's behavior. Changing lifestyles and behaviors at the population level is a difficult, tedious process that requires significant resources. In a society where resources are distributed unevenly, how can we best approach such a task and mitigate these costly and preventable health conditions?

Effective population health management (PHM) must be driven by data from both the healthcare system and the public health system. This chapter examines three key elements of data-driven PHM—electronic heath records, claims data, and big data—that are crucial for understanding and influencing behaviors, improving population health, and lowering healthcare costs.

Electronic Health Records

electronic health record (EHR)
A digital collection of health information about a patient; an EHR allows for the efficient collection of data across multiple organizations and the sharing of that data for informed decision making.

An **electronic health record (EHR)** is a digital collection of health information about a patient. (The term *EHR* is also sometimes used to refer to the software platform through which the records are managed.) EHRs are "real-time, patient-centered records that make information available instantly and securely to authorized users" (HealthIT.gov 2016). Information in an EHR can come from multiple sources and typically includes patient demographics, progress notes, medications, vital signs, past medical history, immunizations, laboratory data, and radiology reports (*HealthcareITNews* 2015).

The use of EHRs can contribute to effective PHM by allowing for the efficient collection of data across multiple healthcare organizations and the sharing of that data for informed decision making. The key benefits of EHRs can be summarized as follows (HealthIT.gov 2013):

- *They can improve public health reporting and surveillance.* EHRs make it easier for organizations to collect standardized, systematic data. HealthIT.gov (2013) writes: "Through syndromic surveillance data submission, immunization registries, and electronic laboratory reporting, providers can transmit public and population health data to public health officials."

- *They can improve disease prevention.* With access to electronic health information about the population served, providers are better able to remind patients about preventive or follow-up care.
- *They can improve communication.* By meaningfully using EHRs, healthcare organizations can expand their communication and collaboration with the public health system.

The Health Information Technology for Economic and Clinical Health (HITECH) Act, part of the American Reinvestment and Recovery Act (ARRA) of 2009, identifies the **meaningful use** of interoperable EHRs as a critical goal for modernizing the nation's healthcare system (CDC 2016b). The CDC (2016b) explains that meaningful use involves "the use of certified EHR technology in a meaningful manner" (e.g., electronic prescribing), ensuring that the technology is "connected in a manner that provides for the electronic exchange of health information to improve the quality of care." Furthermore, providers using EHR technology are expected to submit information about quality of care and other measures to the Department of Health and Human Services (CDC 2016b). Medicare and Medicaid incentive programs encourage providers to meet the meaningful use standards.

meaningful use
The use of certified electronic health record technology to improve quality, safety, and efficiency; to engage patients and families; to improve coordination of care; to advance public health; and to ensure security of health information.

The CDC (2016b) explains that the concept of meaningful use was based on the "five pillars" of health outcomes: (1) improving quality, safety, efficiency, and reducing health disparities; (2) engaging patients and families in their health; (3) improving coordination of care; (4) improving population and public health; and (5) ensuring privacy and security of personal health information.

Claims Data

After a patient meets with a provider, **claims data** are submitted to an insurance company or other payer for reimbursement. This type of data, which includes "information about patient demographics, billable charges, dates of service, diagnosis codes, procedure codes, insurance, and providers" (Brown and Skelley 2015), can be valuable for PHM purposes. The advantages of using claims data are that the data are readily available, provide information about the patient's full continuum of care, and are collected in a standardized fashion. Key limitations of using claims data include lack of clinical detail, a lag between the time of care delivery and the availability of data, and limited insight into the actual process of care (Brown and Skelley 2015). To obtain a more complete picture of the delivery of care and to highlight potential areas for quality improvement and cost containment, claims data can be supplemented with clinical data and patient satisfaction survey data.

claims data
Administrative data that are collected when a patient meets with a provider and are later submitted to an insurance company or other payer for reimbursement.

Big Data

big data
Vast collections of information, both structured and unstructured, that can be mined from various sources.

The term ***big data*** refers to vast collections of information, both structured and unstructured, that can be mined from various sources. According to Frost & Sullivan (2015, 3), the term represents "electronic datasets so large and complex that they are difficult (or impossible) to manage with traditional software and hardware." Big data is overwhelming not only because of the amount of information available, but also because of the variety of data types and the speed with which it must be managed. Hence, volume, velocity, and variety are often called "the three *V*s of big data" (Frost & Sullivan 2015).

Three categories of big data are particularly relevant for healthcare: clinical data, health research, and business/organizational records. Clinical data include information in EHRs, digital images, and data from information-sensing wireless medical devices (Frost & Sullivan 2015). Health research data can cover topics ranging from drug development to biotechnology to public health (Frost & Sullivan 2015). A noteworthy initiative in this category is Big Data to Knowledge (BD2K), from the National Institutes of Health. BD2K aims to enhance the utility of big data to enable biomedical research, facilitate discovery, and maximize community engagement (BD2K 2016). The category of business/organizational records includes scheduling and billing information, demographic data, diagnostic codes, and other information gathered through basic organizational processes (Frost & Sullivan 2015).

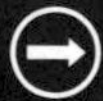
Data Visualization Tools

As we navigate the advancements in data generation and analysis, we need to be able to communicate our findings from big data (and not-so-big data) in a manner that can be understood by both our peers and the communities we serve. A variety of web-based tools are available to help you visualize preloaded data or to input a new data set. Examples include the following:

- Institute for Health Metrics and Evaluation (www.healthdata.org/results/data-visualizations)
- Gapminder (www.gapminder.org)
- PolicyMap (www.policymap.com)
- Tableau Public (https://public.tableau.com/s/)

Key Chapter Points

- Electronic heath records, claims data, and big data all play important roles in population health management efforts to understand health risks, improve population health, and lower healthcare costs.
- An electronic health record (EHR) is a digital collection of health information about a patient. EHRs are "real-time, patient-centered records that make information available instantly and securely to authorized users" (HealthIT.gov 2016).
- EHRs can help improve public health reporting and surveillance, improve disease prevention, and expand communication between the healthcare and public health systems.
- The Health Information Technology for Economic and Clinical Health (HITECH) Act identifies the meaningful use of interoperable EHRs as a critical goal for modernizing the nation's healthcare system.
- Meaningful use involves "the use of certified EHR technology in a meaningful manner," ensuring that the technology is "connected in a manner that provides for the electronic exchange of health information to improve the quality of care" (CDC 2016b).
- After a patient meets with a provider, claims data are submitted to an insurance company or other payer for reimbursement. This type of data includes information about demographics, billable charges, dates of service, diagnosis and procedure codes, insurance, and providers.
- The use of claims data has both advantages and limitations. To obtain a more complete picture of the delivery of care and to highlight potential areas for improvement, claims data are often supplemented with clinical data and patient satisfaction survey data.
- The term *big data* refers to vast collections of information, both structured and unstructured, that can be mined from various sources. It represents "electronic datasets so large and complex that they are difficult (or impossible) to manage with traditional software and hardware" (Frost & Sullivan 2015, 3).
- Three categories of big data are particularly relevant for healthcare: clinical data, health research, and business/organizational records.

Discussion Questions

1. Why do we need a data-driven approach to manage the health of populations?
2. Describe three tools for implementing a data-driven approach.

3. What are those tools' strengths and weaknesses?
4. What areas of big data are most relevant to population health management?

References

Big Data to Knowledge (BD2K). 2016. "About BD2K." Updated July 7. https://datascience.nih.gov/bd2k/about.

Brown, B., and L. Skelley. 2015. "Why Population Health Management Strategies Require Both Clinical and Claims Data." Health Catalyst. Accessed June 30. www.healthcatalyst.com/white-paper/clinical-claims-data-population-health-management/.

Centers for Disease Control and Prevention (CDC). 2016a. "Chronic Disease Overview." Updated February 23. www.cdc.gov/chronicdisease/overview/index.htm.

———. 2016b. "Meaningful Use." Updated May 26. www.cdc.gov/ehrmeaningfuluse/introduction.html.

Cronkite, W. 1990. PBS-TV, December 17.

Frost & Sullivan. 2015. *Drowning in Big Data? Reducing Information Technology Complexities and Costs for Healthcare Organizations*. Accessed June 30. www.emc.com/collateral/analyst-reports/frost-sullivan-reducing-information-technology-complexities-ar.pdf.

HealthcareITNews. 2015. "Electronic Health Record Defined." Accessed June 30. www.healthcareitnews.com/directory/electronic-health-record-ehr.

HealthIT.gov. 2016. "Electronic Health Records: The Basics." Accessed November 3. www.healthit.gov/providers-professionals/frequently-asked-questions/334#id2.

———. 2013. "How Can Electronic Health Records Improve Public and Population Health Outcomes?" Updated January 15. www.healthit.gov/providers-professionals/faqs/how-can-electronic-health-records-improve-public-and-population-health-.

CHAPTER 14

THE MOMENTUM BEHIND POPULATION HEALTH

"Hospitals should challenge themselves to reach beyond their walls and partner with community organizations to implement innovative approaches that sustainably improve total population health."

—Health Research & Educational Trust (2014)

Learning Objectives

After completing this chapter, you should be able to

- explain the momentum that has been building behind population health,
- describe three population health management approaches to carry that momentum forward, and
- name five metrics that are useful in assessing the effectiveness of population health management.

Introduction

In a report titled *The Second Curve of Population Health*, the Health Research & Educational Trust (HRET) discusses the transformation in healthcare in the United States from a "first curve" emphasizing volume of services provided and fee-for-service payment models to a "second curve" that focuses on population health. The report describes the growing needs for healthcare organizations to "actively address a broad array of socioeconomic and environmental factors" and to "provide preventive care, particularly for populations who lack access to care or engage the system at the wrong place and time" (HRET 2014, 3). Such needs are best addressed through population health management (PHM).

During this period of transition and reform, momentum is building behind the population health movement and the greater integration of public health and healthcare. HRET (2014) identifies several key factors:

- Transition from a fee-for-service payment to a value-based system that rewards positive outcomes
- Increased provider accountability for the cost and quality of healthcare
- Improved access to care for underserved and vulnerable populations via the Affordable Care Act
- Demand to reduce fragmentation and improve efficiency in care delivery
- Greater transparency of financial, quality, and community benefit data
- Economic and legislative pressure to limit increases in healthcare spending
- Demographic changes that will increase demand for healthcare, combined with projected provider shortages
- Realization that acute medical care is only one facet of maintaining and improving health

The American Hospital Association (2012) has recognized that a population health focus can improve health by analyzing the distribution of health statuses and outcomes within a population, identifying and evaluating factors that cause certain outcomes, and developing and implementing interventions to modify determinants. HRET (2014, 4) further states that this "ecological model of health" can produce positive results by proactively addressing "upstream factors" that influence health; in turn, "improved population health will ultimately decrease medical costs and allow hospitals to invest in prevention."

Moving Forward with Population Health Management

The following are tactics and strategies recommended by HRET (2014) for organizations transitioning to the "second curve" and implementing a population health approach:

- *Value-based reimbursement.* In shifting from volume-based to value-based reimbursement, hospitals and healthcare systems deliver services to specific populations at predetermined prices and levels of quality, and payment contracts and compensation arrangements are linked to performance results. Models such as accountable care organizations and patient-centered medical homes align organizations across a wide range of services and varying acuity levels. Smaller providers delivering specialized services to target populations work in partnership within networks managed by larger entities functioning as population health managers. Care delivery systems emphasize the goals of the Institute for Healthcare Improvement's Triple Aim—improving the patient experience, improving the health of populations, and reducing cost per capita (HRET 2014).
- *Seamless care across all settings.* The shift toward PHM emphasizes communication and coordination between care settings, with the aim of ensuring proper care, reducing complications and readmissions, and engaging patients and families as patients move from one care setting to another. Preventive services are incorporated across all care settings. Care transition teams or navigators can help manage complicated patient cases, and partnerships between hospitals and care systems can help ensure coordination in community-based settings. Telemedicine can help organizations connect with patients in remote areas (HRET 2014).
- *Proactive and systematic patient education.* Patient education and engagement in matters of disease prevention and management are a key focus of population health. Organizations carry out community outreach programs, education events, and health screenings, with special initiatives targeting at-risk population groups. Providers monitor and report on patient and family engagement, and they use a variety of tools (e.g., advisory councils, wellness programs) to boost such engagement. Multidisciplinary teams coordinate chronic disease cases, set patient goals, and track patient progress (HRET 2014).
- *Workplace competencies and education on population health.* Hospital leadership and staff must be trained in population health competencies and dedicated to population health. Staff members should have defined roles within the

PHM process, and care coordinators, community health workers, and health educators should be employed as needed (HRET 2014).

- *Integrated, comprehensive health information technology (HIT).* HIT systems should have capacity for sophisticated analytics to support clinical and business decisions, with data from various sources combined in health information exchanges and data registries. Providers should have access to timely and local data about health issues in the community, and they should use those data to guide the care of individuals (HRET 2014).
- *Partnerships to collaborate on community-based solutions.* Under a population health approach, hospitals and healthcare systems engage the community, share resources and knowledge, and build relationships to address community health challenges. They partner with the community and public health departments to address such issues as environmental hazards, poverty, unemployment, and inadequate housing and to develop relevant metrics to measure community needs and progress (HRET 2014).

> *"As the public health and provider sectors become better aligned, hospitals will need to engage in challenging but necessary changes to improve the health of the patient and community population as well as the organization's financial bottom line."*
>
> —Health Research & Educational Trust (2014)

Success in population health must be measured using appropriate metrics. For example, in evaluating the effectiveness of a wellness event, success is not determined by the number of people who attend the event but rather by the impact the event has on specific health outcomes (HRET 2014). Metrics applied at both the patient and the community level can focus on descriptive variables (e.g., age, gender, ethnicity, income, education); life in years adjusted for disability and quality; age-adjusted mortality rates; or access to care, including location and types of services provided (Parrish 2010; Healthy People 2016).

Finally, implementation of PHM strategies in an ever-changing healthcare landscape requires continuous engagement with key leaders and organizations in the field. The Internet and social media resources listed in the appendix of this book provide convenient access to emerging ideas, new developments, and useful information.

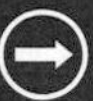

EXERCISE: POPULATION HEALTH CASE REPORTS

This exercise includes excerpts from four population health case reports made available through the National Academy of Medicine. The reports describe the work of communities striving to improve population health. For each case report, complete the following steps:

1. Identify the concepts being addressed, and discuss these concepts with a peer.
2. Consider information *not* presented in the report that might be important for fully understanding the condition of the population.
3. Propose future work that you think should be conducted by the authors of each case.

Population Health Case Report #1: Integrating Clinical Care with Community Health Through New Hampshire's Million Hearts Learning Collaborative

Persson (2016, 1–2) describes a hypertension control strategy modeled after an initiative by Cheshire Medical Center/Dartmouth Hitchcock-Keene (CMC/DHK):

> The approach of CMC/DHK's hypertension control effort was systematic. To start, the implementers established a provider planning team, which developed a four-question, multiple-choice questionnaire to be administered to primary care providers and nurses who supported the specified patient population. Using the survey data, CMC/DHK implemented new strategies to help identify and more aggressively treat patients with hypertension. Although the approach was multifaceted, success could be most directly tied to four specific interventions:
>
> 1. Utilization of a uniform data measure;
> 2. Development of a patient registry;
> 3. Creation of patient engagement information cards; and
> 4. Cultivation of community partnerships.

The full report is available at https://nam.edu/integrating-clinical-care-with-community-health-through-new-hampshires-million-hearts-learning-collaborative-a-population-health-case-report/.

Population Health Case Report #2: Integrating Health Care and Supported Housing to Improve the Health and Well-Being of the Homeless

(continued)

Lovelace (2016, 2) describes an initiative to address the health and well-being of the homeless:

> The goals of Cultivating Health for Success are to reduce unplanned services (i.e., emergency department use and unscheduled hospital admissions and readmissions) and increase planned services (i.e., visits to primary care physicians, including recommended post-acute follow-up; compliance with individual care plans for chronic disease management; and preventive screenings) for eligible members who
>
> - are homeless as defined by [the US Department of Housing and Urban Development];
> - are disabled according to the attestation of a physician;
> - have a medical (as opposed to behavioral) disability, although behavioral health issues do not disqualify a member;
> - are enrolled as UPMC *for You* Medicaid or Special Needs Plan members;
> - have at least 1 year of high total health care expenditures, including unplanned services.
>
> The program is structured to impact the health care of eligible members positively through a collaborative, team-based approach that integrates three interrelated components—permanent supported housing, an assigned medical home, and intensive case management/care coordination. . . . In combination, these components ensure that all program participants have stable housing and social supports, timely and coordinated medical care, in-home assistance with activities of daily living and more consistent medical monitoring, and basic life skills training.

The full report is available at https://nam.edu/wp-content/uploads/2016/03/Integrating-Health-Care-and-Supported-Housing-to-Improve-the-Health-and-Well-Being-of-the-Homeless-A-Population-Health-Case-Report.pdf.

Population Health Case Report #3: Technology-Enabled Transitions of Care in a Collaborative Effort Between Clinical Medicine and Public Health

Ahmed and colleagues (2016, 2) describe a health information technology initiative in Minnesota:

> The initial aim of the Transitions of Care project was to improve the quality of care and to reduce hospital readmissions for public health clients through a health

(continued)

information technology–enabled transition-of-care solution (Marchant et al. 2013). The project required the development of a scalable health information technology architecture with data exchange capabilities across clinical and public health entities. The pilot between Mayo Clinic Rochester and Olmsted County Public Health Services went live in June 2013. The development of real-time connectivity among the Mayo Clinic registration system (Healthquest), the Mayo Clinic G. E. Electronic Medical Record (EMR), and Olmsted County Public Health Services PH-Doc EMR system enabled the following functions: (1) timely alerts to public health case managers each time one of their clients visited the ED, was kept under observation, or was admitted or discharged from the hospital; (2) the management of client consent to share data across entities in real time for public health and inpatient care locations; and (3) timely communications among case managers, inpatient clinicians, and clients to determine care plans, support clinical decisions, utilize community resources, inform follow-up, and reduce the number of readmissions in order to better meet the patient's health care needs (Marchant et al. 2013). Importantly, this technology infrastructure can be scaled up, can be used with multiple vendors, and adheres to HIPAA and other privacy and security regulations and protocols for exchanging protected health information.

The full report is available at https://nam.edu/wp-content/uploads/2016/03/Technology-Enabled-Transitions-of-Care-in-a-Collaborative-Effort-between-Clinical-Medicine-and-Public-Health.pdf.

Population Health Case Report #4: The Olmsted County (MN) Collaborative School-Located Influenza Immunization Program

Brickley and colleagues (2016, 2) describe a school-based vaccination initiative:

In 2011, leaders of the Southeast Minnesota Beacon Program, funded by the US Department of Health and Human Services, expressed an interest in collaborating with the school-located immunization program. With their participation and guidance, the program was able to establish an electronic registration process to supplement the paper registration forms, assist with data analysis for future planning, and increase the use of media outreach and communication for promoting the clinics. Officials from the national Beacon Communities in Washington, DC, visited one of the elementary schools that year and received their influenza vaccines while interacting with program participants. Under the Beacon initiative, the program continued to expand over the subsequent years. Mayo Clinic and Olmsted Medical Center supplied

(continued)

their own influenza vaccines for the first time in 2011, billing individual insurance companies for both the vaccines and administration fees. Both entities utilized state-supplied vaccines from the Vaccines for Children Program to ensure that all children, regardless of socioeconomic status, would have the opportunity to be vaccinated (Santoli et al. 1999).

The full report is available at https://nam.edu/wp-content/uploads/2016/05/The-Olmsted-County-MN-Collaborative-School-Located-Influenza-Immunization-Program-A-Population-Health-Case-Report.pdf.

Key Chapter Points

- The United States is experiencing increasing integration of the public health and healthcare systems, and momentum is building in the shift toward population health.
- The Health Research & Educational Trust (2014) describes a transformation in US healthcare from a "first curve" emphasizing volume of services provided and fee-for-service payment models to a "second curve" that focuses on population health.
- Key tactics and strategies for this shift toward population health include value-based reimbursement; seamless care across all settings; proactive and systematic patient education; workplace competencies and education on population health; integrated, comprehensive health information technology; and partnerships to collaborate on community-based solutions (HRET 2014).

Discussion Questions

1. What are some reasons for the momentum behind population health?
2. Describe three PHM approaches recommended by the Health Research & Educational Trust.
3. Consider the PHM strategies listed in this chapter. Do you believe these approaches are feasible? Provide your rationale. Are there any approaches that should be considered but are not listed here? If so, describe them.

4. What barriers do you think a healthcare system might encounter when trying to improve population health?
5. What are some metrics that are useful in assessing the effectiveness of PHM efforts?

References

Ahmed, L., D. Jensen, L. Klotzbach, G. Huntley, A. Alexander, V. Roger, and L. Finney Rutten. 2016. *Technology-Enabled Transitions of Care in a Collaborative Effort Between Clinical Medicine and Public Health: A Population Health Case Report.* National Academy of Medicine. Published March 31. https://nam.edu/wp-content/uploads/2016/03/Technology-Enabled-Transitions-of-Care-in-a-Collaborative-Effort-between-Clinical-Medicine-and-Public-Health.pdf.

American Hospital Association (AHA). 2012. *Managing Population Health: The Role of the Hospital.* Published April. www.hpoe.org/Reports-HPOE/managing_population_health.pdf.

Brickley, J. L., T. L. Schmit, L. J. Finney Rutten, J. L. St. Sauver, K. L. Ytterberg, and R. M. Jacobson. 2016. *The Olmsted County (MN) Collaborative School-Located Influenza Immunization Program: A Population Health Case Report.* National Academy of Medicine. Published March 29. https://nam.edu/wp-content/uploads/2016/05/The-Olmsted-County-MN-Collaborative-School-Located-Influenza-Immunization-Program-A-Population-Health-Case-Report.pdf.

Health Research & Educational Trust (HRET). 2014. *The Second Curve of Population Health.* Published March. www.hpoe.org/Reports-HPOE/SecondCurvetoPopHealth2014.pdf.

Healthy People. 2016. "Leading Health Indicators." Updated August 25. www.healthypeople.gov/2020/Leading-Health-Indicators.

Lovelace, J. 2016. *Integrating Health Care and Supported Housing to Improve the Health and Well-Being of the Homeless: A Population Health Case Report.* National Academy of Medicine. Published March 29. https://nam.edu/wp-content/uploads/2016/03/Integrating-Health-Care-and-Supported-Housing-to-Improve-the-Health-and-Well-Being-of-the-Homeless-A-Population-Health-Case-Report.pdf.

Marchant, K., D. Jensen, D. Costellanos, D. Eid, and A. Alexander. 2013. "Public Health Based Transitions of Care: ADT Alerts to Reduce Readmissions in Public Health Patients." Unpublished white paper. Southeast Minnesota Beacon Program, Rochester, MN.

Parrish, R. G. 2010. "Measuring Population Health Outcomes." *Prevention of Chronic Disease* 7 (4): A71.

Persson, K. 2016. *Integrating Clinical Care with Community Health Through New Hampshire's Million Hearts Learning Collaborative: A Population Health Case Report*. National Academy of Medicine. Published March 31. https://nam.edu/wp-content/uploads/2016/03/Integrating-Clinical-Care-with-Community-Health-through-New-Hampshires-Million-Hearts-Learning-Collaborative.pdf.

Santoli, J. M., L. E. Rodewald, E. F. Maes, M. P. Battaglia, and V. G. Coronado. 1999. "Vaccines for Children Program, United States, 1997." *Pediatrics* 104 (2): e15.

APPENDIX

INTERNET AND SOCIAL MEDIA RESOURCES

American Medical Association
Website: www.ama-assn.org
Twitter: @AmerMedicalAssn

American Public Health Association
Website: www.apha.org
Twitter: @PublicHealth

Association of State and Territorial Health Officials
Website: www.astho.org
Twitter: @ASTHO

BBC Health News
Website: www.bbc.com/news/us/health
Twitter: @bbchealth

Boston Public Health Commission
Website: www.bphc.org
Twitter: @HealthyBoston

Boston University School of Public Health
Website: www.bu.edu/sph
Twitter: @BUSPH

Centers for Disease Control and Prevention (CDC)
Website: www.cdc.gov
Twitter: @cdcgov

CDC *Morbidity and Mortality Weekly Report*
Website: www.cdc.gov/mmwr
Twitter: @cdcmmwr

Community Catalyst
Website: www.communitycatalyst.org
Twitter: @HealthPolicyHub

County Health Rankings & Roadmaps
Website: www.countyhealthrankings.org
Twitter: @CHRankings

Environmental Protection Agency
Website: www.epa.gov
Twitter: @EPA

Harvard Health
Website: www.health.harvard.edu
Twitter: @HarvardHealth

Harvard School of Public Health Prevention Research Center
Website: www.hsph.harvard.edu/prc
Twitter: @HarvardPRC

Harvard T. H. Chan School of Public Health
Website: www.hsph.harvard.edu
Twitter: @HarvardChanSPH

Health Canada
Website: www.hc-sc.gc.ca
Twitter: @HealthCanada

Healthcare.gov
Website: www.healthcare.gov
Twitter: @HealthcareGov

Healthy People 2020
Website: www.healthypeople.gov
Twitter: @GoHealthyPeople

Johns Hopkins Bloomberg School of Public Health
Website: www.jhsph.edu
Twitter: @JohnsHopkinsSPH

David Kindig
Twitter: @PopHealth

Massachusetts Department of Public Health
Website: www.mass.gov/eohhs/gov/departments/dph
Twitter: @MassDPH

Mayo Clinic
Website: www.mayoclinic.org
Twitter: @Mayoclinic

National Academies of Sciences, Engineering, and Medicine—Health and Medicine Division
Website: http://nationalacademies.org/HMD
Twitter: @NASEM_Health

National Association of County and City Health Officials
Website: www.naccho.org
Twitter: @NACCHOalerts

National Institutes of Health
Website: www.nih.gov
Twitter: @NIH

New Hampshire Public Health Association
Website: http://nhpha.org
Twitter: @NHPHA

***New York Times* Well**
Website: www.nytimes.com/section/well
Twitter: @nytimeswell

NPR Health News
Website: www.npr.org/sections/health
Twitter: @NPRHealth

Partnership for a Healthier America
Website: http://ahealthieramerica.org
Twitter: @PHAnews

Partners in Health
Website: www.pih.org
Twitter: @pih

Policy Map
Website: www.policymap.com
Twitter: @policymap

Public Health Foundation
Website: www.phf.org
Twitter: @ThePHF

ReThink Health
Website: www.rethinkhealth.org
Twitter: @rethinkhealth

Robert Wood Johnson Foundation
Website: www.rwjf.org
Twitter: @RWJF

UNICEF
Website: www.unicef.org
Twitter: @unicef

USAID
Website: www.usaid.gov
Twitter: @usaid

US Department of Health and Human Services
Website: www.hhs.gov
Twitter: @HHSgov

US Department of Health and Human Services Office of Minority Health
Website: http://minorityhealth.hhs.gov
Twitter: @MinorityHealth

US Food and Drug Administration
Website: www.fda.gov
Twitter: @US_FDA

World Health Organization
Website: www.who.int
Twitter: @WHO

GLOSSARY

abstractor bias: A form of information bias related to the way a data abstractor reviews and interprets records.

accountable care organization (ACO): A collaboration of healthcare professionals—including doctors, hospitals, and other providers—that works to provide coordinated, high-quality care to Medicare patients.

active surveillance: Surveillance efforts that involve local public health practitioners collecting information via in-person interviews, phone calls, and other methods.

adjusted rate: A summary measure that has been adjusted or standardized through the use of statistical procedures to account for differences in the composition of populations.

agent: A factor whose presence, excessive presence, or, in some cases, relative absence is necessary for disease to occur; sometimes called a *pathogen*.

age-specific rate: A rate for a particular age group.

analytic epidemiology: The branch of epidemiology that uses studies to examine associations—often, putative or hypothesized causal relationships—concerning the health effects of various risk factors, characteristics, and exposures.

assessment: The public health function that involves systematic collection, analysis, and reporting on the health status of a community.

assurance: The public health function of confirming that agreed-upon health services are provided and effective.

attack rate: A measure of disease occurrence used when a disease increases greatly within a population over a short period.

bias: Systematic deviation from the truth, or any processes that contribute to such deviation.

big data: Vast collections of information, both structured and unstructured, that can be mined from various sources.

blinding: The act of making participants in a study unaware of the group to which subjects have been assigned; also called *masking*.

cancer cluster: Occurrence of a greater-than-expected number of cancer cases within a group of people in a geographic area over a certain period.

cancer registry: A central location that collects information about cancer patients and the treatments they receive.

carcinogen: An agent that can cause cancer.

case-control study: An observational study in which investigators select a case group (with a particular disease or outcome) and a control group and then compare previous exposures between the two groups.

case definition: A set of criteria that must be fulfilled to identify a person as a case of a particular disease.

case fatality rate: The proportion of cases of a particular condition that are fatal within a specified period.

case report: A description of a patient or event that could lead to further investigation based on the case's uniqueness or magnitude; also called a *count*.

case series: A summary of characteristics for a consecutive listing of patients from one or more clinical settings.

cause-specific rate: A kind of rate that describes events, such as deaths, according to their cause.

Census Bureau: A US government agency that provides data about the nation's people and economy. The bureau provides information through a decennial census of population and housing, an economic census, a census of governments, the American Community Survey, and economic indicators.

Centers for Disease Control and Prevention (CDC): A health protection agency in the United States.

cholera: An acute illness caused by infection of the intestine with the bacterium *Vibrio cholerae.*

claims data: Administrative data that are collected when a patient meets with a provider and are later submitted to an insurance company or other payer for reimbursement.

clinical trial: An experimental research activity that involves administering a test regimen to people to evaluate its effectiveness and safety.

cluster: An aggregation of an event or disease in a place or time in an amount greater than would be expected by chance.

cohort: A well-defined group of people who have a common characteristic or experience.

cohort study: An observational study in which participants are classified according to their exposure status and then followed over time to ascertain the outcome.

cold-spotting: A population health management approach that involves identifying population groups who lack access to healthcare or other community supports that influence health.

collective impact: An approach to problem solving that involves organizations from different sectors agreeing to address a specific issue using a common agenda, aligning their efforts, and using the same measures for success.

communicable disease: An illness that arises through the direct or indirect transmission of an infectious agent or its toxic products from an infected person, animal, or reservoir to a susceptible host.

community benefit standard: A set of requirements for nonprofit hospitals in the United States seeking tax-exempt status and federal funding for services provided to the poor.

community health assessment (CHA): A systematic examination of health status indicators for a population, conducted for the purpose of identifying key problems and assets in a community and assisting with the development of strategies to address the community's health issues.

community health improvement process (CHIP): A broad improvement effort that includes a community health assessment, builds from the assessment's findings, and provides a framework for addressing key health issues.

confounding: Distortion that occurs when the outcomes being observed are influenced by associations with factors other than the one being studied.

congenital malformation: A physical anomaly present in a baby at birth.

continuous common source outbreak: A disease outbreak in which people are exposed to the same source for a period of days, weeks, or longer.

cross-sectional study: A study designed to estimate disease prevalence and examine the relationship between health outcomes and other variables in a defined population.

crude birth rate: The number of live births during a certain time period divided by the resident population at the midpoint of that period.

crude death rate: The proportion of a population that dies during a certain period.

crude rate: A summary measure based on the actual number of events in a population over a certain period.

demographic transition: The shift toward lower fertility rates and delayed mortality.

demography: The study of populations in terms of various factors (e.g., numbers, fertility, mortality, growth, vital statistics) and the interaction of these factors with the social and economic environments.

descriptive epidemiology: The branch of epidemiology that helps answer questions of what (health issue of concern), who (person), where (place), when (time), and why/how (causes, risk factors, modes of transmission).

direct transmission: The direct transfer of an infectious agent to a portal of entry.

electronic health record (EHR): A digital collection of health information about a patient; an EHR allows for the efficient collection of data across multiple organizations and the sharing of that data for informed decision making.

endemic: Having a constant presence within a given area or population group.

environment: External conditions, including biological, cultural, physical, social, and other dimensions that influence health.

epidemic: The occurrence of an illness or other health-related event clearly in excess of normal expectancy.

epidemic curve: A graphic plotting of the distribution of cases during an epidemic; sometimes called an "epi curve."

epidemic threshold: The minimum number of cases or deaths required for an event to be considered an epidemic.

epidemiologic transition: A shift in the pattern of morbidity and mortality away from causes related to infectious and communicable diseases and toward causes associated with chronic and degenerative diseases.

epidemiologic triangle: A model that helps to explain the causes and origins of infectious disease. Its vertices are host, environment, and agent.

epidemiology: The science of public health, which studies the distribution and determinants of health-related events in a population and applies the findings to help control health problems.

essential public health services (EPHS): The public health activities that all communities should undertake to prevent disease and promote health.

evidence-based public health: The use of the best available evidence for the development of public health policies and practices.

experimental study: A study in which the researcher determines the exposure for the subjects and then tracks the subjects to observe the effects of the exposure.

field model of health and well-being: A model, developed by Evans and Stoddart, suggesting that determinants such as social and physical environment, genetic endowment, prosperity, healthcare access, and individual behavior all factor into the health of a population.

fomite: A contaminated object capable of carrying an infection to a person.

frequency: The rate of occurrence for a disease.

general fertility rate: The number of live births during a certain time period divided by the number of women of childbearing age.

geographic information systems (GIS): Science and technology tools that relate data to place factors, manage geographic relationships, and provide spatially referenced information to support decision making.

health: A state of complete physical, mental, and social well-being—not merely the absence of disease.

health coaching: An effort to engage people to modify their behaviors and address their health risks.

health determinant: An event, characteristic, or other factor that brings about change in health.

health exchange: A marketplace that helps individuals, families, and small businesses view, compare, and purchase health insurance plans that meet government standards.

health factors: Behaviors and conditions that influence health.

Health in All Policies (HiAP): A collaborative approach to improving population health by incorporating health considerations into decision making across various sectors and policy areas.

Health Insurance Portability and Accountability Act (HIPAA): A US law that provides standards for the exchange, privacy, and security of health information. The HIPAA Privacy Rule protects "individually identifiable health information." The HIPAA Security Rule provides safeguards for electronic protected health information.

health outcomes: Indicators of how healthy a community is.

herd immunity: General immunity in a group or community; it occurs when a large percentage of a group or community has immunity to an agent.

Hill's criteria: A series of epidemiologic criteria for causal association introduced by Sir Austin Bradford Hill in 1965. The criteria are strength, consistency, specificity, temporality, dose–response relationship, biological plausibility, coherence, experiment, and analogy.

host: A living human or animal that, under natural conditions, provides subsistence or lodgment to an infectious agent.

hot-spotting: A population health management approach that involves identifying population groups with particular areas of need and developing interventions to address those needs.

inapparent infection: An infection that lacks recognizable clinical signs or symptoms.

incidence: The number of new cases or illnesses in a given period for a specified population.

incubation period: The length of time between invasion by an infectious agent and the appearance of the first sign of disease.

indirect transmission: The transfer of an infectious agent through an intermediary source.

infant mortality rate: The yearly rate of deaths in children less than one year old.

infectivity: A disease agent's capability to enter a host, survive, and multiply.

information bias: A flaw in the measurement of exposure or outcome data that results in differences in the quality of information between comparison groups.

informed consent: A subject's knowing, voluntary agreement to participate in a study.

International Classification of Diseases (ICD): A classification and coding system for diseases and other health problems, maintained by the World Health Organization and revised on a regular basis.

interviewer bias: A form of information bias related to an interviewer's gathering of data or influencing of responses.

isolation: Separation of infected people from other individuals with the aim of preventing the transmission of an infectious agent.

managerial epidemiology: The application of epidemiologic tools and principles to decision-making processes and the practice of management in healthcare settings.

matching: The process of making sure that the case group and control group have the same characteristics except for the exposure of interest.

maternal mortality rate: A rate that represents the risk of women dying from causes related to pregnancy and childbirth.

meaningful use: The use of certified electronic health record technology to improve quality, safety, and efficiency; to engage patients and families; to improve coordination of care; to advance public health; and to ensure security of health information.

morbidity: Sickness or illness within a population group.

Morbidity and Mortality Weekly Report (MMWR): A series prepared by the Centers for Disease Control and Prevention to provide timely and reliable public health information and recommendations.

mortality: Death within a population group.

natural experiment: An experiment in which the manipulation of a study factor is not under the experimenter's control but rather is a result of natural phenomena or policies.

natural history: A disease's usual manner of progression in the absence of treatment.

notifiable disease: A disease for which frequent and timely information about individual cases is considered necessary for public health.

odds ratio (OR): The measure of association for a case-control study, representing the odds of exposure to a particular disease for the case group relative to the control group.

outbreak: A localized epidemic, with an increase in the incidence of a disease within a limited area.

over-the-counter (OTC) surveillance: A surveillance process driven by analysis of a community's over-the-counter medication purchases.

pandemic: An epidemic occurring worldwide, or over a very wide area, usually affecting large numbers of people.

passive surveillance: Surveillance efforts that largely depend on the submission of standardized reporting forms from healthcare providers and laboratories.

pathogenicity: The extent to which overt disease occurs in a population infected by a disease agent.

patient-centered medical home (PCMH): A model for changing the way primary care is organized and delivered, based on the principles of physician-led practice, whole-person orientation, integrated and coordinated care, focus on quality and safety, and access.

period prevalence: The proportion of people known to have had a condition at any point during a specified period.

person-time: A concept that allows for the combination of people and time in the denominator for incidence or mortality rates when individuals, for varying periods, are at risk of developing disease or dying.

person-time incidence rate: The number of events during a time period divided by the number of person-time units at risk observed during that period.

plan-do-check-act (PDCA) cycle: A process consisting of four phases (*plan*, *do*, *check*, and *act*) for developing, implementing, testing, and refining quality-improvement activities.

point prevalence: The proportion of people who have a particular disease or attribute at a specified point in time.

point source outbreak: A disease outbreak resulting from the exposure of a group to a noxious influence that is common to the members of the group; also called a *common source outbreak*.

policy development: The public health function that uses scientific knowledge and a shared process to create and implement policies that are protective of the public's health.

population-based surveillance: Surveillance that involves the reporting of information from healthcare providers and laboratories about unusual diseases or diseases that are required by law to be reported.

population health: Health as measured by health status indicators within populations and influenced by social, economic, and physical environments; personal health practices; health services; and various other factors. A population health approach focuses on interrelated conditions that influence the health of populations, identifies variations in observed patterns, and uses the resulting knowledge to inform policies to improve the health and well-being of populations.

population health driver diagram: A tool for aligning the efforts of public health and healthcare organizations to address health issues. The diagram links key health aims with broad primary drivers and more specific secondary drivers.

population health management (PHM): The application of management strategies to improve the delivery of healthcare for populations, with an emphasis on achieving the highest quality at the lowest cost.

population pyramid: A graphic presentation of the age and sex structure of a population.

prevalence: The total number of people who have a condition at a particular time, divided by the population at risk of having the condition.

prevarication bias: A form of information bias that occurs when participants answer questions dishonestly.

primary data: Data collected by investigators for their own specific purpose.

primary prevention: Prevention efforts concerned with eliminating risk factors for a disease.

propagated outbreak: An outbreak in which disease spreads from person to person, without a common source.

prophylactic trial: A type of clinical trial seeking to evaluate the effectiveness of a treatment intended to prevent disease.

proportional mortality ratio (PMR): The number of deaths within a population resulting from a specific cause or disease, divided by the total number of deaths in that population.

prospective cohort study: A cohort study that groups participants according to their past or current exposure and then follows them going forward to determine if an outcome occurs.

public health: The field concerned with advancing society's interest in maintaining conditions in which people can be healthy; also, the science and art of preventing disease, prolonging life, and promoting physical health and efficiency through organized community efforts.

public health system: The public, private, and voluntary entities that contribute to the delivery of essential public health services within a jurisdiction. The system may include government, public health departments, physician offices, emergency response personnel, community health clinics, schools, and charity organizations.

qualitative data: Data provided in a verbal or narrative form.

quality improvement (QI): The continuous use of deliberate processes to improve efficiency, effectiveness, outcomes, and other aspects of performance.

quantitative data: Data that can be counted or expressed numerically.

quarantine: Restriction of the activities of people who have been exposed to a communicable disease.

randomization: The assignment of individuals to test and control groups by chance, with the aim of ensuring that the two groups will be comparable except in the regimen that is given to them.

randomized controlled trial (RCT): An epidemiologic experiment in which subjects are randomly assigned to test and control groups, which either receive or do not receive an intervention, and outcomes from the two groups are compared.

rate: A measure of the frequency with which an event occurs in a population over a specified period. Rates are useful for comparing disease frequency for different locations, at different times, or among different groups.

recall bias: Systematic error resulting from differences in the accuracy or completeness of people's memories of past events.

relative risk (RR): The measure of association for a cohort study, expressed as the incidence of disease in the exposed group divided by the incidence of disease in the nonexposed group.

reportable disease: A disease for which an occurrence must, by law, be reported to authorities.

resistance: The ability of a disease agent to survive adverse conditions.

retrospective cohort study: A cohort study that is conducted when both the exposure and the outcomes have already occurred in the past.

secondary data: Data that have already been collected by others.

secondary prevention: Prevention efforts that focus on early detection and treatment of disease.

secular trend: A pattern reflecting change over an extended period, usually years or decades; also called a *temporal trend.*

selection bias: Distortion resulting from systematic differences in characteristics between people who take part in a study and people who do not.

sentinel surveillance: Surveillance conducted on population samples that have been selected to represent the experience of larger groups.

"shoe-leather" epidemiology: Epidemiologic studies conducted by asking questions directly to the people. The name comes from the idea of walking from door to door and wearing out shoe leather in the process.

social gradient of health: The idea that, in general, people with lower socioeconomic positions have worse health.

specific rate: A summary measure based on a particular subgroup of the population. The subgroups may be defined, for instance, in terms of age, race, or sex, or they may refer to the entire population but focus specifically on a single illness or cause of death.

spot map: A map showing the geographic location of people with a specific disease or attribute. Spot maps have proved useful in the investigation of localized disease outbreaks.

stakeholder: An individual or organization that has an interest in a particular issue.

standardized mortality ratio (SMR): The ratio of the number of deaths observed in a study population to the number that would be expected if that population had the same specific rates as the standard population.

surveillance: The ongoing systematic collection, analysis, and interpretation of health data. Surveillance is essential to the planning, implementation, and evaluation of public health practice.

syndromic surveillance: A form of surveillance that uses health and health-related data nearly in real time to provide information about the health of a community.

telemedicine: The exchange of information via electronic communications (e.g., e-mail, two-way video, remote monitoring) for the purpose of improving a patient's health status.

tertiary prevention: Prevention efforts aimed at minimizing disability associated with advanced disease.

therapeutic trial: A type of clinical trial seeking to evaluate the effectiveness of a treatment in improving a patient's health.

three *Ps*: The three parts of the mission of public health: the *promotion* of health in a population, the *prevention* of disease in a population, and the *protection* of the health of a population.

toxigenicity: The capability of an agent to produce a toxin or poison.

Triple Aim: A framework for optimizing health system performance by emphasizing three dimensions: improving the patient experience, improving the health of populations, and reducing cost per capita; developed by the Institute for Healthcare Improvement.

2 × 2 table: A tool for evaluating the association between exposure and disease.

vector-borne transmission: Transmission of an infectious agent via insect.

vehicle-borne transmission: Transmission of an infectious agent through contaminated material or objects.

virulence: The disease-evoking power of an agent in a particular host.

vital records: Legal certificates of births, marriages, divorces, and deaths.

vital statistics: Systematically tabulated data concerning births, marriages, separations, divorces, and deaths.

INDEX

Note: Italicized page locators refer to figures or tables in exhibits.

ABOUT THE AUTHOR

Rosemary M. Caron, PhD, MPH, is a professor and chair of the Department of Health Management and Policy in the College of Health and Human Services (CHHS) at the University of New Hampshire (UNH) in Durham. She previously served as director of the Master of Public Health program and director of undergraduate studies in the department. Dr. Caron is also core faculty in UNH's Community Development Policy and Practice master's program. She was a faculty member in the New Hampshire Leadership Education in Neurodevelopmental Disabilities program and an adjunct associate professor of pediatrics at the Geisel School of Medicine at Dartmouth. She currently teaches population health in the Executive MBA in Health Administration program in the Business School at the University of Colorado in Denver. Dr. Caron received the 2011 Teaching Excellence Award at CHHS and the 2015 Outstanding Associate Professor Award at UNH. Her research on community-based participation in solving complex urban public health issues has been published in peer-reviewed journals, and she has authored and edited several books about the public health workforce and public health issues. She recently completed a management residency with a local community hospital in New Hampshire.

Dr. Caron is a member of several professional organizations, including the American Public Health Association and the American College of Healthcare Executives. She has held several leadership positions in the Association for Prevention Teaching and Research, the American College of Epidemiology, and the Association of University Programs in Health Administration. Prior to entering academia, Dr. Caron was a public health practitioner for several years in a variety of settings. Specifically, she worked as the assistant state epidemiologist in the Bureau of Health Risk Assessment and as the chief of the Bureau of Health Statistics and Data Management for the New Hampshire Department of Health and Human Services. At the state's largest local health department, Dr. Caron worked as a chronic disease epidemiologist and environmental toxicologist.